Disability and Sanctity in the Middle Ages

Disability and Sanctity in the Middle Ages

Edited by
Stephanie Grace-Petinos,
Leah Pope Parker, and
Alicia Spencer-Hall

Routledge
Taylor & Francis Group
LONDON AND NEW YORK

First published in 2025 by Amsterdam University Press Ltd.

Published 2025 by Routledge
4 Park Square, Milton Park, Abingdon, Oxon OX14 4RN
605 Third Avenue, New York, NY 10158

Routledge is an imprint of the Taylor & Francis Group, an informa business

ISBN: 9789463724333 (hbk)
ISBN: 9781041178194 (pbk)
ISBN: 9781003694038 (ebk)
NUR 684

Cover illustration: Corpus from a Crucifix, c. 1130–1140. France, Burgundy, Autun?, 12th century. Polychromed wood; overall: 111.1 × 20.2 × 7.8 cm (43 3/4 × 7 15/16 × 3 1/16 in.). The Cleveland Museum of Art, Leonard C. Hanna, Jr. Fund 1980.1. (CC0.1.0)

Cover design: Coördesign, Leiden

DOI 10.5117/9789463724333

For Product Safety Concerns and Information please contact our EU representative:
GPSR@taylorandfrancis.com
Taylor & Francis Verlag GmbH, Kaufingerstraße 24, 80331 München, Germany

Table of Contents

Part II Saints and the Disability Community

List of Figures

Acknowledgements

It has been a long road to bring this project to fruition. The entire world was remade during this volume's genesis. Our lives have been upended in ways both familiar and disorientingly new. The coronavirus pandemic swept across the globe, at once an agent of connection—compelling shared experiences of disbelief, fear, grief, keeping on keeping on, no matter what—and an agent of dislocation, as we locked down, shifted online, stayed safe. We lost loved ones; we welcomed new babies. We changed jobs, changed careers. We stood still for interminable pauses; we raced to the finish line. The editors would like to thank our contributors for their graciousness and their patience in travelling this long road with us. Likewise, we are grateful to Shannon Cunningham and the entire Amsterdam University Press team for their continued support during this journey.

We put out a call for proposals in the autumn of 2018. We were blown away by the response: so many excellent abstracts by so many excellent scholars. We could easily fill two volumes with this path-breaking work—and that was our excited plan. And yet, this volume stands alone. As the pandemic's effects have rippled ever outwards, as life and professional circumstances have changed, we have lost these scholars' urgent contributions. Our project is diminished by the loss of their voices. We are haunted by our second 'ghost' volume. The editors would like to thank the authors of *that* volume for their vital work, for their collaboration in our collective project, and for travelling with us as far as was feasible. We hope to read your research in future publications.

Stephanie would like to thank Parker and Alicia for this wonderful collaborative experience, for their passion for this project, and for being the most generous and understanding colleagues as a career change and second baby drastically altered her previous workflow. To my parents and in-laws for their unwavering support and willingness to always watch the kids. To Antoni, Mihali, and Sofia, I love you to the moon and back.

Parker is forever grateful for Stephanie and Alicia's enthusiasm for the topics covered here, and their patience, which was crucial for bringing this volume into the world. Thank you also to my mentors and friends at UW-Madison and USM, to my students and their difficult questions, and most of all to Brad, who has allowed me to tell him the stories of many medieval saints.

Alicia would like to thank Stephanie and Parker for being such good-humoured, skilled, and dedicated co-pilots on this project. Big thanks go out also to Amanda J. Langley and Mark Thakkar for their invaluable help in tracking down hard-to-access sources in record-breaking time, amply demonstrating the magic of #MedievalTwitter. To the Triangle Team, you are the joy, the love, the reason that things matter at all. Jon, Peanut—does anyone know who's tickling Tilly?

Introduction: Medieval Disability beyond the Sin-Sanctity Binary

Stephanie Grace-Petinos, Leah Pope Parker, and Alicia Spencer-Hall

Abstract: In the introduction to *Disability and Sanctity in the Middle Ages*, the editors articulate the volume's priorities: to assert the compatibility and nuances relationships between disability and sanctity, and to provide historically specific models for disability and religion in the Middle Ages beyond the widely simplified reading of disability as symbolic of sin. The editors offer a selective overview of prior scholarship about disability and medieval religion, and emphasize the resonance of such scholarly conversations to contemporary experiences of disability and of the COVID-19 pandemic. The collection of essays is offered as a series of efforts to connect present-day members of the disability community and disability scholars to crip ancestors. The introduction concludes with a summary of chapters.

Keywords: medieval disability, hagiography, saints, disability, crip ancestors, crip time

The cover image for this volume shows what remains of a twelfth-century monumental crucifix of polychromed wood.[1] No cross survives, only the corpus Christi, which the Cleveland Museum of Art calls 'fragmentary but finely carved'.[2] Christ's head, torso, right leg, and most of his left leg are wrought in exquisite detail, revealing a golden crown, dark hair and beard, and incised ribs; the body is draped in a loose loincloth below the

1 The corpus is held by the Cleveland Museum of Art (Leonard C. Hanna, Jr. Fund 1980.1). It dates to c. 1130–1140, and was produced in Burgundy (Autun?), France. It measures 111.1 × 20.2 × 7.8 cm.
2 Cleveland Museum of Art, 'Corpus'.

Grace-Petinos, Stephanie, Leah Pope Parker, and Alicia Spencer-Hall, eds. *Disability and Sanctity in the Middle Ages*. Taylor & Francis Group, 2025
DOI 10.5117/9789463724333_INTRO

waist. The familiar body of Christ on the cross is rendered unfamiliar. The expected crucifix, whereon Christ's body hangs upon the intersecting perpendicular beams of the cross, is made linear in the absence of the figure's arms and, indeed, the cross itself. As a medieval object of contemplation, such a monumental crucifix facilitated a devotional interaction between the bodies of medieval Christians and the representative body of Christ, mapping the worshipper's body to the artwork and to the Church. In the faded polychrome, the flesh and clothing of the corpus blend into one, evoking the fusion of the body of the Church and the flesh of the faithful in Christian tradition. Moreover, the tapered stump of Christ's left leg casts a qualitatively medieval shadow, an inversion of the arch of a cathedral window that also follows the iconic shape of Christ's wound in medieval art, a vertical ellipse verging on the vulviform.[3] This figure manifests the polysemy of Christ's body on the cross; in addition to lying beyond binary gender, as scholars of gender and medieval Christianity have often commented, this corpus without a cross troubles any simplistic demarcation between disability and notional able-bodiedness.[4] The corpus in its present-day form forces the viewer to reconcile holiness and the breakdown of the body.

We chose the cover image for this volume as it shows Christ in a physically impaired state not typically seen. The positioning evokes Christ on the cross, though there is no cross included; the missing arms prevent Christ's body from forming a cross shape, and yet, the Cross is ever present despite its 'lack'. Aside from being provocative, this image highlights that bodily fragmentation is not, in fact, antithetical to sanctity. Indeed, it testifies to the extraordinary power of a signifying artefact. Just as the missing limbs in the cover image serve to actually reinforce the symbolism of the cross, the implement of torture that became the singular sign of Christianity, so too does dismemberment render the saint's body more spiritually able than ever before. Disability writ large similarly empowers saints and other holy figures in religions beyond Christianity. Moreover, in the Middle Ages, dismemberment became a necessary process for distributing materialized sanctity, that is, body-part relics. Even an intact saint's body was often fragmented upon their death, with the pieces distributed and circulated widely to promote and reinforce that saint's spiritual worthiness. The relic's

3 For an overview of scholarship on Christ's wound as connotatively vulviform, and a discussion of his body as non-binary, see Sexon, 'Gender-Querying Christ's Wounds', especially pp. 136–50.

4 On bodies exceeding gender binaries in medieval Christianity, see, for example, Sexon, 'Gender-Querying Christ's Wounds'.

symbolic function depends upon the logic of *pars pro toto*: an artefact that is both a singular part of the saint, yet also carries their blessed wholeness in its entirety.[5] Fragmentation actually multiplies and strengthens the saint and their sanctity.

Sanctity has often been presumed to be at odds with disability. In medieval studies, the miraculously whole and undecaying body of the saint stands as a model for the ideal of bodily integrity, a refusal of human corporeal fragility made possible by exceptional piety. Medieval disability studies has in recent years begun to unveil the extensive ties between disability and sanctity: the refusal of disability through healing miracles, but also the embrace of disability through care work and the veneration of saints who were themselves disabled. The prevalence of disability in the construction of sanctity is all the more apparent where disability is defined expansively. Such a definition encompasses, for a start, the experiences of bodies and minds (and bodyminds) that exceed the norms of form and function in a given socio-temporal context. This includes not only the material fact(s) of bodily and mental difference, but also the ways in which such difference impacts an individual in the totality of their life: the kinds of accommodations and affordances, including time and money, necessitated by disability. Following the social model, 'impairment' refers to the bio-medical 'facts' of variation from medically defined norms. 'Disability', by contrast, is produced by society in response to an impaired bodymind. In this way, disability is fundamentally contingent, emerging according to the interaction of specific historical, cultural, and individual factors that are in play in a given individual's context, including shifting social perceptions, available resources, and accommodations.

The current volume extends the nuance of this conversation through multifaceted meditation on the relationship between disability and sanctity in the Middle Ages. The essays included differ in their subject matter, geographical location(s), and timeframe(s), but each underscores the notion that disability and sanctity can coexist with a vast array of connotations: not just those that are fully positive or fully negative, but every inflection in between. The value of this collection is that it shows there are manifold ways to experience and understand disability in relation to holiness that are not simply shame or embarrassment. Instead, the essays recentre the figures and texts discussed as disability history, a lived history that merits exploration and celebration, and that also imagines relationships and futures for disability and faith that go beyond stigma and shame. Recovering these

5 On this, see Bynum's seminal study, *Fragmentation and Redemption*, especially pp. 239–98.

histories is a way of reclaiming crip ancestorship and imagining more radical disability futures going forward.[6]

Disability and Sanctity

Religion is key to understanding the representation and construction of disability in the Middle Ages. Yet for far too long, the assumption has been that this framework mandates the rigid equivalence of disability and sin. The Middle Ages is still frequently characterized by non-medievalists as the 'truly Dark Ages of stigma' for disabled people.[7] In this framing, medieval disability is exclusively presented as bearing 'a *shameful stigma* provoking fear, ridicule and mockery, if not isolation, ostracism and even persecution'.[8] Moral corruption was accepted as a cause of disability in the era, certainly, but so too was moral perfection, such as in the lives of disabled saints, as chapters in this volume amply demonstrate. Similarly, impairment could be part and parcel of the happenings of ordinary life, caused by foul weather, poor diet, accidents, and disease outbreaks. There was no one way of interpreting disability across all of medieval Europe from the fifth through fifteenth centuries, even less so across the hemispheric Middle Ages encompassing the interconnected communities of Afro-Eurasia.

Prior scholarship on disability in the Middle Ages has frequently commented on the multiplicity of models available for interpreting disability within religious contexts, where even mainstream theological understandings of embodiment varied in the ascription of negative moral valences to disability. The foundational work in medieval disability studies, Irina Metzler's *Disability in Medieval Europe*, resists assumptions that disability was exclusively explained as a manifestation of sin, remarking that the 'belief of modern authors that ancient or medieval societies *invariably* saw a link between sin and illness appears to be the dominant historiographical notion on the subject of disability'.[9] Metzler argued that while impairment certainly existed in the Middle Ages, disability as a socially constructed

6 Our use of 'crip' evokes the move in crip theory to describe embodiments and perceptions of embodiment that call upon a relationship to disability, without requiring that the person or body in question self-identify as disabled. See, for example, Kafer, *Feminist, Queer, Crip*; McRuer, *Crip Theory*; Schalk, 'Coming to Claim Crip'.

7 Marin, 'Transforming Disability Welfare Policy', p. 69.

8 Ibid., p. 70 emphases in original.

9 Metzler, *Disability in Medieval Europe*, p. 13. On disability and sin in the Middle Ages, see especially Seal, 'Disabled Devotion'.

identity was rare.[10] More recent work, however, has shown that even without a singular term, people with distinctive or marginalized bodies and minds nonetheless were made socially legible in medieval communities.[11] We thus find 'disability' to be a constructive term for medieval studies, even if no perfectly corresponding term existed in any medieval language.[12]

In addition to establishing the field of medieval disability studies, Metzler's work also inaugurated sanctity as a crucial component of medieval disability, by drawing extensively on miracle narratives for evidence of how disability was recognized, interpreted, and explained. Edward Wheatley, likewise working in part on hagiographic sources, articulated a 'religious model' for medieval disability, in which Christian sources do interpret disability as a sign of sin, and yet it is often also a signifier of divine power and an opportunity to witness that power—sometimes, but not always, through healing.[13] This work has become increasingly specific and nuanced. For instance, Ninon Dubourg's forensic examination of neglected source has significantly shifted our understanding of the Church's attitudes towards disabled clerics.[14] Although the Church had structural mechanisms in place to exclude disabled men from the clergy, many disabled men were nonetheless admitted into the clergy with recognized disabilities that did not preclude them from clerical service, and clerics with acquired disabilities were often offered accommodations to support their continuation in post. The Church legitimized some impairments but excluded others.

Disability was neither only, nor always read as a signifier of sin in the Middle Ages. However, that assumption still circulates. As a 2016 publication asserts, 'The earliest recorded views of disability explained disability as resulting from immorality or sin. [...] This so-called moral view of disability sprang forth from early human cultures and continued to dominate thinking until the end of the Middle Ages.'[15] While the 'moral view of disability' was quite evidently part of medieval thought, as Wheatley and others have shown, the sources dispute its dominance. Reading disability primarily as a marker of sin did not 'dominate thinking until the end of the Middle

10 Metzler, *Disability in the Middle Ages*, p. 190.

11 See, for example, Eyler, 'Breaking Boundaries, Building Bridges'.

12 On proposed contemporary terms that approximate the modern category of disability, see, for example, Mustakallio, Krötzl, and Kuuliala, '*Infirmitas* in Antiquity and the Middle Ages'; Skevington, '*Unhal*'.

13 Wheatley, *Stumbling Blocks*.

14 Dubourg has published widely on this topic, most recently her monograph *Disabled Clerics*. See also 'Clerical Leprosy', '*Deo iudicio percusset*', 'L'incapacité'.

15 Mackelprang and Salsgiver, *Disability*, p. 98.

Ages'; rather, it has dominated references to disability in the Middle Ages made in non-specialist scholarship.

The issue that catalysed medieval disability scholarship continues to perturb us. We offer this volume as an expansive rebuttal to assumptions that medieval disability was exclusively tied to sin. The contributors' close attention to a vast range of sources refutes simplistic pronouncements that point to any singular meaning of disability in the Middle Ages, even in an explicitly religious context. Though our discussion in this introduction is self-awarely Eurocentric, in large part due to the three editors being specialists in literary traditions local to Europe, work in medieval disability studies has also shown the complexities of religious interpretations of disability beyond European Christianity.[16] The chapters in this volume that examine contexts beyond both Europe and Christendom do precisely this work; they demonstrate that, while viewing disability as a moral deficit did occur, it was only one interpretation that existed alongside other negative, neutral, and positive connotations.[17]

Medieval hagiographic texts—that is, the biographies of holy persons—often offer multiple, even conflicting, aetiologies of disability that coexist without any apparent need for explanatory commentary. In the opening to the eighth-century prose *Life of St Cuthbert*, for instance, the Venerable Bede (d. 735) describes a worsening leg condition that the saint experienced as a youth, leading to his mobility impairment:

> For his [Cuthbert's] knee was seized with a sudden pain, and began to swell into a large tumor; the nerves of his thigh became contracted, and he was obliged to walk lamely, dragging after him his diseased leg, until at length the pain increased, and he was unable to walk at all.[18]

In direct speech, Cuthbert diagnoses the cause of his infirmity as his own sin (*exigentibus culpis*).[19] Yet later in the *Life*, the saint emphasizes that '"not only the wicked but the innocent are sometimes permitted by God to be afflicted in body"'.[20] This holds even when the individual in question, in this

16 See, for example, Abrams, *Judaism and Disability*; Ghaly, *Islam and Disability*; Richardson, *Difference and Disability*; Schumm and Stoltfus, *Disability and World Religions*; Schumm and Stoltfus, *Disability in Judaism, Christianity, and Islam*; Shoham-Steiner, *On the Margins*.

17 See chapters by Edwards, pp. 235–63; Jensen, pp. 87–113; and Vargas-O'Bryan, pp. 115–46.

18 Bede, 'Life', 2.194. 'Nam subito dolore genu correptum illius, acri coepit tumore grossescere, ita ut neruis in poplite contractis, pedem primo a terra suspensum claudicans portaret, dehinc ingrauescente molestia, omni poene priuaretur incessu'; Bede, 'Vita', 2.158.

19 Bede, 'Life', 2.194; 'Vita', 2.160.

20 Bede, 'Life', 15.195–96. 'Neque enim tali tormento soli subiciuntur mali, sed occulto Dei iudicio aliquotiens etiam innocentes in hoc saeculo'; Bede, 'Vita', 15.206.

case a woman on the brink of death who displayed signs of madness, has been '"taken captive in spirit by the devil"'.[21] In another vignette, the Abbess Elfled and one of her nuns are cured of serious illness through contact with Cuthbert's linen girdle. The article subsequently disappears:

> For if the girdle had remained, all those who were sick would have gone to it, and whilst some of them would be unworthy of being cured, its efficacy to cure might have been denied, whereas their own unworthiness would have been to blame.[22]

The moral valency of an impairment is determined on a case-by-case basis: to prevent misinterpretation of the saint's denial of intervention for unworthy plaintiffs, the relic itself is withdrawn. The story of Cuthbert and his healing contact relic models what Wheatley describes as the religious model for medieval disability, in which disability could be read as indicative of sin, but in which impairment could also be 'the site where a saint or holy figure was to prove his or her holiness'.[23] Disability both occasioned stigma and served a positive spiritual purpose.

These multiple interpretations of impairment could appear even within a single body. The holy woman Colette of Corbie (d. 1447), for instance, lived with a host of serious illnesses throughout her life, causing her severe pain and disability according to her *vita*. She makes a clear distinction, however, between illnesses that are caused by natural, human means (*venoient naturellement et humainement*), and those of divine origin (*que Dieu luy envoyoit*).[24] Struck with an eye disease by 'natural cause' (*par cause naturelle*), she turns to an unspecified medicine in an effort to stave off blindness. The aggressive treatment saves her sight, though it does not cure the agonizing condition.[25] Elsewhere, a painful throat condition that had rendered Colette involuntarily mute is healed entirely after the Virgin Mary bestows a kiss on the holy woman's mouth in a vision.[26] The Virgin's cure is presented as entirely appropriate, and certainly welcome, though the holy woman had not appealed for such

21 Bede, 'Life', 15.196. '[M]ente captiuantur a diabolo'; Bede, 'Vita', 15.206.

22 Bede, 'Life', 23.196. 'Si enim eadem zona semper adesset, semper ad hanc concurrere uoluissent egroti, et dum forte aliquis ex his non mereretur a sua infirmitate curari, derogaret impotentiae non saluantis, cum ipse potius esset salutis indignus'; Bede, 'Vita', 23.232.

23 Wheatley, *Stumbling Blocks*, p. 11.

24 Pierre de Vaux, 'Vie', 14.121.109; for analysis of this saint and further related examples, see Cohen, *Modulated Scream*, especially pp. 123–28.

25 Pierre de Vaux, 'Vie', 14.126.114.

26 Ibid., 14.127.114–15.

help. This suggests that the throat condition was not sent by God as a means for Colette to demonstrate her piety. By contrast, Colette actively embraces, and glories in, the impairments that God in his grace chose to gift her (*luy envoyant et donnant* [...] *par grace*).[27] These illnesses are framed as instances of martyrdom, opportunities for Colette to engage in *imitatio Christi* through which she demonstrates her love for Christ, her reverence for his suffering, and her own piety.[28] Crucially, this includes conditions that the text ascribes to diabolical persecution. In later life, Colette is often battered by demons for long periods, leaving cuts and bruises on her legs, and, in one instance, causing damage so severe that her legs swell to become bigger than her body.[29] Even in cases of impairment of explicitly diabolical origin, it cannot be unquestioningly assumed that the impaired person's sin was a correlative causative agent.

Colette's *imitatio Christi* gestures towards the central importance of Christ's embodiment in conceptions of saintly embodiment for medieval Christians, though the ties between sanctity and non-normative embodiment do not exclusively originate with Christ. Significantly, the story of Christ cannot be told without disability. According to Christian scripture, he dedicated his ministry to individuals suffering from various afflictions, oftentimes healing them through miraculous means. Medieval care communities, for example leprosaria, were created to imitate the type of care Christ administered during his lifetime. Even more significantly, Christ himself can be read as disabled.[30] With the Resurrection—the conquest of what might be read as the ultimate impairment: death—Christ's body becomes a site at which both impairment and cure coexist. Even as his resurrected body serves as a model for the promised resurrection of all humankind, that same body retains the wounds on his hands, feet, and side that, when Thomas the Apostle doubts, serve as proof of Christ's identity.[31] Even after death and resurrection, the marks of his suffering continue; although Christ eliminates these wounds and transcends their apparent signification of impairment, their persistence witnesses the necessity of suffering for sanctity, setting off centuries of saints 'witnessing' Christ's suffering through their own.

Patterns such as this, the *imitatio Christi*, participate in the narrative habit theorized by David T. Mitchell and Sharon L. Snyder as *narrative prosthesis*,

27 Ibid., 14.123.111–12.

28 Ibid., 17.177.151–52; 17.179.153; 18.185.157–58.

29 Ibid., 16.153.132.

30 The iconic modern theological work reading Christ as disabled is Nancy Eiesland's 1994 book, *The Disabled God*. In a similar vein, see also Cox, *Jesus*; McCloughry and Morris, *Making a World of Difference*, pp. 64–73.

31 This scene is recounted in John 20.19–31.

which reveals that 'disability has been used throughout history as a crutch upon which literary narratives lean for their representational power, disruptive potentiality, and analytical insight'.[32] Hagiographic narratives frequently lean on disability to indicate a holy person's degree of holiness, whether through the compassionate care or miraculous healing of disabled persons or through the patient endurance of their own suffering or impairment. This pattern appears across multiple religious traditions.[33] In medieval Christianity, both miraculous healing and martyrial suffering situate a saint as Christ-like. One of us (Parker) has elsewhere argued that in saints' cults and other realms of Christian theology, the prosthetic effect provided by disabled bodies and experiences goes beyond narrative, supporting Christianity's theological promises of resurrection and salvation in the afterlife.[34] Parker describes the theological support provided by disability in spiritually inflected narratives, especially those like saints' lives and miracle collections that present themselves as truth, as a *spiritual prosthesis*. With particular reference to tenth-century England, but implications for the whole of medieval Christianity, Parker argues that medieval Christianity relied upon disabled bodies, both depictions of holy persons like Christ and the saints and their real-world counterparts, ordinary disabled people going about their daily lives, in order to conceive of the promised Christian afterlife.

In the imitation of Christ, Christian sanctity was intertwined with suffering and bodily affliction. Indeed, visualization of, and meditation upon, Christ's agonies on the Cross became a mainstay of affective piety from the eleventh century, a worship practice for saints and lay believers alike. The fourteenth-century *Meditations on the Life of Christ*, an immensely popular meditation manual, presents Christ as the very embodiment of brokenness:

> Now the Lord hangs on the cross: dead. [...] If you too carefully contemplate your Lord, you will realize that *from the sole of his foot up to the crown of his head, there is no soundness in him* (Is. 1.6). There is not a member or sense in his body that has not felt his affliction, his infirmity, his suffering.[35]

32 Mitchell and Snyder, *Narrative Prosthesis*, p. 49.

33 See, for example, the chapters by Edwards (pp. 235–63), Jensen (pp. 87–113), and Vargas-O'Bryan (pp. 115–46) in this volume.

34 Parker, *Light of the Everlasting Life*.

35 John of Caulibus, *Meditations*, 78.256. 'Ecce igitur pendet Dominus in cruce mortuus. [...] Sed et tu, si bene comtemplaris Dominum tuum, considerare potes quod a planta pedis usque ad uerticem non est in eo sanitas; non enim est in eo membrum nec sensus corporis qui suam affliccionem et infirmitatem siue passionem non senserit'; John of Caulibus, *Meditaciones*, 78.145, 78.149–53. The authorship of this text remains debated, though the cited editions ascribe it to John of Caulibus. It was previously classified as Pseudo-Bonaventuran. Our thanks to Mark Thakkar for his invaluable help in sourcing the Latin text.

Readers are urged to meditate upon and internalize an impaired Christ, and in so doing to absorb and restage his bodily torments in their own bodies. In this way, Christ's impairment flows into the collective body of Christianity, ceaseless authentication of his glory as the Saviour.

Pushing back against simplistic readings is a particularly complex, and urgent, task for scholars of medieval hagiography. This is, in large part, due to the prominence of cure in such texts.[36] In a typical miracle tale, disability is invoked explicitly to be annihilated. Take, for example, the following example from the twelfth-century *Life and Miracles of William of Norwich*, composed by Thomas of Monmouth:

> In those days a certain woman called Goldeburga, who had been ill for many days, trusted in the power of the martyr [William of Norwich] and—her limbs hardly supporting her—came to his tomb with a candle, and spending some time in prayer with tears, begged for a remedy for her persistent illness. There, as the grace of merciful God operated through the merits of the blessed martyr [William], she sensed the celestial cure spreading slowly through her limbs, and so within a few days, recovering her strength, she obtained full health.[37]

Goldeburga is stripped of her personhood, reduced to little more than an emblem of bodily non-normativity, an unspecified condition that must be 'fixed'. In receipt of 'full health' (*plenam* [...] *sospitatem*), she disappears entirely from the narrative.[38] This, too, is a feature of narrative prosthesis, that the disabled figure is eliminated from the narrative. Similarly, Jay Dolmage describes the options for resolving disability in narrative as the

36 On this, see Kudlick, 'Social History of Medicine', pp. 112–18; Kuuliala, 'Physical Disability'; Spencer-Hall, 'Chronic Pain', especially pp. 56–59. On the ideology of cure more generally, see Clare, *Brilliant Imperfection*, especially pp. 5–17; Clare and Lau, 'Conversation'; Garland-Thomson, 'Integrating Disability', pp. 13–17; Moore, 'I'm Tired'; Wendell, 'Unhealthy Disabled', and *Rejected Body*, pp. 19–22.

37 Thomas of Monmouth, *Life and Passion*, 3.24. 'Diebus illis mulier quedam Goldeburga nomine, cum multis egrotasset diebus, de uirtute martiris confisa, membris uix se sustentantibus, ad sepulcrum eius cum candela uenit, et cumlacrimis aliquamdiu in oratione persistens egritudini sue remedium postulauit. Vbi dementis dei cooperante gratia meritis beati martiris celestem medelam paulatim membris sensit infundi, atque infra dies paucos refectis uiribus plenam optinuit sospitatem.' Thomas of Monmouth, *Life and Miracles*, 3.24.156–57.

38 Accounts of cures kept at saints' shrines do shed light on the historical lives of cure-seekers, despite providing them little narrative space outside the articulation of complaint, cure-seeking behaviour, and cure (or lack of cure); a valuable recent study that includes Thomas of Monmouth's *Vita et Passio S. Willelmi Martyris Norwiciensis* in its analysis is Salter, *Saints*.

'kill-or-cure' motif, a 'myth' about the possible outcomes of disablement: the only way to remain in the narrative and alive is to be cured.[39] Yet for some medieval devotees, cure is only the beginning. We find episodes of partial, temporary, and even failed miraculous healing in hagiography.[40] If we return to Bede's *Life of St Cuthbert*, for example, we discover that the Abbess Elfled undergoes two cures. Before her healing by Cuthbert's girdle, she experienced a spontaneous and partial cure on her deathbed through the workings of 'Divine grace' (*diuina gratia*) within her.[41] The text emphasizes that, whilst this miracle saved her life, Elfled 'was not fully cured' (*nec tamen plene sanata*):

> The pain in her inside left her, the strength of her limbs returned, but the power of standing and walking was still denied her, for she could not support herself on her feet, nor move from place to place, save on all fours.[42]

The cure bestowed by divine grace does not eradicate Elfled's disability; this is achieved only later, by contact with Cuthbert's girdle. The saint's healing prowess is situated as superior even to the miraculous power of divine grace, and certainly better than anything a believer could access themselves. Such vignettes challenge modern assumptions about cure itself, understood as a decisive, final, permanent—and often framed by modern models of disability as an ideologically neutral—'solution' to non-normativity. By contrast, medieval texts show that cure is integrally ideological, a transactional exchange between the healer and the healed body that does not necessarily demand the annihilation of disability itself.[43]

In the archetypal miracle tale, the disabled body is instrumentalized as an object of the saint's miraculous healing, thereby demonstrating the latter's holiness and privileged access to the divine. Douceline of Digne's

39 Dolmage, *Disability Rhetoric*, p. 39.

40 On partial healing, see Kuuliala, 'Heavenly Healing'; Salter, *Saints*; Spencer-Hall, 'Chronic Pain'. On the persistence of disability beyond death in the Middle Ages, see Parker, 'Crip Eschatological Anticipation'. On the ideology of cure, see the references in n. 36.

41 Bede, 'Life', 23.196. 'Cui cum nil curationis possent adhibere medici, subito diuina intrinsecus gratia curante paulatim morti subtracta est, nec tamen plene sanata'; Bede, 'Vita', 23.230.

42 Bede, 'Life', 23.196. 'Nam dolor quidem interaneorum abscessit, membrorum uigor rediit, sed facultas standi uel ambulandi prorsus defuit, quia nee ad standum erigi, nec nisi quadrupes ualebat ingredi'; Bede, 'Vita', 23.230–32.

43 On the incomplete removal of disability, see the chapter in this volume by Holtan (pp. 147–63). On medieval texts that did endorse the elimination of disability, see the chapter by Parker (pp. 265–89).

hagiographer, for instance, emphasizes the direct link between miraculous healing and the holy woman's prestige:

> And the Saint [Douceline] began to shine through her miracles, for large numbers of sick people came with great faith and reverence to her place of burial and there, because of her worthiness, they received the healing they had been seeking. Many people with different kinds of illness were cured when they turned to her for help.[44]

Saints' holiness inversely maps onto the presence of disability in their hagiography, and in their community: the more holy a saint becomes, the less disability is visible. Such depictions, and the power dynamics at play, hew all too closely to the medical model of disability. This model pathologizes impairment as a bodily defect that must be corrected, with disabled bodies the object of curative therapy conducted by expert medical practitioners who know more, know better than their patients.[45] At the same time, the saint's reputation for sanctity—their spiritual 'visibility'—depends upon the presence, the availability, of disabled bodies.[46] Disability is integral to the constitution of sanctity.

It is imperative that researchers adopt a 'source-critical' approach to miracle tales, as Jenni Kuuliala asserts.[47] This includes acknowledging, and interrogating, 'the narrative structure of a miracle, which required emphasis on the negative consequences of a condition being healed, as well as the need to provide proofs of the beneficiary's physical state'.[48] Such analytical circumspection does not limit the utility of such tales in developing our understanding of medieval disability. 'The narrative pattern of miracles was not disconnected from everyday life', as Kuuliala notes, 'but rather was culturally internalized'.[49] In an epistemological feedback loop,

44 Phillipine of Porcellet, *Life*, 14.2.94. 'E comenset li Sancta resplandir per miracles; car venian am gran fe motz malautes sobre son moniment, am mot gran reverencia, e recobravan aqui, per los siens meritis, la salut ques avian dezirada. Car motz de diversas malautias garian, cant si tornavan az ella'; Phillipine of Porcellet, *Vida*, 14.2.200. On disability in Douceline's biography, see Spencer-Hall, 'Chronic Pain', pp. 58–66; 'Stopping the Clock(s)'.

45 Spencer-Hall, 'Chronic Pain', pp. 56–66.

46 In this way, the typical structure of the miracle tale is an example of 'narrative prosthesis', as theorized by Mitchell and Snyder, as discussed above (pp. 18–19) in which disability is both essential to the narrative, and annihilated by it; *Narrative Prosthesis*, pp. 56–57. On narrative prosthesis in medieval miracle tales, see Parker, *Light of the Everlasting Life*, Chapter 2; Spencer-Hall, 'Chronic Pain', p. 59.

47 Kuuliala, 'Physical Disability', p. 205.

48 Ibid.

49 Ibid.

the 'emphases and details' of miracle tales 'stemmed from everyday life and influenced it as well'.[50]

Not all of the essays in this volume deal primarily with healing miracles, but they are all source-critical, in that they contextualize primary sources and question assumptions about what they say about disability and sanctity. Rather than beginning from the expectation that disability will be stigmatized or associated with sin, they interrogate what the sources actually indicate. Sometimes they do indeed find that disability was associated with sin, as in Christopher Jensen's chapter on references to sensory impairments in Buddhist *Eminent Monks* literature, or in the premodern eugenic logic Leah Pope Parker's chapter observes in an eleventh-century English manuscript. The reality of stigma is not one we wish to dispute; rather, we assert the reality of other models in addition to the stigmatization of disability, by foregrounding as well histories that accepted, cared for, and even valorized disability.

Crip Ancestorship, Crip Time, and the Coronavirus Pandemic

For too long, the historical record has erased disabled lives. 'History frequently has not found our lives valuable enough to record-keep or tell our stories', observes disability activist Stacey Milbern, 'and if it does, the narratives do not look like us, and if they by some miracle chance do, they are riddled with so much ableism that it is hard to separate out how the person with impairment felt about their life and what is the story keeper's ableist projections onto them'.[51] We know, as Milbern underscores, that 'disabled people have been surviving, resisting, and leading communities from the beginning of time', and so we 'seek[] ourselves out across time and planes'.[52] Filled with longing to locate ourselves in the present, we travel to the past to find fellowship with our crip ancestors—and with them, build affirmative crip futures, futures that embrace embodiments because of and through their relationship to disability. 'It is radical to articulate that we have a past and lineages and cultures, in a world that says we are individual medical defects to be eliminated': this is the political work of claiming crip ancestorship.[53] All of the essays in this volume perform the

50 Ibid.

51 Milbern and Piepzna-Samarasinha, 'Crip Lineages', p. 243.

52 Ibid.

53 Ibid., p. 249.

work of recognizing crip ancestors and reclaiming what voices the historical record permits, even though only a few explicitly claim community with such ancestors.

It is crucial, as Leah Lakshmi Piepzna-Samarasinha asserts, that we resist the urge to 'pedestalize ancestors as saints'—even if they really were (medieval) saints.[54] It is all too easy for scholarship on disabled medieval saints to slide into inspiration porn.[55] In such readings, disabled saints become supercrips: the 'worthy' disabled people we should all want to emulate, who shoulder any and all challenges with humility and patience, achieving literally superhuman feats of religiosity 'despite' their disability.[56] If, as Rosemarie Garland-Thomson asserts, '[m]odernity secularized wonder into the stereotype of the supercrip', the disabled medieval saint is revealed as the trope's crip ancestor.[57] Indeed, the supercrip paradigm is central to the utility of hagiographical texts as *de facto* marketing for God and the power of his grace, with the Church as his representative on earth. If you, too, held as staunchly to your faith as the disabled saint, perhaps you could 'overcome' the limitations of your bodily condition and become one of God's chosen. Likewise, emblematized as a supercrip, the disabled saint becomes currency in the contemporary spiritual marketplace. The saint's cult rests upon the symbolism of overcoming, bearing with their disability, of bearing the almost unbearable with humility. After death, the disabled saint becomes the supercrip *par excellence*. Entering the heavenly paradise, the saint's earthly disability is entirely erased, even as what remains of their mortal body is broken down into ever smaller parts. Their relics, used as conduits for miraculous healing for other disabled bodies, signify both an intensification and an erasure of disability. Further complicating matters, some theologies of saintly afterlife affirmed that the marks of saints' wounds would remain apparent upon their resurrected bodies; the marked bodies of the most blessed would not find these to

54 Ibid., p. 250.

55 On inspiration porn, see Young, 'I'm Not Your Inspiration'.

56 On the figure of the supercrip, see in particular: Kama, 'Supercrips'; Schalk, 'Reevaluating'. Kama proposes two types of supercrip: the 'regular' and the 'glorified' (p. 450). Whilst the former 'excels' at doing 'mundane, taken-for-granted tasks as if they were great accomplishments', the latter 'performs highly extraordinary deeds'. Schalk expands Kama's typology to include the 'superpowered' supercrip, with 'abilities or "powers" that operate in direct relationship with or contrast to their disability', and at times even erase it entirely (p. 81). There is much slippage, as Schalk notes, between the categories of the 'glorified' and 'superpowered' supercrip. All three of these narrative types are relevant to medieval hagiography featuring disabled protagonists.

57 Garland-Thomson, 'Politics of Staring', pp. 60–61.

be blemishes, but badges of honour.[58] Crip saints were complex beings, as are we.

The goal of crip ancestorship is not to retroactively 'discover', or apply, a unity of disability experience across time. Milbern notes:

> I don't know if these ancestors feel the same way about disability and ableism as I do. I don't know. Probably not! It's likely they had some wicked internalized ableism and isolation. Or maybe they thought all the same shit I do but it didn't get passed down or recorded/they didn't have anyone to speak it to/no one who cared was listening. Maybe they experienced disability in fundamentally different ways than I did that aren't just internalized ableism. I don't know. I am making it up as I go along.[59]

The point is to allow for the endless possibilities of disabled lives, to choose to imagine with our crip ancestors what disability was, is, and could be in future. Milbern recounts how she found her own crip ancestors: 'I stumbled upon them. I dug them up. I fought to find them. I dreamed them. Others shared them. I remembered them'.[60] This is an active task of recovery, a willingness to 'dig through' the historical record to find the traces of disabled life that have been made invisible. The issue of authenticity is a particularly acute problem for scholars of medieval hagiography. Saints' lives are not straightforward biography. These texts were written, usually by male clerics, for specific ideological and political purposes. The vision of disabled life they offer is partial, filtered. But traces of the disability experience remain, if only we dig in the right places. Crip ancestorship, above all, is a choice to acknowledge, connect with, and honour the disabled people that came before us.[61] If we choose to turn our eyes away from our crip heritage, we elect 'only to see a glimpse of who we are'.[62]

Connecting with our crip ancestors enacts a kind of reciprocal, cross-temporal communion:

> [Crip ancestors] learn as we are learning, just as we learn from them. We grow knowledge and movements with them. We crip futurism with them. We demand and entice the world to change the way things have

58 See, for example, the selections in Augustine, '*City of God*'.

59 Milbern and Piepzna-Samarasinha, 'Crip Lineages', pp. 248–49.

60 Ibid., p. 248.

61 Milbern, 'On the Ancestral Plane'.

62 Ibid.

> always been done, with them. We change ourselves with them. They learn through us.[63]

In this way, crip ancestorship rests upon the logic, and lived experience, of crip time, which describes the time zones of disability, the ways in which disabled bodies demand more time, less time, different kinds of time.[64] As a politics, crip temporality is a rejection—voluntary or not, as the case may be—of the narrative of linear progression that structures contemporary capitalist society, of the hetero-patriarchal, ableist temporal scripts offered as standard. As an embodied methodology for medieval scholarship, crip time is a refusal to keep time with the teleological compulsion of history written by the able-bodied.[65] It means looking back, to move forward. It means looking to the present, to better understand our past, and ultimately to imagine manifold crip futures. It means collapsing boundaries installed between periodic compartments, analytically dwelling in the messiness that remains when we allow ourselves, as disabled people, to meet ourselves—our crip ancestors—here, there, and everywhere. This is a medievalist methodology which demands radical temporal accessibility.

This volume offers an example of the productivity of crip time, of crip ancestorship, as a methodology, a sometimes-tacit practice of recovery that underscores the reclaiming of disability experience from the medieval past. But our foray into crip time goes beyond a methodological intervention. We have skin in this game. This project is a collaboration of disabled scholars and our allies. We foreground not just our crip ancestors in the Middle Ages, but our crip peers and our crip selves in present time, researchers who are structurally marginalized by the ableist Academy. This collection is a direct product, and further expansion, of our cripistemologies, of the ways of knowing and being opened up by the experience(s) of disability.[66] Disabled scholars live in crip time, all the time. Our experience of crip temporality structures our professional trajectory, and all too often compromises our

63 Ibid.

64 On crip time, see Godden, 'Getting Medieval'; Kafer, 'After Crip' and *Feminist, Queer, Crip*, pp. 25–46; McRuer, *Crip Times*; Samuels, 'Sick and Well Time' and 'Six Ways'; Samuels and Freedman, *Crip Temporalities* and 'Introduction'; Sheppard, *Chronic Pain*, pp. 65–83, and 'Performing Normal'; Spencer-Hall, 'Chronic Pain', 'Stopping the Clock(s)', and 'Body Talk'. On specifically medieval forms of crip time, see Kennedy, 'Crip Time'; Parker, 'Crip Eschatological Anticipation' and *Light of the Everlasting Life*.

65 On crip time as a medievalist methodology, see Godden and Hsy, 'Analytical Survey', pp. 330–34; Spencer-Hall, 'Body Talk', 'Chronic Pain', pp. 64–66, 'Stopping the Clock(s)'.

66 On cripistemologies—epistemologies of cripness—see Johnson and McRuer, 'Cripistemologies'.

presence in the academy altogether.[67] We are the authors that require extensions, flexibility with deadlines. On bad days, we may write very, very slowly; and on good days, very, very fast. Disability admin clogs our calendar, the business of existing as a disabled person in a trenchantly ableist society, and industry, fills our hours.[68] We are deemed less productive, and thus less academically valuable. The punishing pace, the crushing workloads of neoliberal academia threaten our survival, professionally and literally.[69]

For reasons both personal and methodological, then, crip time has been a central touchstone to this project since its earliest inception in the autumn of 2017. We envisaged working in a hybridized temporality, at the intersection of crip and academic time zones. And then came the pandemic. The coronavirus cripped the world, and time itself.[70]

We need our crip ancestors more than ever. The coronavirus pandemic has been a 'mass disabling event'.[71] As of August 2024, more than 776 million cases of COVID-19 have been reported to the World Health Organization (WHO) since the virus's emergence in 2019; the WHO also estimates that 10–20% of people infected with COVID-19 go on to develop post-COVID-19 condition, also known as 'long COVID'.[72] This is a 'multisystemic illness', comprising elements of myalgic encephalomyelitis/chronic fatigue syndrome and dysautonomia, 'vascular and clotting abnormalities', with significant 'impacts on multiple organ systems'.[73] The work of 'crip doulaship' becomes more important than ever, 'supporting people rebirthing themselves as

67 On crip time in the academy, see Spencer-Hall, 'Stopping the Clock(s)'.

68 Margaret Price describes the compounding work of being a disabled academic as an 'accommodations loop'; Price, 'Time Harms'.

69 Likewise, disabled scholars are disproportionately likely to be disadvantaged by academic precarity: Bailey, 'Ethics of Pace'; Cepeda, 'Thrice Unseen'; Price, 'Time Harms'; Spencer-Hall, 'Stopping the Clock(s)'.

70 For more on the genesis of this volume and the impact of the pandemic, see the Acknowledgments, p. 9. On the pandemic and/as crip time, see Spencer-Hall, 'Body Talk', and 'Stopping the Clock(s)'; Samuels and Freeman, 'Introduction'. On the pandemic as cripping the world, see in particular: Piepzna-Samarasinha, *Future is Disabled*. The contents of this volume in its final form witness the vagaries of pandemic-era academia. That the chapters unintentionally skew towards the study of England may reflect the relatively higher availability and stability of jobs in English programmes in Anglophone countries, rather than the higher resiliency of such scholars in maintaining a research output during the pandemic. See the Medieval Academy of America report on medieval studies hiring across the peak pandemic years, available in Fleming, 'Job-Market Data'.

71 While this phrase has since become widespread, the earliest naming of the Covid-19 pandemic as a 'mass disabling event' was, to our knowledge, first articulated in Barbarin, TikTok post.

72 World Health Organization, 'COVID-19 Cases' and 'Post COVID-19 Condition'.

73 Davis, McCorkell, Vogel, and Topol, 'Long COVID', p. 143.

disabled (or more disabled)'.[74] This involves '[n]aming disability as a space we can be born into, not alone but supported and welcomed by other people' so that we can 'view coming into disability identity as a birth, not a death'.[75] Here, again, we point to the role of medieval saints, and their texts, as crip ancestors engaged in the act of doulaship. With the reclamation of these ancestors, we demonstrate the temporal expansiveness of the disability community, and the diversity of disabled lives across and within time.

Overview of Chapters

The chapters in this volume explore relationships between disability and sanctity first within saintly figures themselves and then in interactions between saints and the disability community. The variety of approaches herein is both intentionally and fortuitously eclectic; the medieval saintly figures for whom disability is relevant are too many to be fully represented here, and no volume could hope to perfectly, equitably, and evenly represent them all. In particular, we note the absence in this collection of non-Christian monotheisms (Judaism and Islam) and Hinduism, and of many intersectionalities of identity categories with bodily inflections: while intersections of disability and gender are repeatedly explored here, intersections between disability and race or sexuality are conspicuously underdeveloped.[76] We hope that the essays in this collection form only the beginnings of a subfield in medieval disability studies that explores the mutual construction of disability and sanctity—across languages, regions, and religions. Taking one small step in this direction, we refuse to demarcate geographical categories in the order of these chapters, and instead venture back and forth between continents with studies that, while examined in historically and geographically specific contexts, nonetheless illuminate one another through juxtaposition.

The essays in Part One, 'Disabled Saints', examine saintly figures who experience disabling conditions. Donna Trembinski articulates the strategic emphasis and de-emphasis of St Francis of Assisi's disabilities as ways of constructing saintly masculinity in a thirteenth-century life of the saint. Also

74 Milbern and Piepzna-Samarasinha, 'Crip Lineages', pp. 240–41.

75 Ibid., p. 241.

76 For studies of disability in the premodern world with greater attention to religions other than Christianity, see above, n. 16. For a recent example of scholarship on the intersection of crip and trans embodiment, with reference to a medieval saintly figure, see Gutt, 'Holy Queer and Holy Cure'.

looking at the thirteenth century, Joshua S. Easterling considers 'Margareta contracta', Margaret the Lame of Madgeburg, who reimagined suffering as a blessed experience and leveraged pain and impairment as an authorizing measure to co-produce her own narrative. Ivette Vargas-O'Bryan's essay brings our attention beyond Europe, to consider the hagiographic representation of Gelongma Palmo, a scholarly monastic who refigured leprosy to resist notions of embodied perfection in tenth-century Tibet. Similarly resistant to perfection in saintly embodiments, Aidan Holtan examines the signifying power not only of whole saintly bodies but of individual marks on those bodies, through the representations of St Æthelthryth and St Edmund in tenth-century English homiletic saints' lives. Closing out this section, Rachael Gillibrand examines the representational trope of Christian saints, particularly the Evangelists, wearing anachronistic spectacles as a shorthand for extensive pious reading and writing—even at the risk of suggesting inappropriate behaviour as the source of vision impairment—in Western European visual culture from the fourteenth century.

The essays in Part Two, 'Saints and the Disability Community', consider the ways in which saintly figures interacted with and impacted larger disability communities. Elizabeth A. Wiedenheft examines the socio-economic consequences of both healing miracles and punitive miracles in the cult of St Foy for the local communities of eleventh-century Aquitaine. Libby Karlinger Escobedo then brings our attention to a particular scene common in Books of Hours from northern France in the fifteenth century—the withered hand of a midwife who attended the Virgin Mary—in order to articulate some of the ways these manuscripts reflect the devotional interests of their owners, which made disability and healing part of conversations about the medical profession. Working cross-culturally and cross-temporally, Jennifer C. Edwards considers the collection of conditions understood as leprosy in the Middle Ages, observing a pattern in the emphasis on care, not cure, that emerges in accounts of European noblewomen and a Japanese empress in the sixth through fourteenth centuries, all of whom were seen as saintly because of their care work. Christopher Jensen articulates possibilities for a 'Buddhist approach' to disability, exploring references to sensory and communication-related disabilities in *Eminent Monks* literature from the sixth and seventh centuries, and advocates for more attention to nuances in Buddhist attitudes towards disability, which could be negative, but were also sometimes neutral or even positive. Finally, Leah Pope Parker examines texts across genres in a single eleventh-century English manuscript centred on a life of St Margaret of Antioch, which witness a collective investment in eliminating disability from a 'Holy Society' through prognosis and the healing cult of the saint, even as the manuscript also reveals a sense of community identity across forms of disability that is typically not expected in premodern contexts.

Following the crip temporal rhythm, we end this book where we have started—and indeed, we have started where we will end. The volume concludes with an epilogue by Richard H. Godden that returns to, and further expands upon, the conversation we begin here, on the methodology and lived experience of crip time. Godden reflects upon the crip-temporal refrain that echoes through the volume as a whole, emphasizing the vital productivity of the study of disability and/as sanctity as a means to explore crip time in the Middle Ages. Collectively, the essays in this collection assert the crucial function of disability in formulations of sanctity during the Middle Ages, within and beyond Christianity, within and beyond Europe, and in continuous conversation with other forms of marked embodiments. Our medieval crip ancestors were never only read one way. At times, they were stigmatized as sinful, at other times, they were integral to the workings of faiths; often, they were both.

Bibliography

Primary Sources

Augustine of Hippo, '*City of God Against the Pagans*: Book XXII, Chapter 19', in *The Medieval Disability Sourcebook*, ed. by Cameron Hunt McNabb, trans. by Leah Pope Parker (Earth, Milky Way: punctum books, 2020), pp. 157–61

Bede, 'The Prose Life of Cuthbert (ca. 721)', in *Medieval Disability Sourcebook: Western Europe*, ed. by Cameron Hunt McNabb, trans. by Marit Ronen (New York: punctum books, 2020), pp. 190–205

Bede, 'Vita sancti Cuthberti auctore Beda', ed. and trans. by Bertram Colgrave, in *Two Lives of St Cuthbert* (Cambridge: Cambridge University Press, 1940; repr. 2017), pp. 141–307

John of Caulibus, *Meditaciones vite Christi olim S. Bonaventurae attributae*, ed. by C. Mary Stallings-Taney (Turnhout: Brepols, 1997). In Library of Latin Texts (database), Brepolis <http://clt.brepolis.net/LLTA/pages/TextSearch.aspx?key=MIOCAC153_>

John of Caulibus, *Meditations on the Life of Christ*, ed. and trans. by Francis X. Taney, Anne Miller, and C. Mary Stallings-Taney (Asheville, NC: Pegasus Press, 2000)

Phillipine of Porcellet, *La Vie de Sainte Douceline: fondatrice des béguines de Marseille, composée au treizième siècle en langue provençale*, ed. by Joseph Mathias Hyacinthe Albanés (Marseille: Étienne Camoin, 1879)

Phillipine of Porcellet, *The Life of Saint Douceline, a Beguine of Provence: Translated from the Occitan with Introduction, Notes, and Interpretive Essay*, ed. and trans. by Kathleen Garay and Madeleine Jeay (Cambridge: D. S. Brewer, 2001)

Pierre de Vaux, 'Vie de sainte Colette', in *Les vies de Ste. Colette Boylet de Corbie, réformatrice des fréres mineurs et des Clarisses (1381–1447)*, ed. by P. Ubald D'Alençon (Paris: A. Picard, 1911), pp. 7–201

Thomas of Monmouth, *The Life and Miracles of St William of Norwich*, trans. and ed. by Augustus Jessop and Montague Rhodes James (Cambridge: Cambridge University Press, 1896)

Thomas of Monmouth, *The Life and Passion of William of Norwich*, trans. and ed. by Miri Rubin (London: Penguin, 2014), ebook

Secondary Sources

Abrams, Judith, *Judaism and Disability: Portrayals in Ancient Texts from the Tanach through the Bavli* (Washington, DC: Gallaudet University Press, 1998)

Bailey, Moya, 'The Ethics of Pace', *South Atlantic Quarterly*, 120.2 (2021), 285–99

Barbarin, Imani, (@crutches_and_spice), TikTok post, 13 December 2020, <https://www.tiktok.com/@crutches_and_spice/video/6905830183601769733> [accessed 16 May 2023]

Bynum, Caroline Walker, *Fragmentation and Redemption: Essays on Gender and the Human Body in Medieval Religion* (New York: Zone Books, 1992)

Cepeda, María Elena, 'Thrice Unseen, Forever on Borrowed Time: Latina Feminist Reflections on Mental Disability and the Neoliberal Academy', *South Atlantic Quarterly*, 120.2 (2021), 301–20

Clare, Eli, *Brilliant Imperfection: Grappling with Cure* (Durham, NC: Duke University Press, 2017)

Clare, Eli, and Travis Chi Wing Lau, '*Brilliant Imperfection*: A Conversation Between Eli Clare and Travis Chi Wing Lau', *The Deaf Poets Society*, 5 (August 2017), <https://www.deafpoetssociety.com/eli-clare-ideas-issue-5> [accessed 12 May 2023]

The Cleveland Museum of Art, 'Corpus from a Crucifix', <https://www.clevelandart.org/art/1980.1> [accessed 16 April 2024]

Cohen, Esther, *The Modulated Scream: Pain in Late Medieval Culture* (Chicago: Chicago University Press, 2010)

Cox, Jennifer Anne, *Jesus the Disabled God* (Eugene, OR: Resource, 2017)

Davis, Hannah E., Lisa McCorkell, Julia Moore Vogel, and Eric J. Topol, 'Long COVID: Major Findings, Mechanisms and Recommendations', *Nature Reviews Microbiology*, 21 (March 2023), 133–46, <https://doi.org/10.1038/s41579-022-00846-2>

Dolmage, Jay Timothy, *Disability Rhetoric* (Syracuse, NY: Syracuse University Press, 2014)

Dubourg, Ninon, 'Clerical Leprosy and the Ecclesiastical Office: Dis/Ability and Canon Law', in *New Approaches to Disease, Disability and Medicine in Medieval Europe*, ed. by Erin Connelly and Stefanie Künzel (Oxford: Archaeopress, 2018), pp. 62–77

Dubourg, Ninon, '*Deo iudicio percusset*: L'idée de contamination d'après les suppliques et les lettres pontificales', in *Alter-habilitas: Perception of Disability among People*, ed. by Silvia Carraro (Verona: Alteritas, 2018), pp. 89–114

Dubourg, Ninon, *Disabled Clerics in the Middle Ages: Un/Suitable for Divine Service?* (Amsterdam: Amsterdam University Press, 2023)

Dubourg, Ninon, 'L'incapacité dans les lettres de dispenses pontificales: aller à l'encontre de la réglementation ecclésiastique médiévale pour franchir la clôture', in *L'exception et la Règle, les pratiques d'entrée et de sortie des couvents, de la fin du Moyen Âge au XIXe siècle*, ed. by Albrecht Burkardt and Alexandra Roger (Rennes: Presse universitaire de Rennes, 2022), pp. 41–54

Eiesland, Nancy L., *The Disabled God: Toward a Liberatory Theology of Disability* (Nashville: Abingdon Press, 1994)

Eyler, Joshua R., 'Introduction: Breaking Boundaries, Building Bridges', in *Disability in the Middle Ages: Reconsiderations and Reverberations*, ed. by Joshua R. Eyler (Burlington, VT: Ashgate, 2010), pp. 1–8

Fleming, Robin, 'Job-Market Data for Medieval Studies', *The Medieval Academy Blog*, 30 May 2023 <https://www.themedievalacademyblog.org/job-market-data-for-medieval-studies/> [accessed 30 April 2024]

Garland-Thomson, Rosemarie, 'Integrating Disability, Transforming Feminist Theory', *NWSA Journal*, 14.3 (2002), 1–32

Garland-Thomson, Rosemarie, 'The Politics of Staring: Visual Rhetorics of Disability in Popular Photography', in *Disability Studies: Enabling the Humanities*, ed. by Sharon L. Snyder (New York: Modern Language Association of America, 2002), pp. 56–75

Ghaly, Mohammed, *Islam and Disability: Perspectives in Theology and Jurisprudence* (London: Routledge, 2010)

Godden, Richard H., 'Getting Medieval in Real Time', *postmedieval: a journal of medieval cultural studies*, 2 (2011), 267–77

Godden, Richard H., and Jonathan Hsy, 'Analytical Survey: Encountering Disability in the Middle Ages', *New Medieval Literatures*, 15 (2013), 313–39

Gutt, Blake, 'Holy Queer and Holy Cure: Sanctity, Disability, and Transgender Embodiment in *Tristan de Nanteuil*', in *Trans and Genderqueer Subjects in Medieval Hagiography*, ed. by Alicia Spencer-Hall and Blake Gutt, (Amsterdam: Amsterdam University Press, 2021), pp. 223–44

Johnson, Merri Lisa, and Robert McRuer, 'Cripistemologies: Introduction', *Journal of Literary & Cultural Disability Studies*, 8.2 (2014), 127–47

Kafer, Alison, 'After Crip, Crip Afters', *The South Atlantic Quarterly*, 20.2 (2021), 415–34

Kafer, Alison, *Feminist, Queer, Crip* (Bloomington: Indiana University Press, 2013)

Kama, Amit, 'Supercrips versus The Pitiful Handicapped: Reception of Disabling Images by Disabled Audience Members', *Communications*, 29.4 (2004), 447–66

Kennedy, Amelia, 'Crip Time in the Medieval Monastery: Cistercian Writers on the Time-Scapes of Infirmity, c. 1150–1250', *Journal of Medieval Monastic Studies*, 10 (2021), 67–87

Kudlick, Catherine, 'Social History of Medicine and Disability History', in *The Oxford Handbook of Disability History*, ed. by Michael A. Rembis, Catherine Kudlick, and Kim Nielsen (Oxford: Oxford University Press, 2018), pp. 105–24

Kuuliala, Jenni, 'Heavenly Healing or Failure of Faith?: Partial Cures in Later Medieval Canonization Processes', in *Church and Belief in the Middle Ages: Popes, Saints, and Crusaders*, ed. by Kirsi Salonen and Sari Katajala-Peltomaa (Amsterdam: Amsterdam University Press, 2016), pp. 171–98

Kuuliala, Jenni, 'Physical Disability and Bodily Difference', in *A Companion to Medieval Miracle Collections*, ed. by Sari Katajala-Peltomaa, Jenni Kuuliala, and Iona McCleery (Leiden: Brill, 2021), pp. 196–205

Mackelprang, Romel W., and Richard O. Salsgiver, *Disability: A Diversity Model Approach in Human Service Practice* (Oxford: Oxford University Press, 2016)

Marin, Bernd, 'Transforming Disability Welfare Policy: Completing A Paradigm Shift', in *European Disability Pension Policies: 11 Country Trends 1970–2002*, ed. by Christopher Prinz (London: Routledge, 2003; repr. 2018), pp. 23–76

McCloughry, Roy, and Wayne Morris, *Making a World of Difference: Christian Reflections on Disability* (London: Society for Promoting Christian Knowledge, 2002)

McRuer, Robert, *Crip Theory: Cultural Signs of Queerness and Disability* (New York: New York University Press, 2006)

McRuer, Robert, *Crip Times: Disability, Globalization, and Resistance* (New York: New York University Press, 2018)

Metzler, Irina, *Disability in Medieval Europe: Thinking about Physical Impairment During the High Middle Ages, c. 1100–1400* (London: Routledge, 2006)

Milbern, Stacey, 'On the Ancestral Plane: Crip Hand Me Downs and the Legacy of Our Movements', *Disability Visibility Project*, 10 March 2019 <https://disability-visibilityproject.com/2019/03/10/on-the-ancestral-plane-crip-hand-me-downs-and-the-legacy-of-our-movements/> [accessed 15 May 2023]

Milbern, Stacey, and Leah Lakshmi Piepzna-Samarasinha, 'Crip Lineages, Crip Futures: A Conversation', in Leah Lakshmi Piepzna-Samarasinha, *Care Work: Dreaming Disability Justice* (Vancouver: Arsenal Pulp Press, 2018), pp. 240–56

Mitchell, David T., and Sharon L. Snyder, *Narrative Prosthesis: Disability and the Dependencies of Discourse* (Ann Arbor: University of Michigan Press, 2000)

Moore, Liz, 'I'm Tired of Chasing a Cure' in *Disability Visibility: First-Person Stories from the Twenty-First Century*, ed. by Alice Wong (New York: Vintage Books, 2020), pp. 75–81

Mustakallio, Katariina, Christian Krötzl, and Jenni Kuuliala, 'Introduction: *Infirmitas* in Antiquity and the Middle Ages', in *Infirmity in Antiquity and the Middle Ages: Social and Cultural Approaches to Health, Weakness and Care*, ed. by Katariina Mustakallio, Christian Krötzl, and Jenni Kuuliala (Farnham, Surrey: Ashgate, 2015), pp. 1–11

Parker, Leah Pope, 'Crip Eschatological Anticipation: The Body in *The Grave*', *Early Middle English*, 4.2 (2022), pp. 1–21

Parker, Leah Pope, *Light of the Everlasting Life: Disability and Crip Eschatology in Old English Literature* (Ann Arbor: University of Michigan Press, forthcoming 2025)

Piepzna-Samarasinha, Leah Lakshmi, *The Future is Disabled: Prophecies, Love Notes, and Mourning Songs* (Vancouver: Arsenal Pulp Press, 2022)

Price, Margaret, 'Time Harms: Disabled Faculty Navigating the Accommodations Loop', *South Atlantic Quarterly*, 120.2 (2021), 257–80

Richardson, Kristina L., *Difference and Disability in the Medieval Islamic World: Blighted Bodies* (Edinburgh: Edinburgh University Press, 2012)

Salter, Ruth J., *Saints, Cure-Seekers and Miraculous Healing in Twelfth-Century England* (Woodbridge, Suffolk: Boydell Press and York Medieval Press, 2021)

Samuels, Ellen, 'Sick and Well Time', *Brevity*, 65 (2020), <https://brevitymag.com/nonfiction/sick-and-well-time/>

Samuels, Ellen, 'Six Ways of Looking at Crip Time', *Disability Studies Quarterly*, 37.3 (2017), <https://dsq-sds.org/article/view/5824/4684>

Samuels, Ellen, and Elizabeth Freeman, eds, *Crip Temporalities*. Special edition of *South Atlantic Quarterly*, 120.2 (2021)

Samuels, Ellen, and Elizabeth Freeman, 'Introduction: Crip Temporalities', *South Atlantic Quarterly*, 120. 2 (2021), 245–54

Schalk, Sami, 'Coming to Claim Crip: Disidentification with/in Disability Studies', *Disability Studies Quarterly*, 33.2 (2013), n.p.

Schalk, Sami, 'Reevaluating the Supercrip', *Journal of Literary & Cultural Disability Studies*, 10.1 (2016), 71–86

Schumm, Darla Y., and Michael Stoltfus, eds., *Disability and World Religions: An Introduction* (Waco: Baylor University Press, 2016)

Schumm, Darla, and Michael Stoltzfus, eds., *Disability in Judaism, Christianity, and Islam: Sacred Texts, Historical Traditions, and Social Analysis* (New York: Palgrave Macmillan, 2011)

Seal, Samantha Katz, 'Disabled Devotion: Original Sin and Universal Disability in the *Prik of Conscience*', in *Rethinking Medieval Margins and Marginality*, ed. by Ann E. Zimo, Debra Blumenthal, Kathryn Reyerson, and Tiffany D. Vann Sprecher (London: Routledge, 2020), pp. 226–42

Sexon, Sophie, 'Gender-Querying Christ's Wounds: A Non-Binary Interpretation of Christ's Body in Late Medieval Imagery', in *Trans and Genderqueer Subjects in Medieval Hagiography*, ed. by Alicia Spencer-Hall and Blake Gutt (Amsterdam: Amsterdam University Press, 2021), pp. 133–54.

Sheppard, Emma, *Chronic Pain, BDSM and Crip Time* (London: Routledge, 2023)

Sheppard, Emma, 'Performing Normal but Becoming Crip: Living with Chronic Pain', *Scandinavian Journal of Disability Research*, 22.1 (2020), 39–47

Shoham-Steiner, Ephraim, *On the Margins of a Minority: Leprosy, Madness, and Disability among the Jews of Medieval Europe* (Detroit: Wayne State University Press, 2014)

Skevington, Fay, 'The *Unhal* and the Semantics of Anglo-Saxon Disability', in *Social Dimensions of Medieval Disease and Disability*, ed. by Sally Crawford and Christina Lee (Oxford: Archaeopress, 2014), pp. 7–13

Spencer-Hall, Alicia, 'Body Talk: The Semiosomatics of Chronic Pain', keynote lecture presented at Voice and Vulnerability, 4th Annual Medieval and Modern Languages Graduate Network Conference, University of Oxford, 5 February 2021 <https://www.youtube.com/watch?v=kPpuCYxEtIU>

Spencer-Hall, Alicia, 'Chronic Pain and Illness: Reinstating Chronic-Crip Histories to Forge Affirmative Disability Futures', in *A Cultural History of Disability in the Middle Ages*, ed. by Jonathan Hsy, Tory V. Pearman, and Joshua R. Eyler (London: Bloomsbury, 2020), pp. 51–66

Spencer-Hall, Alicia, 'Stopping the Clock(s): Precarious Times in the Academy', in *Towards an Accessible Academy: Perspectives from Disabled Medievalists*, ed. by Alexandra R. A. Lee, Hope Doherty-Harrison, and E. R. P. Champion (Kalamazoo, MI: Medieval Institute Press, 2025), pp. 71–113

Young, Stella, 'I'm Not Your Inspiration, Thank You Very Much', Talk at TEDxSydney, 26 April 2014 <https://www.ted.com/talks/stella_young_i_m_not_your_inspiration_thank_you_very_much> [accessed 15 May 2023]

Wendell, Susan, *The Rejected Body: Feminist Philosophical Reflections on Disability* (New York: Routledge, 1996)

Wendell, Susan, 'Unhealthy Disabled: Treating Chronic Illnesses as Disabilities', *Hypatia*, 16.4 (2001), 17–33

Wheatley, Edward, *Stumbling Blocks before the Blind: Medieval Constructions of a Disability* (Ann Arbor: University of Michigan Press, 2010)

World Health Organization, 'COVID-19 Cases | WHO COVID-19 Dashboard' <https://data.who.int/dashboards/covid19/cases> [accessed 30 August 2024]

World Health Organization, 'Post COVID-19 Condition (Long COVID)', *WHO Fact Sheets*, 2022 <https://www.who.int/europe/news-room/fact-sheets/item/post-covid-19-condition> [accessed 30 August 2024]

About the Authors

Stephanie Grace-Petinos is Assistant Editor of the Film and Media list at Bloomsbury Academic Publishing. She received her PhD in 2016 from the City University of New York Graduate Center and is the former Outreach Chair for the Hagiography Society. Her research interests include medieval hagiography, medieval spirituality, disability, dismemberment, and materiality.

Leah Pope Parker is Assistant Professor of English and English Undergraduate Coordinator at the University of Southern Mississippi. Parker's research explores disability and religion in medieval English literature and has been published in the *Journal of English and Germanic Philology* and *Early Middle English*. Her monograph, *Light of the Everlasting Life: Disability and Crip Eschatology in Old English Literature*, is forthcoming in 2025 from University of Michigan Press.

Alicia Spencer-Hall is an Honorary Senior Research Fellow at University College London. Their research interests include: medieval hagiography, disability, gender, digital culture, and film and media studies. Her first monograph, *Medieval Saints and Modern Screens: Divine Visions as Cinematic Experience* was published by Amsterdam University Press in 2018, and is now available Open Access. *Trans and Genderqueer Subjects in Medieval Hagiography*, a collection co-edited with Blake Gutt, was published in 2021 and shortlisted for the Transgender Non-Fiction award at the 34th Lambda Literary Awards; the volume is now also available in Open Access. Alicia's second monograph, *Medieval Twitter*, was published by Arc Humanities Press in 2024.

Part I

Disabled Saints

1. Francis's Disappearing Infirmities: Disability and the Expectations of Masculine Sanctity in the Thirteenth Century

Donna Trembinski

Abstract: This essay explores Bonaventure's *Legenda maior* as a site of negotiation. Completed in 1266, the hagiography presents a Francis intended to unite the factions in his Order: those who wanted the Order to hold property and be led by educated clerics and those who believed that Francis' vision of an Order dedicated to apostolic poverty was being compromised. In doing so, Bonaventure had to contend with the disparate views of these factions, which vacillated between seeing Francis an active founder and seeing him as a man dedicated to apostolic poverty who was ill for most of his converted life. The *Legenda maior* threads the needle between these views, by presenting an active, less infirm Francis who passively receives God's direction and love.

Keywords: Francis of Assisi, Bonaventure, *Legenda maior* of St Francis, disability, hagiography

St Francis of Assisi experienced chronic illness and impairment throughout his entire life.[1] For those familiar with the broad outlines of the saint's life,

1 As much as possible, this essay uses terminology found in early hagiographies of St Francis. The most commonly used term to describe Francis's experiences of chronic illness and physiological distress is *infirmitas*, which I have most often translated as its cognate 'infirmity', and on occasion, when the circumstances of the discussion suggest it, 'illness' or 'impairment'. There is slippage between the language in the chapter because there is slippage in the texts themselves. Finally, I avoid using the term *disability* to describe Francis's experiences since I find the distinction made by proponents of the social model of disability helpful. On the multiplicity of ways *infirmitas* was

Grace-Petinos, Stephanie, Leah Pope Parker, and Alicia Spencer-Hall, eds. *Disability and Sanctity in the Middle Ages*. Taylor & Francis Group, 2025
DOI 10.5117/9789463724333_CH01

this short statement about him may come as a surprise. Today, Francis (c. 1180–1226 CE) is rarely described in such terms. Instead, he is known as the man who created the first crèche at Greccio, the lover of animals who preached to birds and one of the few holy people who received the stigmata. He is the saint who is remembered for changing how people connected to God, though what has come to be called experiential piety, and the founder of the mendicant Order of the Friars Minor.[2] But as a careful analysis of his early *Lives* show, Francis experienced periods of illness from before his conversion to religious life, circa 1208, until his death in 1226. At the end of his life, his sight was seriously impaired, he was suffering from an internal disorder that affected his organs, and he was unable to walk. While Francis's experiences were often presented to medieval audiences as the actions of a future saint devoted to imitating Christ, a close reading of early sources suggest that his infirmities created difficulties for Francis's ability to lead his new and growing order.

Francis's experiences of disability—that is, the barriers Francis experienced due to his increasing illnesses—also perplexed some of his hagiographers, especially Bonaventure, who was tasked with writing a new official *Life* circa 1260. Francis's lived experience did not easily fit into the established and expected patterns of a founder-saint. As this essay will demonstrate, Bonaventure's *Legenda maior* minimized discussions of infirmities found in earlier hagiographies of the saint to mould his story into a more acceptable portrait, one that more closely conformed to medieval social expectations of what a male religious founder looked like. Yet Bonaventure could not entirely ignore earlier narratives about Francis's illnesses and infirmities and their impact on his life—impacts which, as will be demonstrated below, served to feminize him in Aristotelian terms. As a result, Bonaventure crafted a narrative that presented a version of Francis that both conformed to and challenged the thirteenth-century ideal of a male religious leader and founder-saint. In doing so, Bonaventure served two distinct audiences within the Order: the educated Franciscans who were taking over its organization and leadership, and other Franciscans who believed that Francis would have vehemently opposed the growing number of educated clerics in leadership positions within the Order.

understood in the Middle Ages, see Kuuliala, Mustakallio, and Krötzl, 'Introduction', pp. 5–6. On the social model of disability and other models that have been suggested for the study of disability in the past and present, see, recently, Retief and Letšosa, 'Models of Disability'.

2 Traditionally Francis founded two other Orders as well, the Sisters of St Clare and a lay Franciscan Order.

Francis and his Biographers

The son of a wealthy merchant from Assisi, Francis lived a life of luxury and pleasure until he was sent to war in the ongoing skirmishes between Assisi and Perugia. Around 1204 he was captured and spent time as a prisoner of war. It is possible, though unproven, that Francis contracted a severe illness in prison, which nudged him towards converting to religious life. In the early years of his conversion, he repaired churches and ministered to lepers. His way of living gathered followers, and the Franciscan Order was formally founded circa 1209–1210. The Order grew quickly and numbered more than three thousand by 1221, when Francis resigned from leading the Order. Francis is traditionally said to have received the stigmata in 1224, two years before his death. The years between 1224 and 1226 are customarily held to be a period of contemplative isolation for Francis, until he died of an unspecified illness of the 'liver, spleen and stomach' and dropsy. By that time, Francis could no longer walk and was living with significant vision loss.

This summary of Francis's life is pieced together using early sources written by and about the saint, though precisely which sources should be considered the most accurate has been the source of extensive debate.[3] While this so-called 'Franciscan Question' is far from resolved, this essay will explore the differences in how Francis's illnesses and infirmities are described in earlier sources and Bonaventure's *Legenda maior*, which became the official *Life* of Francis when it was adopted by the Franciscan Order in 1266, whereupon all earlier *Lives* of Francis were ordered destroyed.[4] In particular, the chapter compares Bonaventure's Francis with the version presented in Thomas of Celano's *Vita prima*, written circa 1228, and his *Remembrance of the Desire of a Soul* (formerly known as the *Vita secunda*), completed circa 1244.[5] The more informal *Assisi Compilation*, written circa 1311 but reflecting traditions from the 1240s, is also examined.[6] Francis also left a small body of his own work, including sermons, songs, letters and a

3 For a relatively recent introduction to the Franciscan Question, see Blastic, Constable, Dalarun, and Johnson, 'Towards a Resolution of the Franciscan Question'.

4 Bonaventure, *Legenda maior sancti Francisci* (henceforth LM), in *Fontes Franciscana* (henceforth FF), pp. 778–962. The English translation may be found in *Francis of Assisi: Early Documents* (henceforth FA:ED), II, pp. 525–683.

5 Thomas of Celano, *Vita prima* (henceforth VP) in FF, pp. 276–425; English translation found in FA:ED, I, pp. 180–308. Thomas of Celano, *Remembrance of the Desire of a Soul* (the so-called *Vita secunda*) (henceforth RDS), in FF, pp. 444–640; English translation found in FA:ED, II, pp. 239–393.

6 *Assisi Compilation* (henceforth AC), in FF, pp. 1472–1691; English translation found in FA:ED, II, pp. 118–230.

series of rules written for the Order over time. Perhaps the most important of these works for this essay is his *Testament*, dictated on his deathbed, which reflects profoundly on his legacy and vision for the Order.[7]

Illness and Impairment in Francis's Lived Experience

That Francis experienced different illnesses and suffered from temporary and more permanent impairments cannot be seriously questioned by scholars who have examined the early sources of his life closely. The *Vita prima* notes that Francis suffered an illness that hampered his ability to walk for a time even before his conversion to religious life, and that it was during a brief respite, while he was 'supporting [himself] with a [walking] stick' that he began to contemplate his conversion.[8] While the trope of an illness leading to a conversion was common in the lives of saints of both genders by the thirteenth century, the details provided in the *Vita prima* about Francis's slow recovery suggest that this illness may have been a significant turning point in the saint's life. As corroboration, the *Assisi Compilation* notes that Francis was 'fragile' (*fragilis*) even before his turn to religious life.[9]

Once Francis had fully embraced his converted life, he experienced periodic bouts of illness, like the one that forced him to turn back from a planned preaching trip to Morocco or the one that left him lying ill in the bishop's palace at Assisi.[10] While descriptions of these illnesses provide context for the *Assisi Compilation*'s repeated descriptions of Francis as moving between periods of sickness and health, it appears that his infirmities did not seriously impact his ability to preach or lead the Order until after his return from a missionary trip to Egypt, circa 1219. In Egypt, the *Assisi Compilation* tells us, Francis contracted a serious disease of the eye that would eventually diminish his vision significantly.[11] Francis's visual impairment, in particular, alarmed those in positions of authority in the Franciscan Order and the hierarchy of the Church, who ordered Francis

7 Francis of Assisi, *Testament*, 3.27–3.28, in *Francisci Assisiensi: Scripta*, p. 400; FA:ED, I, p. 126.

8 'Sicque diu infirmitate attritus, ut meretur pervicacia hominum quae vix nisi suppliciis emendatur, coepit intra se alia solito cogitare. Cumque iam paululum respirasset et baculo sustentatus'. VP 1.2.3; FF, p. 280; FA:ED, I, p. 185. On Francis and sickness, see also Easterling, pp. 67–68, in the present volume.

9 AC, 117; FF, p. 1682; FA:ED, II, p. 225.

10 VP, 1.20.56; FF, pp. 331–32; FA:ED, I, p. 230; AC 70; FF, pp. 1573–74; FA:ED, II, p. 174.

11 AC, 77; FF, pp. 1588; FA:ED, II, p. 181.

to seek out treatment, probably against the wishes of the saint himself, who may well have seen his visual impairment as a gift from God and an opportunity for spiritual growth.[12] None of the treatments restored Francis's sight. By early 1226, the saint's ability to walk was steadily declining, and in the last six months of his life, he also suffered from illnesses of the stomach, spleen, and liver. This period of Francis's life is most often described in modern biographies as the period after he had received the stigmata, a frame which has allowed readers and scholars to compartmentalize Francis's experiences as *imitatio Christi* rather than exploring how Francis and those in positions of authority within the Franciscan Order responded to his impairment. Indeed, Francis's position as a founder and saint has allowed tensions related to his infirmities, which are present in the source material for his life, to be overlooked by both medieval hagiographers and modern scholars in favour of reading such episodes as evidence of Francis's trust in and devotion to God.

However, reading the early *vitae* of Francis against the grain demonstrates that Francis's illnesses and infirmities impacted the way he lived. From the beginning of his converted life, Francis dedicated himself to living a life of absolute poverty, begging for food and shelter as he travelled. He set a high bar for himself in terms of asceticism, engaging in the physical labour of rebuilding churches and living for a short time in a cave. Yet even the earliest formal *Life* of Francis, Thomas of Celano's *Vita prima*, notes that Francis was sometimes forced to relax the rigours of his ascetic life due to illness.[13]

The early *vitae* also suggest that Francis's illnesses and impairments became a barrier to leading his Order. Francis resigned his leadership role within the Order by 1221 at the latest. In perhaps the most reliable source about Francis's later life, the *Assisi Compilation*, there is debate about the reasons behind Francis's so-called resignation. The episode is discussed three times and Francis's illnesses are twice mentioned as the cause of his departure. However, in the third discussion, the text notes in words reported to have come directly from Francis, that although he renounced his office because he was

> no longer able to have care and concern for [the brothers] on account of [his] infirmity, if the brothers walked and had walked according to Francis's will, for the sake of comforting them, [he] would not have wished

12 VP, 2.5.101; AC, 83; RDS, 2.125.166.

13 VP, 2.6.103; FF, p. 381; FA:ED, 1, p. 273.

> them to have any minister except [himself], up until the day of [his] death.[14]

This suggests that Francis may have resigned more out of frustration about the direction of the Order rather than because of his illness. However, despite the different narratives surrounding Francis's resignation in the *Assisi Compilation*, all three episodes note that Francis's worsening health was a factor in his withdrawal from leadership.

Francis's separation from secular authority runs deeper than his stepping away from formal positions of power within the Order he founded. At times, Francis appeared unable even to exercise choice over the care of his own body. In the *Testament*, dictated by Francis himself at the end of his life, he tells us that he had asked the Minister-General of his own Order for a guardian whom he wished to obey, subsuming his own will to his caretaker's.[15] This desire for a guardian is most often constructed by medieval hagiographers and modern biographers as Francis seeking a method of practising humility. However, it is clear from the early *Lives* that one of the roles the guardian had in Francis's life, and possibly the primary one, was to care for the saint and ensure he took care of himself in times of illness. Francis's guardian acted in his client's physical self-interest even when his decisions did not accord with the saint's, as, for instance, in the famous story where Francis would not extinguish his trousers (which were on fire) until his guardian told him to do so.[16] This story demonstrates that, at times, Francis's wishes conflicted with those whom he had sworn to obey.

Asking for a guardian (Latin: *gardianus* and *custodes*) can be understood an act of self-determination on Francis's part. It was also a very unusual request. In medieval practice, guardians provided protection and were most commonly appointed in cases where a person was perceived to be unable to care for themselves either by age or incapacity. Individuals did not seek out guardians for themselves. The term *guardian* was, then, a surprising linguistic choice for Francis and/or his hagiographers to make, but in asking for such a guardian, Francis was, in some way, expressing agency and,

14 'Quoniam licet tempore quo renuntiavi et dimisi officium fratrum, coram fratribus me excusarem in capitulo generali, quod propter infirmitatem meam de ipsis curam et sollicitudinem habere non possem, tamen modo, si secundum voluntatem meam fratres ambularent et ambulassent, propter ipsorum consolationem nollem, quod alium ministrum haberent preter me, usque in diem mortis mee.' AC, 106; FF, pp. 1648–49. This anecdote likely reflects the growing concern about the clericalization of the Order on the part of the authors or editors of the text.

15 Francis of Assisi, *Testament*, 3.27–28, in *Francisci Assisiensi: Scripta*, p. 400; FA:ED, I, p. 126.

16 AC, 86; FF, pp. 1608–09; FA:ED, II, p. 192.

perhaps, a desire for care.[17] However, there is no direct evidence for this in the early sources of Francis's life. Rather the texts emphasize that Francis wished to obey his guardian out of desire to practise perfect obedience. And yet, in many episodes in which the guardian is present in the early *vitae* of Francis, he acts to care for Francis's health, precisely what an appointed guardian was expected to do.

Despite Francis's desire for and willingness to accept a guardian, he often chafed at the restrictions his guardian imposed. The *Assisi Compilation* describes times when Francis actively worked to subvert his guardian's intentions. For instance, when Francis was suffering from illnesses of the stomach and spleen, his guardian ordered him to wear fox fur on the inside of his tunic to keep the area warm. Francis agreed, unhappily, and only if he could also sew the fur on the outside his tunic so people would know that he was relaxing his ascetic practice. His guardian agreed, but even this did not make the saint happy, for, the *Assisi Compilation* tells us, he did not wear the fox fur for very long.[18] In another even more perplexing instance, Francis was ordered by his guardian not to give away any pieces of his tunic so that his body could be fully protected from the cold. Yet when a poor man came by asking for a piece of cloth, Francis cut a piece of his tunic to give away. He did this secretly, knowing that his guardian would order him not to cut his clothing. Francis was caught in the act, and, as he had expected, his guardian forbade him to give away the cloth.[19] Episodes such as these suggest a tension between Francis's own desires and those of his guardian. The promise to obey meant that although Francis had willingly conceded authority to his guardian, in moments of disagreement, the future saint could not act of his own accord. Ultimate authority for Francis's body and well-being rested with the saint's guardian, no longer with Francis himself. As should be clear from the above narratives, although Francis appeared to have chosen to limit his own authority, he also struggled against these limitations—sometimes exhibiting outright disobedience.

Whether by choice or through encouragement from others in positions of authority within the Franciscan Order or the Church hierarchy or both, Francis's leadership role within the Order and the Church seems to have been diminished as his illnesses became more acute. Yet he worked hard to retain as much informal authority within the Order as he could, by writing letters

17 I appreciate the comments of the editors of this volume who pushed me to think a bit more deeply about Francis's relationship with his chosen guardians.

18 AC, 81; FF, pp. 1592–93; FA:ED, II, p. 184.

19 AC, 91; FF, p. 1616; FA:ED, II, pp. 195–96.

and telling those near him his own positions on debates occurring within the Order. Indeed, nearly all the writings we have that can be attributed to Francis were written after his resignation. But this was, ultimately, a lost cause. In his writings, Francis repeatedly tried to return the Order to the vision he had for it, one of itinerancy and mendicancy, even down to the *Testament*, which was written on his death bed, but he was unable to exert the necessary pressure on the Order to enact such change. While Francis remained a moral exemplar to Franciscans and the Catholic Church as a whole, his lack of formal power diminished his influence over the Order he had founded.

A Feminine Francis? Disability and Francis's Fragile Masculinity

As others before me have noted, Francis's gender expression is complicated. Catherine Mooney has suggested that we might best understand Francis as androgenous, since he exhibits both masculine and feminine characteristics at different times.[20] Jacques Dalarun has traced many threads of Francis's devotion that seem to have feminine attributes in his *Francis of Assisi and the Feminine*.[21] Bynum understood Francis to sometimes exhibit modes of piety coded as feminine in the Middle Ages, yet did not see Francis as part of the larger trend of embodied experiential piety so commonly practised by late medieval mystics.[22] Clearly, Francis's gender identity is complex, multifaceted, queer.[23]

What constituted normative expressions of secular and religious masculinity in the High Middle Ages has been the subject of much debate in the last fifteen years or so. Of course, masculinity was experienced in medieval Europe in a variety of ways but there were also some commonalities. For instance, a key signifier of many types of masculinity in the Middle Ages was agency.[24] The more agency a person had in both their personal and private lives, the more masculine that person was perceived to be. This

20 Mooney, 'Francis of Assisi'.

21 Dalarun, *Francis of Assisi.*

22 Bynum, *Holy Feast and Holy Fast*, loc. 1279–1364.

23 Although Francis was not an object of study in this edited collection, see the 'Introduction' and 'Appendix' for a broad introduction to transgender and genderqueer saints, along with many excellent essays, in Spencer-Hall and Gutt, *Trans and Genderqueer Subjects.*

24 On the general subject of medieval masculinities see Cohen and Wheeler, *Becoming Male in the Middle Ages*; Lees, *Medieval Masculinities*; Hadley, *Masculinity in Medieval Europe*; Karras, *From Boys to Men*; Neal, *The Masculine*; Murray; *Conflicted Identities.*

agency was expressed in various ways, as scholars have noted—one way was violence; another was ongoing governance over oneself, one's household and, with more economic prosperity and power, one's neighbours; a third was taking an active part in sex and procreation.[25] In various ways, perceptions of medieval masculinity intersected with class and economic power; nobles and those who controlled substantial wealth, as was the case for Francis's family, had more agency and thus were understood to exude more clearly masculine characteristics than those of lesser economic status. Conversely, the less agency a person had, the less masculine the individual might seem.[26] In very real ways this reflects the dichotomy presented in Aristotle's perceptions of male and female characteristics: men were active and productive, women were passive and receptive. This idea, found in Aristotle's biological works and his *Politics*, was discussed and debated in medieval universities, but filtered from there to many different aspects of art, literature, and life itself.[27]

The Aristotelian focus on masculine ability, activity, and productivity posed a problem for medieval perceptions of clerics, religious, and especially friars in the Middle Ages. After the Gregorian Reforms of the eleventh century, religious were not supposed to engage in sex or procreate, and they were also forbidden from participating in worldly economic endeavours. Jo Ann McNamara recognizes the difficulties such expectations placed on clerics, suggesting that the newly required celibacy of clerics encouraged the restructuring of the gender system in ways that highlighted women's sexuality and the necessity of keeping clerics, who valiantly fought their desires, separate from women. Such strict separation and control of women demonstrated the virility of clerics even as they practised their newly imposed celibacy.[28] While initially supporting McNamara's position, in later work Jacqueline Murray has challenged the assumption that clerics

25 On the link between violence and masculinity in medieval Europe, see Kaeuper, *Chivalry and Violence*. The link between violence and masculinity has been questioned by recent scholars who focus on the importance of controlled or governed violence as the hallmark of masculinity. On this subject, see Meyerson, Thierry, and Falk, 'Conclusion'; and Christie, 'Self-Mastery and Submission'.

26 On agency and governance as key signifiers of masculinity, see McSheffrey, 'Men and Masculinity'.

27 The longest and most clear discussion of Aristotle's perception of differences between males and females can be found in his *On the Generation of Animals*, Book II. It is in this text that Aristotle famously likens women to malformed males. Aristotle, *On the Generation of Animals*, 737a, I, p. 1144. In *The Politics* (1254b, II, p. 1990), Aristotle argues that men are naturally superior, while women are naturally inferior—thus men ought to govern women.

28 McNamara, 'The *Herrenfrage*'.

necessarily performed or were expected to perform normative masculinity by suggesting that we might best understand clerics as neither male nor female, but as a third gender in the Middle Ages.[29] Perhaps they might be best understood as ungendered.[30] Yet, as Robert Swanson has argued, medieval priests were physiologically male, though they may have hoped to progress beyond the markers of their gender to become something Swanson terms 'emasculine'.[31] More recent work has pointed to the possibility that active priests and preachers or active lay brothers may have been perceived to have different gendered characteristics from those men who lived contemplative lives. Martha Newman has noted that in Cistercian monasteries, lay brothers were described as imitating a clearly masculine Christ through labour and asceticism even as Cistercian monks framed their own devotion to God in feminine terms suggested by Bernard of Clairvaux's commentary on the Song of Songs.[32] Moving from community to individual, Alison More notes that in the hagiographies of both holy men and women of Liège, the apparent desired trajectory for contemplatives of both sexes was to move beyond the limitations of a sexed body and societal expectations of gender.[33]

While there is still much debate about how clerical and religious gender was conceived, what is clear is that their notions of masculinity often reflected or related to those performed by secular men who operated in the same society.[34] For, while masculinities varied, there is clear evidence that clerics were expected to be physiologically male. How precisely disability intersected with expectations of gender in the Middle Ages is an ongoing question. Based on the seminal work of Rosemarie Garland-Thompson, a subset of medieval disability studies locates medieval femininity as a perceived disability in the Middle Ages. Thompson argues that the Aristotelian perception of women as 'malformed males' outlined in *On the Generation of Animals* ensures that for much of Western history, women were in some

29 For her earlier position, see 'Masculinizing Religious Life'. For an analysis of the ideas of a third gender being applied to medieval Western clergy and religious see Murray, 'One Flesh, Two Sexes, Three Genders'.

30 Since Bynum's *Holy Feast and Holy Fast* there has been much discussion problematizing the notion of feminine or masculine religious piety. While it is impossible to include an entire bibliography here, some notable works are Kuefler's *Manly Eunuch* and Murray's important work on the gender of clerics, developed in essays such as 'Masculinizing Religious Life', 'Mystical Castration', and 'One Flesh, Two Sexes, Three Genders'.

31 Swanson, 'Angels Incarnate', p. 161.

32 Newman, 'Crucified by the Virtues'.

33 More, 'Convergence, Conversion, and Transformation'.

34 See Thibodeaux, 'Introduction', p. 4.

sense perceived to be disabled by virtue of their very femaleness.[35] One might wonder, then, whether in the Middle Ages infirmity or illness in men to some extent rendered their masculinity somehow other, and perhaps more feminine. Certainly, since Bynum wrote her influential *Holy Feast and Holy Fast*, embodied suffering, often from illness, has been largely perceived as a feminine trait, especially amongst mystics of the High Middle Ages.[36]

The study of how disability impacted perceptions of masculinity in the Middle Ages is in its infancy. Where such studies do exist, they tend to focus on the intersections of disability, masculinity, and knighthood. For example, Kathleen Kelly has suggested that in Arthurian romance, at least, men on the battlefield managed potential identification and empathy with their combatants by understanding a wounded body as passive, penetrated, and feminine: entirely alien from the active bodies of unwounded knights.[37] Tory Pearman agrees, suggesting that the bleeding body of a wounded knight is both Christ-like and feminized, and that wounded knights tend to disappear from tales of chivalry.[38]

Amongst religious, too, there was an idealized expectation that clerics be active, able-bodied and healthy. Canon law, as outlined in Gratian's eleventh-century rationalization the *Decretum*, also stipulated that such a man must be physically perfect and whole (that is, not in any way infirm, disabled, or castrated) in order to be ordained.[39] However, the chapters within the distinction suggest that the prohibition was not absolute and depended upon several factors, such as an individual's volition in the act of creating a imperfect body and the ability of the person to say the mass. Ninon Dubourg's recent work has suggested that in some cases, at least, it was also possible to petition the papacy for a dispensation to continue in a clerical role in spite of a bodily impairment.[40]

35 Garland-Thomson, 'Integrating Disability', p. 6, and *Extraordinary Bodies*, p. 27. See also Pearman, *Woman and Disability*. For a discussion of Aristotle's humoral hierarchy and its impact on his discussions of sex, see Cadden, *Meanings of Sex Difference*, pp. 22–24.

36 Bynum, *Holy Feast and Holy Fast*.

37 Kelly, 'Malory's Body Chivalric'. This position has been contested by Hodges ('Wounded Masculinity'), who argues that knights who overcame their wounds were able to assert their masculinity that much more strongly.

38 Pearman, *Disability and Knighthood*.

39 Gratian, *Decretum*. The prohibition itself is quite direct: 'Corpore uero uitiati similiter a sacris offitiis prohibentur' ('That those who are damaged with respect to the body are similarly prohibited from sacred offices'; my translation). On the discussion of disability in Gratian's *Decretum* see Parlopiano, '"*Propter deformitatem*"', p. 85. On the possibility of papal dispensations, see Dubourg, '"*Ad obsequium divimum inhabilem*"', and especially 'La reconnaissance'.

40 Dubourg, '"*Ad obsequium divimum inhabilem*"' and 'La reconnaissance'.

With respect to Franciscan masculinity, in particular, much more work needs to be done. Derek Neal makes some cursory observations in his book *The Masculine Self in Late Medieval England*, noting that friars were sometimes perceived as 'less than men' due to their lack of property and descendants.[41] Katherine Lindeman's 2015 doctoral thesis on the subject of Dominican masculinity presents some important conclusions about how masculinity was understood in the other extremely popular mendicant order founded in the early 1200s. Lindeman suggests that Dominican friars generally took on aspects of secular masculinity, such as governance and agency, and reframed them in ways that linked to their own vocation: according to this interpretation, the model Dominican was one who preached, engaged in theological debates, and governed himself spiritually, sexually, and in terms of bodily asceticism.[42] Dominican masculinity required a public life and governance over those who lived secluded lives of prayer and practised a more affective life of piety—generally women and less educated men of lower status within the Order.[43]

While it is possible that Franciscan masculinity was structured entirely differently than early Dominican masculinity, this seems unlikely, especially as the Franciscan Order became more clericalized and more like the Dominican Order in the years after 1220. If normative Franciscan masculinity was constructed similarly, Francis as the founder of this Order presented a potential problem for some. The earliest hagiographies of Francis very clearly suggested that he did not conform to the expectations of a male religious leader and the founder of a popular Order. In fact, while Francis's early preaching was in line with the expectations of an active male religious, Francis's inactivity in later life due to illness appeared shockingly passive, even feminine in Aristotelian terms. While such inactivity may have fit medieval people's expectations of contemplative religious, it was almost certainly read as problematic for the founder-saint of a large and popular medicant preaching order.

In the first place, Francis lacked personal property. He had given up his patrimony in spectacular fashion before his father and the Bishop of Assisi.[44] Of course, the rejection of personal and institutional property was the premise for the whole Order, but the link between holding property and masculinity allows us to see the ongoing debate amongst Franciscans and

41 Neal, *The Masculine Self*, p. 115.

42 Lindeman, '"Go Manfully"', pp. 263–65.

43 Ibid., p. 261.

44 VP, 1.6.15; FF, p. 291; FA:ED, I, pp. 194–95.

the Church hierarchy about the necessity of the Order itself holding and governing its own property in a slightly different light. Francis's position on the Order not holding property was radical and new, and placed his followers in a position of potential passivity. Shelter had to be given; it could not be taken for granted. Such a lack of property also had the potential to limit the preaching and other good works the Order could accomplish, another way the agency of Francis and early Franciscans was curtailed; early Franciscans could also be read as non-normatively masculine and, in their lack of property and agency, even feminine.

Francis himself also appeared to lack the expected masculine agency of a founder-saint in the final years of his life. As outlined above, hagiographies of the saint written before the *Legenda maior* suggested that after 1221 Francis stopped most of his preaching programme, withdrew to live a more eremitic life, and stepped down from leading his Order due to illness and infirmity. In all of these actions, Francis became more passive, a feminine trait by Aristotelian logic. Thus, he contested the normative masculinity expected of an active founder-saint and cleric.

Even more challenging to expectations of masculine behaviour was the fact that Francis often could not reliably act according to his own will in this later period of his life. As we have seen, especially in questions of self-care, Francis's own desires were overruled by his guardian and by leaders of the Order. Francis took better care of his body than he wished—his guardian saw to that—and he saw many doctors for his visual impairment at the insistence of Elias of Cortona, the leader of the Order, and Cardinal Hugolino, the Protector of the Order. This too was seemingly against Francis's wishes, since he believed God's plan for a person was to be accepted rather than challenged.[45]

Especially in the last years of his life, Francis's failing eyesight and body ensured that he could not conform to people's expectations of a male religious leader and founder. This was less of a problem during Francis's lifetime,

45 Francis's position on whether doctors ought to be consulted in cases of illness is complex and changed over the course of his life. All known versions of the *Regula non bullata*, written c. 1210, states that a sick brother should 'desire to be whatever God wishes him to be, whether that is healthy or sick' and 'should not seek out medical treatment too precipitously, for that desire is born of the flesh (*carnalis est*)'. Yet this stipulation is entirely left out of the *Regula bullata*, the papally approved rule that the Franciscan Order came to adopt in 1223. The injunction is included in Hugh of Digne's *Exposition of the 'Rule' of the Friars Minor* and in the fragmented parts of the *Regula non bullata* included in Thomas of Celano's *Remembrance of the Desire of a Soul*. See *Fragmenta inserta in Hugo de Digne* and in *Francisci Assisiensis Scripta*, p. 310; and *Fragmenta in Thomas de Celano, Vita secunda sancto Francisci Conservata*, in *Francisci Assisiensis Scripta*, p. 316.

when, by all accounts, the saint's charisma appeared to draw people to him; but by the time Bonaventure wrote his *Legenda maior*, circa 1260, Francis had been dead for more than thirty years, and the Order had fundamentally changed. While Francis had initially conceived of his Order as a group of religious who were not formally educated and did not take on secular orders, the character of those who joined the Order was changing even during Francis's lifetime. Franciscans were becoming more educated and more tied to the secular Church. By 1260, clericalized intellectuals made up the bulk of Franciscans who lived in friaries governed, if not yet owned outright, by the Order.[46] By then, it had also become clear that some members of the Order believed it was becoming too worldly and was diverging too greatly from Francis's vision. Bonaventure, it seems, was faced with the difficult task of creating an image of Francis that spoke to all factions within the Order—those seeking a more conventional religious life and those who believed the saint's vision had been lost in the make-up and direction of the current Order. Outside the Order, the *Life* also needed to make Francis more understandable as a founder and religious leader. In trying to create a Francis for all, Bonaventure reshaped the saint's lived experience into a narrative that was more normative for a male founder. One of the ways he did this was by diminishing the impact Francis's impairments had on his ability to govern himself and his Order.

Bonaventure's Balancing Act

Even a cursory glance at Bonaventure's *Legenda maior* makes clear that Bonaventure downplayed Francis's illnesses and infirmities. Scott Wells has noted that Francis's blindness all but disappeared from Bonaventure's *Legenda maior*—in this work, any blindness the saint may have experienced was potential, rather than actual.[47] It was also described as a choice in Bonaventure's text; doctors told the saint that *if* he did not stop weeping in

46 This is suggested in Landini, *The Causes of Clericalization* (p. 119), but, more recently, Senocak, in *The Poor and the Perfect*, has questioned whether it is true (p. 158). Nonetheless, a general trend towards recruiting educated friars who would be clerics as well as friars began to emerge in the years after 1230. On these changes within the Order, see Landini, *The Causes of Clericalization*; Manselli, 'S. Bonaventure and the Clericalization of the Friars Minor'; and, more recently, Senocak, *The Poor and the Perfect*, pp. 153–59. On the arrangement that Franciscans may manage but not own property and Pope John XXII's argument that having dominion over property was functionally owing property, see Burr, *The Spiritual Franciscans*, pp. 275–76.

47 See Wells's excellent piece 'Exemplary Blindness'.

adoration and devotion, he *might* lose his eyesight.[48] In spite of this warning, Francis continued to weep, though Bonaventure never acknowledges that Francis's ocular impairment was a reality.

Bonaventure also downplayed the amount of care Francis received for his infirmities. In at least two different cases where earlier source texts included the fact that Francis was in the company of doctors, Bonaventure disappears the doctors. Perhaps the most important example of this is the retelling of Francis's encounter with Lady Poverty in the *Legenda maior*. The earliest account of this now-famous vision is found in Thomas of Celano's *Remembrance of a Soul*. In the *Remembrance*, Francis was travelling from Rieti to Siena for the purpose of visiting a physician to cure his eyes. According to the *Remembrance*, Francis was travelling with a doctor as a companion, one who was bound to the Order.[49] When Bonaventure retold this story, however, Francis appeared to be travelling alone. Nor did Bonaventure relate the reason for Francis's trip to Siena, instead writing that Francis 'was conveying himself to Siena, driven there for a pressing cause'.[50] Bonaventure's diversion from his source text seems a deliberate attempt to obfuscate both the reason for Francis's travel and the fact that Francis was travelling with, and was perhaps even in the care of, a doctor.

In a second example, Bonaventure borrows a story told in both Thomas of Celano's *Remembrance of the Desire of a Soul* and his *Treatise on Miracles*.[51] In both narratives, a noble had given Francis a live pheasant while the saint was ill. Not wanting to eat the pheasant, Francis asked that the bird be taken out of his cell and returned to the countryside. Twice the pheasant returned to Francis. Seeing the bird constantly returning, a doctor (*medicus*) who was devoted to Francis offered to take it home and care for it. The pheasant had other ideas, however, refusing to eat until it was returned to Francis's side. Bonaventure retold this story, but the doctor who offered to care for the pheasant is described simply as 'a man who was accustomed to visit God's servant out of devotion'.[52] Bonaventure's decision to conceal the presence of doctors in his narrative of Francis's life appears to have been calculated.

48 LM, 5.8; FF, p. 820; FA:ED, II, pp. 566–67. Wells, 'Exemplary Blindness', pp. 77–78.

49 RDS, 2.60.93; FF, p. 530; FA:ED, II, p. 307.

50 'Accidit post haec quiddam mirabile viro sancto, dum se ad civitatem Senensem, causa exigente, transferret.' LM, 7.6; FF, p. 837; FA:ED, II, p. 581.

51 RDS, 2.129.170; FF, pp. 594–596; FA:ED, II, pp. 357–58; Thomas of Celano, *Tractatus de Miraculis*, 4.26; FF, pp. 644–755 (pp. 666–67); FA:ED, II, pp. 400–69 (p. 414).

52 'Deinde cuidam collatus viro, qui ex devotione servum Dei visitare solebat, velut sibi molestum foret a pii patris absentari conspectu, escam recusavit omnino.' LM, 8.10; FF, p. 852; FA:ED, II, pp. 594.

Where he could, Bonaventure erased the presence of doctors found in earlier *Lives*. In doing so, Bonaventure diminished the reality of Francis's impairments and the amount of care he was receiving for them. He thus bolstered Francis's individual agency at the expense of acknowledging some of the doctors who were entrusted to care for the infirm saint.

Bonaventure also had to deal with how earlier *Lives* portrayed Francis's lack of agency and formal authority, a problematic reality given late medieval expectations of masculine behaviour, with its emphasis on agency and self-governance. Bonaventure dealt with it by providing descriptions of the saint's behaviour that explained his actions without reference to loss of autonomy or power. Perhaps the most obvious example of this is Bonaventure's choice to ignore earlier source texts that suggested Francis resigned due to illness. Rather, Bonaventure insists that the resignation was linked to Francis's desire for humility, his desire *for* a lack of power.[53] Francis wished to submit his will to God's and did so, in part, by requesting a guardian to obey. By linking Francis's withdrawal from leadership to a voluntary desire for humility, Bonaventure returned agency to Francis himself, agency that was absent in earlier *Lives* due to the saint's illnesses.

Yet, while Bonaventure eliminated discussions of Francis's illnesses and reframed other episodes to emphasize the agency Francis expressed, he also presented Francis as deriving his authority not from his position as a founder-saint but from his nearness to God, as demonstrated through Francis's imitative suffering and reception of the stigmata. For instance, Bonaventure's work spends much more time describing Francis's personal spirituality rather than his role as a founder. This directly contrasts with the early *Lives* of St Dominic written by Jordan of Saxony, Peter Ferrand, Constantine of Orvieto, and Humbert of Romans, which present Dominic absolutely as the founder of his Order— a fellow preacher and not a saint, in the view of David Haseldine.[54] Like Dominic, Francis also founded an enormously popular Order, yet this reality is never central in Bonaventure's *Legenda maior*. While Francis's role as a founder is perhaps not deliberately positioned as incidental to his life, Bonaventure presents Francis as founding a *religio* that developed into an

53 Bonaventure includes his only discussion of Francis's resignation in Chapter 6, which is dedicated to the saint's humility.

54 Jordan of Saxony, *Libellus de principiis Ordinis Praedicatorum*, in Santi Patris Nostri Dominici, Monumenta Ordinis Praedicatorum Historica (MOPH) 16, fasc. 2, 25–88; Peter Ferrand, *Legenda sancti Dominici*, MOPH 16, 209–60; Constantine of Orvieto, *Legenda sancti Dominici*, MOPH 16, 286–352; Humbert of Romans, *Legenda sancta Dominici*, MOPH 16, 355–443. See also Haseldine, 'Early Dominican Hagiography', p. 407.

ordo.[55] In making this contrast, Bonaventure suggests that for Francis the way of living was more important than the institutional foundation. Bonaventure describes the foundation as a group of like-minded men coming together, until Francis realized that he should probably put something together so that they lived according to a Rule—there is initially little intentionality on Francis's part concerning the establishment of an Order as outlined in Bonaventure's *Legenda maior*.[56] Rather than gaining followers through his work as a secular founder, the Francis of the *Legenda maior* grows his Order though the presence of the Holy Spirit, which is working through Francis.[57] Francis is a passive vessel for God's mission, even as he expresses more agency and appears to need less medical care in Bonaventure's *Legenda maior*.

Linked to this is Bonaventure's presentation of Francis as an individual who dedicated himself to living a spiritual life. Unlike the earliest *Lives* of St Dominic, Bonaventure's *Life* presents a Francis who imitated Christ's suffering so thoroughly that he received the stigmata. Most of Bonaventure's thematic chapters deal with Francis's personal piety, humility, obedience, poverty, and charity. As Katherine Lindeman notes, these are typically qualities that Dominicans, at least, associated with the women of their Order, not the men.[58] Thus, while much of Bonaventure's recrafting of Francis's life masked his infirmities and insisted on Francis's ability to enact the expected masculine behaviours of governing self and others, there was room, too, for a spirituality based on devotion to God and somatic experiences of the divine, a spirituality that was coded by his contemporaries as considerably more feminine. Perhaps the early hagiographers of Francis, like those of the contemplatives of Liège examined by Alison More, understood that Francis had inhabited characteristics common in both genders before leaving human sexuality and biological sex aside in his perfect contemplation of God.[59] Had Francis been only a contemplative and not a founder, this would not have been the problem it was for Bonaventure.

When Bonaventure was commissioned to create an official *Life* of St Francis, one that would replace the many different *vitae* that were circulating in the decades after Francis's death, he faced a monumentally difficult task. He

55 Bonaventure begins by calling Francis's group a *religio*, but as more people join and a rule comes into being and is approved, he turns to calling the group an *ordo*. LM, Chapters 3 and 4; FF, pp. 795–814; FA:ED, II, pp. 542–59. The editors of FA:ED suggest that the contrast is deliberate: see note a, II, p. 542.

56 LM, 3.3–3.7; FF, pp. 797–800; FA:ED, II, p. 543–46.

57 See LM, 3.3–4; FF, pp. 797–98; FA:ED, II, pp. 545–46.

58 Lindeman, '"Go Manfully"', p. 174.

59 More, 'Convergence, Conversion and Transformation', p. 44.

had been asked to create a portrait of Francis that satisfied those individuals who remembered or venerated Francis as a sometimes ill and increasingly infirm individual devoted to God. At the same time, it was necessary to create a portrait of the saint that appeared to the medieval world and Church hierarchy as a fitting model for the founder of a large and increasingly powerful Order. Part of that balancing act was trying to fit Francis's character and the events of his life into medieval social expectations of a founder-saint. Bonaventure did this in part by modifying events in Francis's life that would otherwise seem to diminish his agency and his inability to govern his own body, thus making Francis conform to high medieval notions of masculine clerical agency. Yet his portrait of a saint also challenged social preconceptions of clerical masculinity by presenting a Francis who practised a kind of affective, somatic, experiential piety that was more often associated with the feminine than the masculine. In this way, Bonaventure intentionally navigated the needs of two audiences within the Order: those who sought an active founder-saint for the Franciscan founder and those who believed both Francis and his Order advocated a more contemplative life of devotion.

Abbreviations

AC	*Assisi Compilation*, in *Fontes Franciscana,* ed. by E. Menestò and Stefano Brufani (Assisi: Porziuncula, 1995), pp. 1472–1691
FA:ED	Regis Armstrong, J. A. Wayne Hellmann, and William Short, eds, *Francis of Assisi: Early Documents*, 3 vols (New York: New City Press, 1999–2001)
FF	E. Menestò and Stefano Brufani, eds, *Fontes Franciscana* (Assisi: Porziuncula, 1995)
LM	Bonaventure, *Legenda maior sancti Francisci*, in *Fontes Franciscana*, ed. by E. Menestò and Stefano Brufani (Assisi: Porziuncula, 1995), pp. 778–962
MOPH	*Monumenta Ordinis Praedicatorum Historica*
RDS	Thomas of Celano, *Vita secunda*, or Remembrance of the Desire of a Soul in *Fontes Franciscana*, ed. by E. Menestò and Stefano Brufani (Assisi: Porziuncula, 1995), pp. 442–641
VP	Thomas of Celano, *Vita prima*, in *Fontes Franciscana,* ed. by E. Menestò and Stefano Brufani (Assisi: Porziuncula, 1995), pp. 274–425

Bibliography

Primary Sources

Aristotle, *On the Generation of Animals*, in *The Complete Works of Aristotle: The Revised Oxford Translation*, ed. by Jonathan Barnes, 2 vols (Princeton: Princeton University Press, 1984), I, 1111–1218

Aristotle, *Politics*, in *The Complete Works of Aristotle: The Revised Oxford Translation*, ed. by J. Barnes, 2 vols (Princeton: Princeton University Press, 2014), II, 1986–2129

Armstrong, Regis, J. A. Wayne Hellmann, and William Short, eds, *Francis of Assisi: Early Documents*, 3 vols (New York: New City Press, 1999–2001)

Assisi Compilation, in *Fontes Franciscana*, ed. by E. Menestò and Stefano Brufani (Assisi: Porziuncula, 1995), pp. 1472–1691

Assisi Compilation, in *Francis of Assisi: Early Documents*, ed. and trans. by Regis Armstrong, J. A. Wayne Hellmann, and William Short, 3 vols (New York: New City Press, 1999–2001), II, 118–230

Bonaventure, *Legenda maior sancti Francisci*, in *Fontes Franciscana*, ed. by E. Menestò and Stefano Brufani (Assisi: Porziuncula, 1995), pp. 778–962

Bonaventure, *The Major Legend of St Francis of Assisi* in *Francis of Assisi: Early Documents*, ed. and trans. by Regis Armstrong, J. A. Wayne Hellmann, and William Short, 3 vols (New York: New City Press, 1999–2001), II, 525–683

Constantine of Orvieto, *Legenda sancti Dominici*, in *Santi Patris Nostri Dominici*, ed. by M. H. Laurent, Monumenta Ordinis Praedicatorum Historica 16, fasc. 2 (Rome: Institutum Historicum Fratres Praedicatorum, 1935), 286–352

Ferrand, Peter, *Legenda sancti Dominici*, in *Santi Patris Nostri Dominici*, ed. by M. H. Laurent, Monumenta Ordinis Praedicatorum Historica 16, fasc. 2 (Rome: Institutum Historicum Fratres Praedicatorum, 1935), 209–260

Francis of Assisi, *Fragmenta in Thomas de Celano, Vita secunda sancto Francisci Conservata*, in *Francisci Assisiensis Scripta*, ed. by Carolus Paolazzi (Grottaferrata: Collegi S. Bonaventurae, 2009), pp. 314–16

Francis of Assisi, *Fragmenta inserta in Hugo de Digne in Francisci Assisiensis Scripta*, ed. by Carolus Paolazzi (Grottaferrata: Collegi S. Bonaventurae, 2009), pp. 304–14

Francis of Assisi, *Testament*, in *Francisci Assisiensi: Scripta*, ed. by Carolus Paolazzi (Grottaferrata: Collegi S. Bonaventurae, 2009), pp. 394–405

Gratian, *Decretum*, Münchener DigitalisierungsZentrum <http://geschichte.digitale-sammlungen.de/decretum-gratiani/online/angebot> [accessed 16 February 2023]

Humbert of Romans, *Legenda sancta Dominici*, in *Santi Patris Nostri Dominici*, ed. by M. H. Laurent, Monumenta Ordinis Praedicatorum Historica 16, fasc. 2 (Rome: Institutum Historicum Fratres Praedicatorum, 1935), pp. 355–443

Jordan of Saxony, *Libellus de principiis Ordinis Praedicatorum*, in *Santi Patris Nostri Dominici*, ed. by M. H. Laurent, Monumenta Ordinis Praedicatorum Historica 16, fasc. 2 (Rome: Institutum Historicum Fratres Praedicatorum, 1935), pp. 25–88

Thomas of Celano, *Remembrance of the Desire of a Soul* (*the Vita secunda*), in *Francis of Assisi: Early Documents*, ed and trans. by Regis Armstrong, J. A. Wayne Hellmann, and William Short, 3 vols (New York: New City Press, 1999–2001), II, 239–393

Thomas of Celano, *Tractatus de Miraculis,* in *Fontes Franciscana,* ed. by E. Menestò and Stefano Brufani (Assisi: Porziuncula, 1995), pp. 644–755

Thomas of Celano, *The Treatise on Miracles*, in *Francis of Assisi: Early Documents*, ed. and trans. by Regis Armstrong, J. A. Wayne Hellmann, and William Short, 3 vols (New York: New City Press, 1999–2001), II, 400–69

Thomas of Celano, *Vita prima*, in *Fontes Franciscana*, ed. by E. Menestò and Stefano Brufani (Assisi: Porziuncula, 1995), pp. 274–425

Thomas of Celano, *Vita prima*, in *Francis of Assisi: Early Documents*, ed. and trans. by Regis Armstrong, J. A. Wayne Hellmann, and William Short, 3 vols (New York: New City Press, 1999–2001), I, 180–308

Thomas of Celano, *Vita secunda* or Remembrance of the Desire of a Soul, in *Fontes Franciscana*, ed. by E. Menestò and Stefano Brufani (Assisi: Porziuncula, 1995), pp. 442–641

Secondary Sources

Blastic, Michael, Giles Constable, Jacques Dalarun, and Timothy Johnson, 'Towards a Resolution of the Franciscan Question: The Umbrian Legend of Thomas of Celano', *Franciscan Studies*, 66 (2008), 479–510

Broomhall, Susan, and Jacqueline van Gent, eds, *Governing Masculinities in the Early Modern Period: Regulating Selves and Others* (London: Ashgate, 2011)

Burr, David, *The Spiritual Franciscans: From Protest to Persecution in the Century after St Francis* (Philadelphia: University of Pennsylvania Press, 2001)

Bynum, Caroline Walker, *Holy Feast and Holy Fast: The Religious Significance of Food to Religious Women* (Berkeley: University of California Press, 1987)

Cadden, Joan, *Meanings of Sex Differences in the Middle Ages: Medicine, Science and Culture* (Cambridge: Cambridge University Press, 1993)

Callum, Patricia, 'Clergy, Masculinity and Transgression in Late Medieval England', in *Masculinity in Medieval Europe*, ed. by Dawn Hadley (London: Longman, 1999), pp. 178–96

Callum, P. H., and Katherine Lewis, eds, *Holiness and Masculinity in the Middle Ages* (Cardiff: University of Wales Press, 2004)

Christie, Edward, 'Self-Mastery and Submission: Holiness and Masculinity in the *Lives* of Anglo-Saxon Martyr Kings', in *Holiness and Masculinity in the Middle Ages*, ed. by P. H. Callum and Katherine Lewis (Cardiff: University of Wales Press, 2004), pp. 143–57

Cohen, Jeffrey Jerome, and Bonnie Wheeler, eds, *Becoming Male in the Middle Ages* (New York: Garland, 1997; repr. 2000)

Dalarun, Jacques, *Francis of Assisi and the Feminine* (St Bonaventure, NY: The Franciscan Institute, 2006)

Dubourg, Ninon, '"*Ad obsequium divimum inhabilem*": la reconnaissance de la condition de personne infirme par la chancellerie pontificale (XIIe-XIVe siècles)', *Alter: European Journal of Disability Research*, 14.3 (2020), 226–35

Dubourg, Ninon, 'La reconnaissance de la condition de personne infirme par la Chancellerie pontificale (XIIe-XIVe siècles)', (unpublished doctoral thesis, University of Paris Diderot, 2019)

Flood, David, *Fragmenta inserta in Hugo de Digne: Expositio super Regulam fratrum minorum* (Grottaferrata: Editiones Collegii S. Bonaventurae, 1979)

Garland Thomson, Rosemarie, *Extraordinary Bodies: Figuring Physical Disability in American Culture and Literature* (New York: Columbia University Press, 1997)

Garland Thomson, Rosemarie, 'Integrating Disability, Transforming Feminist Theory', *NWSA Journal*, 14.3 (2002), 1–32

Hadley, Dawn, ed., *Masculinity in Medieval Europe* (London: Longman, 1999)

Haseldine, David, 'Early Dominican Hagiography', *New Blackfriars*, 75 (1994), 400–14

Hodges, Kenneth, 'Wounded Masculinity: Injury and Gender in Sir Thomas Malory's *Le Morte d'Arthur*', *Studies in Philology*, 106 (2009), 14–31

Karras, Ruth Mazzo, *From Boys to Men: Formations of Masculinity in Late Medieval Europe* (Philadelphia, University of Pennsylvania Press, 2002)

Kaeuper, Richard, *Chivalry and Violence in Medieval Europe* (Oxford: Oxford University Press, 2001)

Kelly, Kathleen Coyne, 'Malory's Body Chivalric', *Arthuriana*, 6.4 (1996), 52–57

Kuefler, Matthew, *The Manly Eunuch: Masculinity, Gender Ambiguity and Christian Ideology in Late Antiquity* (Chicago: University of Chicago Press, 2001)

Kuuliala, Jenni, Katariina Mustakallio, and Christian Krötzl, 'Introduction: *Infirmitas* in Antiquity and the Middle Ages', in *Infirmity in Antiquity and the Middle Ages*, ed. by Jenni Kuuliala, Katariina Mustakallio, and Christian Krötzl (Abingdon: Routledge, 2016), pp. 1–11

Landini, Laurence, *The Causes of Clericalization of the Order of Friars Minor: 1209–1260, in the Light of Early Franciscan Sources* (Chicago: Pontifica Universitas Gregoriana, 1968)

Lees, Claire, ed., *Medieval Masculinities: Reading Men in the Middle Ages* (Minneapolis: University of Minnesota Press, 1994)

Lindeman, Katherine, '"Go Manfully": Masculine Self-Fashioning in Late Medieval Dominican Sources' (unpublished doctoral dissertation, University of Toronto, 2015)

Manselli, Raoul, 'St Bonaventure and the Clericalization of the Friars Minor', trans. by P. Colborne, *Greyfriars Review*, 4 (1990), 83–98

McNamara, Jo Ann, 'The *Herrenfrage*: The Restructuring of the Gender System, 1050–1150', in *Medieval Masculinities: Regarding Men in the Middle Ages*, ed. by Clare A. Lees, Thelma Fenster, and Jo Ann McNamara (Minneapolis: University of Minnesota Press, 1994), pp. 3–29

McSheffrey, Shannon, 'Men and Masculinity in Late Medieval London Civic Culture', in *Conflicted Identities and Multiple Masculinities: Men in the Medieval West*, ed. by Jacqueline Murray (London: Garland, 2011), pp. 243–278

Metzler, Irina, *Disability in Medieval Europe: Thinking About Physical Impairment in the High Middle Ages c. 1100–1400* (Abingdon: Routledge, 2006)

Metzler, Irina, *A Social History of Disability in the Middle Ages* (Abingdon: Routledge, 2013)

Meyerson, Mark D., Daniel Thierry, and Oren Falk, 'Conclusion', in *A Great Effusion of Blood: Interpreting Medieval Violence*, ed. by Mark. D. Merson, Daniel Thierry, and Oren Falk (Toronto: University of Toronto Press, 2004), pp. 315–19

Mooney, Catherine, 'Francis of Assisi as Mother, Father and Androgynous Figure', in *The Boswell Thesis: Essays on Christianity, Social Tolerance and Homosexuality*, ed. by Matthew Kuefler (Chicago: University of Chicago Press, 2006), pp. 301–332

More, Alison, 'Convergence, Conversion, and Transformation: Gender and Sanctity in Thirteenth-Century Liège', in *Representing Genders and Sexualities in Europe: Construction, Transformation and Subversion, 600–1530*, ed. by Elizabeth L'Estrange and Alison More (Aldershot: Ashgate, 2011), pp. 33–48

Murray, Jacqueline, ed., *Conflicted Identities and Multiple Masculinities: Men in the Medieval West* (London: Garland, 2011)

Murray, Jacqueline, 'Masculinizing Religious Life: Sexual Prowess, the Battle for Chastity and Monastic Identity', in *Holiness and Masculinity*, ed. by Katherine Lewis and P. H. Callum (Cardiff: University of Wales Press, 2004), pp. 24–42

Murray, Jacqueline, 'Mystical Castration: Some Reflections on Peter Abelard, Hugh of Lincoln and Sexual Control', in *Conflicted Identities and Multiple Masculinities: Men in the Medieval West*, ed. by Jacqueline Murray (New York: Garland Press, 2011), pp. 73–91

Murray, Jacqueline, 'One Flesh, Two Sexes, Three Genders', in *Gender and Christianity in Medieval Europe: New Perspectives*, ed. by Lisa Bitel and Felice Lifshitz (Philadelphia: University of Pennsylvania Press, 2008), pp. 34–51

Neal, Derek, *The Masculine Self in Late Medieval England* (Chicago: University of Chicago Press, 2008)

Newman, Martha G., 'Crucified by the Virtues: Monks, Lay Brothers and Women in Thirteenth-Century Cistercian Saints' Lives', in *Gender and Difference in the Middle Ages*, ed. by Sharon Farmer and Carol Braun Pasternack, Medieval Cultures, 32 (Minneapolis: University of Minnesota Press, 2003), pp. 182–209

Pearman, Tory Vandeventer, *Disability and Knighthood in Malory's* Morte d'Arthur (Abingdon: Routledge, 2018)

Pearman, Tory Vandeventer, *Women and Disability in Medieval Literature* (New York: Palgrave Macmillan, 2010)

Parlopiano, Brandon, '"*Propter deformitatem*": Towards a Concept of Disability in Medieval Canon Law', *Canadian Journal of Disability Studies*, 4.3 (2015), 72–102

Retief, Marno, and Rantoa Letšosa, 'Models of Disability: A Brief Overview', *HTS Teologiese Studies/Theological Studies*, 74 (2018), 1–8

Senocak, Neslihan, *The Poor and the Perfect: The Rise of Learning in the Franciscan Order, 1209–1310* (Ithaca, NY: Cornell University Press, 2012)

Singer, Julie, 'Towards a Transhuman Model of Medieval Disability', *postmedieval: a journal of medieval cultural studies*, 1 (2010), 173–79

Spencer-Hall, Alicia, and Blake Gutt, eds, *Trans and Genderqueer Subjects in Medieval Hagiography*, Hagiography Beyond Tradition (Amsterdam: Amsterdam University Press, 2021)

Swanson, Robert N., 'Angels Incarnate: Clergy and Masculinity from the Gregorian Reform to the Reformation', in *Masculinity in Medieval Europe*, ed. by Dawn Hadley (London: Longman, 1999), pp. 160–77

Thibodeaux, Jennifer D., 'Introduction: Rethinking the Medieval Clergy and Masculinity', in *Negotiating Clerical Identities: Priests, Monks and Masculinities in the Middle Ages*, ed. by Jennifer D. Thibodeaux (Houndmills, Basingstoke: Palgrave MacMillan, 2010), pp. 1–15

Thompson, Augustine, *Francis of Assisi: A New Biography* (Ithaca, NY: Cornell University Press, 2012)

Trembinski, Donna, *Illness and Authority in the Life and Lives of Francis of Assisi* (Toronto: University of Toronto Press, 2020)

Vauchez, André, *Francis of Assisi: The Life and Afterlife of a Medieval Saint*, trans. by Michael Cusato (New Haven, CT: Yale University Press, 2012)

Wells, Scott, 'The Exemplary Blindness of Francis of Assisi', in *Disability in the Middle Ages: Rehabilitations, Reconsiderations and Reverberations*, ed. by Joshua Eyler (Abingdon: Routledge, 2010), pp. 67–80

Wheatley, Edward, *Stumbling Blocks Before the Blind: Medieval Constructions of a Disability* (Ann Arbor: University of Michigan Press, 2010

About the Author

Donna Trembinski is a Professor of History at St. Francis Xavier University in Antigonish, Nova Scotia, Canada. Her research areas include the history of disability and medicine and the use of trauma and disability as categories of historical analysis. In 2020, she published *Illness and Authority: Disability in the Life and Lives of Francis of Assisi* (University of Toronto Press). Her current project, Digitized Medieval Medicine of the Eye, examines transmissions of intellectual and practical knowledge about eyecare in medieval Europe between 1050 and 1350.

2. The Paradoxes of Margaret the Lame: Disability and Authorial Work in Thirteenth-Century Magdeburg

Joshua S. Easterling

Abstract: The *Life* of Margaret the Lame, a thirteenth-century anchoress from Magdeburg, is structured by the powerfully internalized and paradoxical spirituality that became the hallmark of her teachings. Though disabled by acute lameness, Margaret came through her interactions with her confessor and lay associates not only to embrace suffering and its attendant limitations, but to transform both into new forms of agency. This essay argues that such forms included her 'authorial work', which emerged through the anchoress's own labour and, more essentially, though the non-economy of privation. Paradoxically, the losses of personal (and bodily) agency that Margaret suffered already contain within them her gains as spiritual teacher to others, and even as authorial collaborator in the making of her text.

Keywords: anchoress, Magdeburg, authorship, lameness, paradox, interiority

The *Life* of the German anchoress Margaret the Lame of Magdeburg (d. c. 1250) ranks among the many treasures of women's mystical piety and writing in thirteenth-century Europe. Composed during Margaret's own lifetime, the work is remarkable on several accounts, and as such deserves far more attention than it has heretofore received. First, the *Life* inhabits an indeterminate space between mystical treatise and *vita*. Within late medieval religious culture, human channels of divine grace were generally either written about, as in hagiographical writings, or actively authored the written text, but did not serve both functions within one and the same

Grace-Petinos, Stephanie, Leah Pope Parker, and Alicia Spencer-Hall, eds. *Disability and Sanctity in the Middle Ages.* Taylor & Francis Group, 2025
DOI 10.5117/9789463724333_CH02

work.[1] Margaret's *Life* operates quite differently in this regard, representing in addition an extended reflection on, and revision of, the very notion of authorial work. More precisely, Margaret's confessor and amanuensis, a Dominican friar named John of Magdeburg, affords the holy woman—styled *contracta* in the Latin original—a status as both subject *and* collaborating author of a work that thereby merges otherwise distinct textual fields.[2]

It is in fact the idea of work—text, labour, and their intersections—that governs another of the *Life*'s central themes: Margaret's physical disability.[3] She obtains the epithet *contracta* because of acute lameness, which she bore from early childhood, and which made it difficult for her to walk, perform manual labour without extreme bodily pain, or even to appear in public, where her disability met with open ridicule. While the precise nature of her disability is unclear—the term *contractus/a* can refer to various physical impairments—for Margaret it remained a source of both physical and emotional pain.[4]

Partly for these reasons, she determines from an early point in her life to become enclosed as a recluse in her hometown, the urban centre of thirteenth-century Magdeburg. In her vocation as anchoress, however, Margaret also struggles with the spiritual and physical demands that such a life requires. As they are presented in this work, none of the saint's many challenges are separable from the question of disability, which becomes the focal point of several paradoxes within the text.[5] In fact, the *Life* is shaped throughout by paradox, including the perception of limitation as enrichment, disability as ability, and privation as a kind of gift. In this sense,

1 Exceptions to this general tendency include what has insightfully been called 'autohagiography'; see Kieckhefer, *Unquiet Souls*, p. 6. It is useful to view the *Life* as an instance of such generic blending, though the specific form that this takes in Margaret's case is in some ways distinct from Kieckhefer's examples (see following note).

2 The *Life* is best understood as the product of what might be called 'collaborative authorship': see Kestemont, Deploigne, and Moens, 'Collaborative Authorship', pp. 199–224. Taking this collaboration seriously, I refer to both Margaret and John as authors throughout this essay.

3 On texts and cultural phenomena related to the disabled or impaired body, see especially Metzler, *Disability* and *Social History*; and Eyler, *Disability in the Middle Ages*. Prior to these studies, disability in the Middle Ages had frequently been given cursory critical treatment, often without reference to saints at all; see for example, Winzer, *History*, pp. 22–26.

4 Vauchez, *Sainthood*, pp. 469–72.

5 Here and throughout the essay I refer to Margaret as 'saint' although she was never officially canonized, nor do we have evidence that anyone, aside from her confessor, was convinced of her sanctity; her *Life* was, accordingly, never included in the *Acta Sanctorum* compiled by the Bollandists. For discussion of such saints or otherwise venerated figures and their communities, see Mulder-Bakker, *Living Saints*, pp. 1–45; and Simons, *Cities of Ladies*; see also Mulder-Bakker, *Living Saints* (p. 305), and *Lives* (p. 161). She nonetheless ranks among the many late medieval saints whose lives were 'represented in hagiographic fashion [...] despite total absence of cult'; Kieckhefer, *Unquiet Souls*, p. 16.

the work ranks among the 'many medieval texts [wherein] disability can be read as an enhancement, as an addition rather than [as] a diminishing of capacities'.[6] This feature of Margaret's experience also relates to the intersections, explored by Irina Metzler, between liminality, disability, and space—relations that guide us to imagine how the restriction of movement caused by one enclosure (the body) interacted with an analogous space of vocational confinement (the anchorhold).[7]

While Margaret's physical lameness forms the centre of the *Life*, it is also one of several points of experience through which the work elaborates her deeply paradoxical spirituality. Her several identities (saint, recluse, teacher, and collaborating author) become vivid expressions of the subjective flexibility afforded in, and through, the various relations that structure her inner development, which includes the interactions between her agency as spiritual instructor to her confessor and lay associates, on the one hand, and her chronic impairment, on the other.[8] Like the other 'gifts' (suffering, rejection, and poverty) that she receives, Margaret's lameness informs her teachings, which reinterpret joy and pain, consolation and suffering, in a way that dissolves the boundary between such oppositions. This essay argues that her loss in the physical arena does not finally operate as loss, as already noted, but as a redirection or transformation of the inner self, which thereby acquires new forms of agency. In fact, the most prominent paradox running throughout the *Life* relates to agency itself, spiritual as well as authorial. The teachings at the heart of the work are in this way channelled through her disability, which becomes a kind of stage for an expansive notion of labour, even as her physical experience of privation similarly establishes the conditions necessary for the making of this text. My reading ultimately takes the *Life* on its own terms, which insist that the paradoxes of agency internal to the saint herself also structure the spiritual, including authorial, work that proceeds through her.

Poverty, Sanctity, and Disability

The *Life* opens by describing Margaret's lameness as 'a sign of her chosenness' (*cuius electionis signum*), a sign acquired when she was only a small

6 Singer, 'Toward a Transhuman', p. 176.

7 Metzler, 'Liminality and Disability', pp. 273–96 and especially pp. 280–94.

8 On the relationship between holy women and their confessors, see especially Griffiths and Hotchin, *Partners in Spirit*; Coakley, *Women, Men, and Spiritual Power*; Morgan, 'Spiritual Autobiographies', pp. 35–51; Hollywood, 'Inside Out', pp. 78–98; and Benedict, *Empowering Collaborations*.

child.[9] Quite unlike her near contemporary and fellow mystic Mechthild of Magdeburg (d. 1282), who went blind near the end of her life, Margaret bore her disability from her early childhood.[10] Throughout the text, embodiment, enclosure, and disability collectively represent the re-evaluation and reversal of her desires; after entering the cell and enduring the 'weakness' (*debilitas/fragilitas*) caused by her impairment, she comes to prefer suffering to consolation. This development stages a reorientation and internalization of value: suffering, abjection, and poverty are presented as gifts, even as her body is figured as an 'ugly sack' (*sacco vili*) that contains and conceals a treasure—Margaret herself. The suffering (*pena*) that Margaret took to be the 'greatest gift' (*donum maximum*) is mentioned so frequently in the text—the term appears roughly 250 times!—that it effectively becomes the one gift to which all others are ultimately referred. From the outset, the transfigured relations of gift and privation, treasure and worthlessness, become the hallmark of her life and work.

> In the city of Magdeburg lived a woman called Margaret, whom God had especially chosen for himself when she was barely one year old. At that age, as a sign of her chosenness, God mortified her in her limbs. God did so, however, to protect her securely, like a precious treasure hidden in an ugly sack. [...] God had chosen her for himself as an heir on earth and bestowed upon her abundant gifts, namely, suffering, rejection, and poverty.[11]

John's description of Margaret as a 'precious treasure' (*preciosum thesaurum*; cf. 2 Cor. 4.7) deploys a common motif, one used, for example, by Bernard of Clairvaux (d. 1153) to describe internal worth concealed by an external form.[12] Such images also set the stage for Margaret's association with various saints, including the Virgin Mary, who, the *Life* affirms, later teaches Margaret to

9 Here and throughout, the *vita* (John of Magdeburg, ed. by Schmidt) and its English translation (John of Magdeburg, *Life*, ed. by Mulder-Bakker) will be cited as *VMC* and *LML*, respectively; citations are given by chapter (*LML*) and page number.

10 Mechthild of Magdeburg, *Flowing Light*, p. 334.

11 *LML*, 1.313; *VMC*, p. 3: 'Fuit in civitate Partenopolis quedam persona, nomine Margareta, quam Deus specialiter sibi preeligit, cum non esset etatis unius anni. Cuius electionis signum fuit, quia in eadem etate eam in membris Deus mortificavit. Fecit autem Deus sicut, qui preciosum thesaurum vult abscondere sacco vili, ut securius servetur. [...] Deus, qui eam elegerat, de hereditate, quam sibimet in terries elegerat, illi tribuit habundanter; hoc fuit: pena, abiectio et paupertas'.

12 Bernard of Clairvaux, *Sancti Bernardi Opera*, Homily III.3.

read and write.[13] It is here, moreover, that attention is directed away from her disability; what is declared as valuable is not the bodily enclosure but the precious treasure that it contains. Value is relocated from corporeality to the spirit, and from the 'ugly' surface to the saint that resides beneath it.

The *Life* positions Margaret at the intersection of poverty and sainthood by assimilating her to mendicant ideals and effectively ranking her among those 'living saints' of the thirteenth century who flourished in central Europe, particularly within the Low Countries. The text survives in over a dozen Latin and vernacular copies from the late thirteenth to the seventeenth centuries. Written largely in Middle Dutch, the vernacular *vitae* demonstrate that Margaret was above all 'a well-known figure in the Low Countries'.[14] In contrast to her near-contemporary St Francis of Assisi (d. 1226), however, Margaret's form of sanctity and poverty are almost entirely restricted to the inner life.[15] Her confessor concludes the *Life* by observing as much, with respect to the 'inner' (rather than outer) miracles by which she distinguished herself: 'may [the reader], in Margaret, praise God, who deigned to work these inner miracles in her in our time. The Lord is glorified in many saints in our time through exterior miracles, but now he wants to reveal his glory through wonders that he works on the inside'.[16] In a common leitmotif of medieval sainthood, Margaret exemplified humility by resisting any such association with miracles, or with those spiritual graces that might invest her with the odour of sanctity.[17] Yet, for John, her sanctity was admirably demonstrated both in her virtues, including poverty, and in the miracles that were performed through her 'on the inside'.[18]

Margaret just as recognizably embodies the widespread linkage between sanctity and disability.[19] In tracing this association and its cultural contexts,

13 *LML*, 3.314; *VMC*, p. 4.

14 Mulder-Bakker, 'Lame Margaret', p. 156. For analyses of the work and of Margaret's life generally, see ibid., pp. 155–69 and Mulder-Bakker, *Lives*, pp. 148–73. For discussion of the extant *vitae* of Margaret, see *VMC*, pp. xv–xviii; and Mulder-Bakker, *Lives*, pp. 171–72, n. 88. On Margaret's status as saint, see note 5 above.

15 On poverty as a Dominican virtue, see Holloway, 'Performing Poverty', pp. 151–63; on the poverty of saints, albeit in a fourteenth-century context, see also Kieckhefer, *Unquiet Souls*, p. 140 and passim.

16 *LML*, 396 (epilogue); *VMC*, p. 101: 'Laudet Deum in Margareta, qui ista interiora miracula in ea operari nostris temporibus est dignatus. In multis sanctis nostris temporibus per exteriora miracula est Dominus glorificatus, modo autem vult suam gloriam revelare per interiora mirabilia, que interius operatur'.

17 See also Mulder-Bakker, *Living Saints*, p. 306.

18 After all, these were the two features of sainthood that Innocent III had outlined just decades earlier. See Vauchez, *Sainthood*, pp. 36–49.

19 Wheatley, 'Monsters, Saints, and Sinners', pp. 22–25.

Edward Wheatley has argued for the importance of a religious model of disability alongside the otherwise dominant social and biological models.[20] The most obvious link between disability and the saints lies of course in the latter's power to heal maladies and physical impairments.[21] Margaret stands among the multitude of disabled saints like the Dominican tertiary Margaret of Castello (d. 1320) and St Francis, who towards the end of his life suffered a form of blindness.[22] To be sure, there were important tensions between disability and sainthood. Just as not all disabled holy people became saints, not all saints were equally enthusiastic about associating with the disabled. Upon encountering a leper, for instance, Francis felt palpable disgust.[23] It is unclear whether the saint was unsettled by the physical deformity, or perhaps shared in a widespread tendency to moralize disability in a rejection of the ill, malformed, or otherwise impaired body. After all, the association of physical or mental defects with a form of presumed moral corruption flourished throughout the later Middle Ages, including in visionary works of the sort not far removed from the *Life*.[24]

That association derives from an ambivalence towards bodily impairment and suffering. In her *Scivias*, for example, the twelfth-century Benedictine nun Hildegard of Bingen (d. 1179) assumes that bodily disfigurement owed first and foremost to God's judgment. She writes that sometimes a weak nature is expressed bodily 'in various deformities' (*in diversitatem formationis contrariae formae*) as when a person's 'limbs are distorted and misshapen and he is a cripple' (*membra hominis divisa sunt non recte ordinata ut debilium*).[25] As we have seen, at its outset Margaret's *Life* asserts that God rendered her lame and so follows Hildegard and others in identifying the cause of disability with divine authority. In similar ways, Old and New Testament narratives served to frame this cultural ambivalence in terms of divine judgment and the compassionate power to heal, respectively.[26] The

20 Ibid., pp. 18–19.

21 Metzler, *Disability*, pp. 126–85. For a compendious list of such miracle narratives, see ibid., pp. 191–259.

22 Vauchez, *Sainthood*, pp. 209–10. On Francis, see Wells, 'Exemplary Blindness', pp. 67–80; and Trembinski's chapter in the present volume, pp. 39–62.

23 Orlemanski, 'How to Kiss a Leper', p. 151.

24 Metzler, *Disability*, pp. 88–89.

25 Hildegard of Bingen, *Scivias*, p. 315, and PL 197 col. 571B. See also Metzler, *Disability*, pp. 38–64. The idea was widespread; Gerald of Wales (d. 1223) makes a similar point about the blind and lame in *The Topography of Ireland*, where such disabilities are 'just punishment from God' (p. 118); quoted in Wheatley, 'Monsters, Saints, and Sinners', p. 20. For discussion of the 'stigmatized body', see also Gilchrist, 'Medieval Bodies', pp. 46–49.

26 Metzler, *Disability*, pp. 133–38; see also Pearman, *Women and Disability*, pp. 30–31.

presentation of disability through 'a narrative explanation of its origin or a narrative of its eradication, whether through cure or social exclusion' is reflected in the *Life* only marginally, however.[27] Both Wheatley and Metzler have also shown that physical impairment was not always and invariably associated with sin.[28] The *Life* in fact represents Margaret's lameness in a way that challenges those aetiologies, which account for disability by linking it to one or several moral transgressions committed by an individual's ancestors (cf. John 9.1–3). After all, her physical condition is understood as an extension of *her* spiritual development, as already noted, and in this sense has far more to do with Margaret's relationship with God than with her social, ancestral, or cultural environments.

Margaret's text, then, moves beyond such moralizations and develops the paradoxes of inner experience already present in its opening description of her. Foremost among these is the 'gift' of personal loss, or poverty, that disability (itself a major experience of privation) brought in its wake. At many points, the *Life* affirms poverty's status as such a gift, and nowhere more eloquently than in its pronouncement that poverty is valuable 'because someone who owns nothing can lose nothing' ([*v*]*alet autem paupertas* [...] *quia, qui nichil habet, amittere nichil potest*).[29] Yet this representation of poverty also underscores that 'nothing' is *not* exactly nothing. While the ownership of nothing renders loss impossible, that fact does not entirely erase the implicit gain: though it is the condition of having nothing, poverty *has value*, and so it is not nothing after all, but a means of radically redefining value as conventionally understood. Both the purpose and effect of such reflections, which fill Margaret's text, are in large part to establish linkages between her own qualities and (physical) privations, on the one hand, and the teachings contained in the *Life*, on the other. Both are fundamentally structured by experiences of bodily loss that, in a reversal, become examples of the saint's many 'treasures'.

Identity and the Paradoxical Body

Framing Margaret's disability not as loss or privation but as enhancement and 'gift', the *Life* proceeds to recast her experience still further by relocating

27 Wheatley, 'Monsters, Saints, and Sinners', p. 17, summarizing Mitchell and Snyder, *Narrative Prosthesis*, pp. 1–10.

28 Wheatley, *Stumbling Blocks*, p. 14; and Metzler, *Disability*, pp. 11–13.

29 *LML*, 59.374; *VMC*, p. 75.

it beyond such oppositions altogether. The development hardly seems intuitive. In a recent reflection, Julie Singer has observed that physical impairment has a way of adding 'another layer of identity instead of stripping away the rest'.[30] At one level, this reading of disability as supplement or addition to subjective identities accords with the unfolding of Margaret's life and vocation: her cell affords Margaret a social presence through which she acquires the identities of anchoress, penitent, spiritual counsellor, and saint.[31] These and other functions that may have accrued to Margaret over the course of her career, however, have no essential or intrinsic relation to her disability. Nor is it clear that the addition of identities rather than the removal of those 'layers' necessarily disrupts the narratives of corporeal normativity that serve to marginalize those with disabilities.[32]

The *Life* negotiates this shifting territory by merging separate identities, though without cancelling out their individual distinctiveness. What effectively becomes a paradoxical image is first treated in relation to another disability—namely, blindness. Prior to its elaboration within the work as an inner or spiritual deficiency, blindness emerges in terms every bit as embodied as Margaret's lameness. Early on, she befriends a 'poor blind woman' (*pauperculam* [...] *cecam*) with whom she travels to church.[33]

> There was a poor blind woman in her mother's house who often accompanied Margaret to church, the lame one guiding the blind, the blind supporting the lame. On the street, people would look at this lame child as if she were a monster, alternately laughing and shouting: 'Look, look, a great miracle! The lame leads the blind!' Quite stunned, workers would stand around and neglect their duties, staring at her while carrying their heavy sandbags.[34]

30 Singer, 'Toward a Transhuman', p. 175.

31 For discussion of Margaret's various social functions, see also Mulder-Bakker, 'Lame Margaret', pp. 163–68.

32 Singer, 'Toward a Transhuman', pp. 175–76; and for what Singer refers to as 'enabling identities', see 'Disability', pp. 138–40.

33 For general theoretical treatment of blindness in the Middle Ages, see Wheatley, *Stumbling Blocks*, pp. 1–28.

34 *LML*, 2.313–14; *VMC*, p. 3: 'Mater eius habuit in domo pauperculam quondam cecam, que cum ista solebat ecclesiam frequentare. Ista contracta cecam duxit, ceca autem contractam sustentavit. Quando iverunt per plateam, respexerunt istam contractam homines sicut monstrum et exclamaverunt ad invicem ridentes; "Videte, videte magnum mirum, contracta ducit cecam." Pre magna ammiratione negligentes viam suam stabant portitores aspicientes eam, qui graves saccos in humeris deportabant'. On this passage, see also Mulder-Bakker, 'Lame Margaret', p. 157.

As the blind woman and the lame child together meet with ridicule, the encounter represents a striking and troubling instance of what Susan Wendell has called the 'rejected body'.[35] Linking this rejection with gender, Wendell's analysis defines such challenges and rejection as 'those aspects of bodily life (such as illness, disability, weakness, and dying) [...] and bodily experience (including most forms of bodily suffering) that are feared, ignored, despised, and/or rejected in a society and its culture'.[36] Yet the scene is also very moving, despite the abusive response to Margaret and her friend by onlookers, as an image of the solidarity and collaborating support the two share. The narrative is not without its analogues elsewhere in medieval texts; in one such account, told in Jacob of Voragine's thirteenth-century *Golden Legend*, a blind man agrees to carry his lame companion on his back, and the two discover a new form of physical mobility despite the fact that both suffer from impairments.[37] Margaret's arrangement with her blind friend so that the two may attend Mass serves a largely similar function.

Meanwhile, by exploiting the semantic flexibility of the term *monstrum*, which denotes at once 'monster' and 'marvel' or 'miracle', the *Life* once again situates Margaret at the intersection of two forms of social alterity—disability and sanctity.[38] The derisive exclamation by onlookers that Margaret had become, or effected, a 'great miracle' (*magnum mirum*) is a critical feature of this effect, as is the presence of the blind woman.[39] While blindness, like Margaret's disability, takes on increasingly internal and spiritual associations as the *Life* progresses, here it underscores how the addition of a physical disability does not necessarily render the individuals in question further impaired, or indeed increase their dependence on those without such impairments. In this scene, two individuals, both physically impaired, are not thereby doubly impeded in their effort to attend church. Quite the contrary, blindness and lameness have the effect of enhancing their physical mobility. Disability is neither exacerbated nor eliminated through the women's cooperation (after all, both retain their disabilities), but is rather negotiated through a form of mutual support that permits them together

35 Wendell, *Rejected Body*. Similar examples of such abusive rejection in late medieval narratives are far too numerous to cite here. For a start, see Wheatley, *Stumbling Blocks*, p. 36 and passim.
36 Wendell, *Rejected Body*, p. 85. See also Bynum, *Fragmentation*, pp. 181–238; and Wisbey, 'Die Darstellung', pp. 9–34.
37 Wheatley, *Stumbling Blocks*, p. 114.
38 Wheatley, 'Monsters, Saints, and Sinners', pp. 17–31; see also Williams, *Deformed Discourse*, especially pp. 107–77; and Thurber, 'Disability and Monstrosity', passim.
39 On the subjection of the blind to ridicule, see especially Wheatley, *Stumbling Blocks*, pp. 90–128.

what they could not accomplish alone. This scene operates as an image of what can only be called a paradoxical body—indeed, a *monstrum*—as the multiplying of disabilities diminishes rather than exacerbates impairment. This thoroughly embodied collaboration is a physical image of what Margaret experiences on the levels of both body and spirit: namely, that loss and privation are potential forms of enhancement.

Margaret is represented as embracing suffering regardless of its form, with her lameness being one of many ways by which debility and pain organized her inner and outer experience. Her bodily pains, which ranged beyond those caused by her lameness, are framed as 'the greatest gift' (*donum maximum*) through her own capacity for embracing rather than resisting such suffering.[40] It again seems strange to frame as a gift the 'immeasurable bodily suffering' (*penalis corpori supra modum*) that doubtless resulted in part from Margaret's disability.[41] But as the *Life* underscores repeatedly, while her disability was permanent, suffering itself, far from being a permanent condition, was subject to transformation. Here it is appropriate to speak of her disabilities, in the plural; for example, her debilitating headaches, which, to modern readers, might seem to resemble intense migraines, at times incapacitated her both physically and spiritually. At one point, she suffers 'such a headache that she could no longer sustain the thought of [God's] goodness'.[42] Though framed from the outset as a 'gift', her pain was clearly felt as a challenge with potentially negative consequences, in this case rendering her incapable of thinking of God's goodness. At times, too, God becomes the agent of her suffering; since she 'desired' (*in desiderio ferventi*) it, God acquiesced to her wishes in this regard.

> After five years of suffering, Margaret was in such fervent desire that she feared the loss of her senses because her body was too fragile to endure such great suffering. Through it, certainly, God satisfied her desires, for she had desired great suffering and few consolations. He therefore gave her a headache that made the suffering even harder to bear. [...] Often she became so anxious that she said: 'God, my God, why have you forsaken me?'[43]

40 *LML*, 4.318; *VMC*, p. 7.

41 *LML*, 3.314; *VMC*, p. 4.

42 *LML*, 59.371; *VMC*, p. 72: 'Semel punivit in capite Deus eam, quod cogitationem de bonitate sua non poterat sustinere'.

43 *LML*, 44.349; *VMC*, p. 46: 'Quinque annis penam habuit Margareta, quando fuit in desiderio ferventi, quod timuit amittere sensus suos. Hoc fuit ex eo, quod pena magna et corpus eius fragile nimis fuit; suo enim Deus in hoc desiderio satisfecit. Desideraverat enim magnas penas

Although Margaret fears that she would eventually lose the use of her senses, Christ assures her that this will not happen. Here the text operates through a recurrent ambivalence: while she desires and welcomes the suffering that she experiences, that very suffering causes her the fear and anxiety—that is, further suffering—that she clearly does not want, at least not wholeheartedly. Echoing the words of Christ (Matt. 27.46), she signals her experience as both the voluntary embrace of (more) suffering and as comprising a particular form of suffering from which she seeks release.

It is in her resemblance with Christ, as well as in her description of herself, that Margaret's identity undergoes both an expansion and a kind of collapse into 'nothing'. While she is compared with Christ at various points throughout the *Life*, through bodily suffering the two merge in a manner that challenges the terms of identification. Her own subjective experience is in a sense both supplemented and elided through that merging as Margaret becomes at once more and less than what she had been previously. The debilitating experiences that have thus intensified her resemblance with Christ at the same time allow her to underscore her nothingness. Her repeated description of herself as 'nothing' (*ego nichil sum*) eliminates her identity altogether.[44] Yet it also registers the internal level of experience wherein personal nothingness, or spiritual poverty, becomes a form of enrichment. She becomes nothing, and yet, always having been nothing, she is also divested of nothing; the process of personal diminishment transforms into spiritual enhancement as she comes to resemble Christ. Here too, the nothingness of inner poverty 'is valuable because those who own nothing can lose nothing'. In this way, then, once Margaret's disability redirects bodily experience to the level of the spirit, the discourses of gain and loss are reorganized—and radically so.

Debilitas and *Fragilitas*: Suffering Transformed

The levels of identification that structure Margaret's relation to her blind companion and Christ remain fluid and elastic, not least because physical impairment itself witnesses to the essential impermanence of *any* bodily condition. The *Life* further implies, through the likewise shifting terminology

et consolationes paucas. Et propter hoc dedit ei flagellum in capite, ut pena esset graior ad portandum. [...] Et sepe ita fuit anxiata, quod dixit: "Deus, Deus meus, ut quid me dereliquisti?" (Matt. 27.46)'.

44 *LML*, 45.351–52, and 60.377; *VMC*, pp. 49–50 and 79.

used to describe disability, a potentially wide range of signifying possibilities. Metzler has addressed the diverse references to disability within medieval writings. As she suggests, the 'vagueness' of such language (*deformans*, *decrepitus*, etc.) argues for a theoretical model of medieval disability that more precisely distinguishes between 'impairment' and 'disability'.[45] However, much of what we might learn about medieval responses to embodied challenges and their spiritual contexts is obscured by an Anglo-American social and cultural model that rigorously contrasts biological and cultural notions of disability.[46] So too does the flexibility of textual language and representations in the terms (*debilitas* and *fragilitas*), used throughout the *Life* to designate 'weakness', show that idea's instability: weakness and strength, impairment and empowerment, function in complementary rather than oppositional ways.[47]

The distinction that John frequently makes between *debilitas* and *fragilitas* (that is, human 'frailty' with respect to sin) also shifts in a way that underscores both the conceptual and lexical flexibility of 'weakness'. Thus the collocation *debilitas corporis* (bodily impairment) appears with regularity throughout the work.[48] In its descriptions of Margaret's physical condition, however, the *Life* does not confine itself to that term exclusively and at times uses *fragilitas*. John writes, for example, of her release 'from all the weakness (*fragilitatibus*) of her body.[49] This usage in fact forms part of two distinct but closely related tendencies in the *Life*. With increasing frequency John favours the term *fragilitas* over *debilitas*, a preference motivated largely by a tendency to perceive disability in spiritual rather than in physical terms. The repeated allusions to blindness in the text, for example, have little to do with the eyes of the body; John and Margaret are concerned primarily with spiritual blindness.[50] Linked to the image of Margaret's companion

45 Metzler, *Disability*, p. 5 and passim. For discussion of the absence of the modern term *disability* from medieval texts, see also Wheatley, 'Monsters, Saints, and Sinners', p. 17; for general theoretical contexts of medieval disability, see also Metzler, *Disability*, pp. 11–37.

46 See especially Metzler, *Disability*, pp. 1–10; and Singer, 'Toward a Transhuman'. That model also at times marginalizes understandings of disability oriented around religious experience. See Wendell, 'Toward a Feminist Theory', passim.

47 Intriguingly, the *Life* does not often use the otherwise common term *infirmitas* to describe bodily impairment. For an exception, see *LML*, 67.390; *VMC*, p. 94. On defining *infirmitas*, see Kuuliala, Mustakallio, and Krötzl, 'Introduction', pp. 5–7.

48 *LML*, 3.314; *VMC*, p. 4; and *LML*, 5.318; *VMC*, p. 8. She is described as pious 'even in her worst bodily weakness [*in maxima quoque debilitate corporis fuit*]', and as suffering 'from extreme bodily weakness [*ex nimia corporis debilitate*]'.

49 *LML*, 31.340; *VMC*, p. 34.

50 On the 'allegorical meanings' that are ascribed to particular disabilities, see Davis, *Enforcing Normalcy*, p. 82.

from the text's opening, blindness far more commonly refers to failures in spiritual sight, or a lack of spiritual wisdom. At one point, Margaret shares her hope that others would be freed 'from great weakness' (*fragilitate*), and that God would lead them 'from great blindness [*a magna cecitate*] to great wisdom and awareness'; elsewhere, spiritual temptations make up for a person's having been 'constituted in great blindness and with many weaknesses' (*in magna cecitate et in pluribus fragilitatibus constitutus*).[51]

Through the flexibility of the term *fragilitas*, Margaret's bodily condition acquires an inner, spiritual relevance, so much so that the borderline between inner and outer modes of experience grows indistinct. Her capacity for enduring suffering is described as a miracle, for example, since 'given the weakness of her body, it should have been impossible' (*quia secundum fragilitatem corporis impossibile hoc fuisset*).[52] The spiritual resonance of *fragilitas* here, as elsewhere, merges with its bodily associations; the point is that, in order to know the power of God and Christ's own suffering, she must suffer the loss or limitation of her spiritual *and* bodily strength, not simply the one or the other. The miracle of divine support thus becomes all the more striking. Meanwhile, this tendency to read disability in spiritual terms transmutes even the term *debilitas*, which otherwise refers strictly to Margaret's experience of the body. The *Life*, which again is as much Margaret's work as it is John's, expresses this in the following terms:

> From extreme weakness [*pre nimia debilitate*], the beloved no longer appeals to the soul as before. Yet in this great weakness [*in illa magna debilitate*], if the soul is capable of anything, she thinks of her beloved. She could never fall so low, but her bodily weakness [*corporis debilitas*] destroyed her in the same way.[53]

What takes precedence in these reflections on Margaret's *debilitas* is her spiritual challenge, a mirror of her physical challenges. In general, the whole notion of 'weakness' as a physical condition seems to disappear from the text entirely as all of Margaret's bodily 'weaknesses' are referred to the level of her spiritual devotion. In discussing her sins, she writes, that whenever a 'soul is united with God so as to be one with him' (*anima in tantum unitur Deo, quod*

51 *LML*, 33.341; *VMC*, p. 36; and *LML*, 60.379; *VMC*, p. 82.

52 *LML*, 50.356; *VMC*, p. 55.

53 *LML*, 45.350; *VMC*, p. 47: 'Pre nimia debilitate non sapit ei dilectus sicut ante. Tamen in illa magna debilitate, quando aliquid potest, cogitat de dilecto. Ipsa numquam sic posset occidi, sed corporis debilitas interficit eam ita'.

unum est cum eo), it reflects only lightly on its 'weaknesses' (*fragilitates*).[54] In this experience, she comes to identify with the spiritual shortcomings of others. Here again, the breakdown of subjective boundaries is occasioned by Margaret's recognition of the inner rather than outer bonds that she shares with others. On the other hand, her *debilitas* remains even when at another level her *fragilitas*, or incapacity of the spirit, has been eliminated, since such *fragilitates* are in effect mere catalysts for her spiritual agency (prayer) and power. She argues throughout that, paradoxically, the loss of virtuous agency only reveals the divine power to eliminate the weaknesses of humans and thereby to reinvest them with the ability to serve God.

This transformation of 'weakness' resembles yet another transformation—that of labour or work. If one of the most persistently repeated themes throughout the *Life* is its insistence that absence or privation is not in fact what it appears to be—for Margaret, weakness *is* strength—it should not surprise us that her intensely painful experience of the body does not entirely prevent her from performing work. Rather than being directed externally to manual tasks, Margaret's work becomes internal and spiritual. Her disability is not eliminated, and indeed suffering remains a constant throughout her life. Yet its presence does not eliminate her potential to perform work, but rather redirects and transforms it. Margaret's work becomes spiritual and in fact textual, as we shall see. In short, her disability becomes *this* ability—her work as counsellor and teacher to others, and as the author of this text. That transformation is also marked by the same paradoxical structure that governs the rest of the *Life*. While she continually experiences privations at the level of her body, these do not cumulatively add up to loss. Loss becomes gain as the physical is redirected to the spiritual.

Work of Praise: Labour and the Transformation of Disability

Margaret's engagement in physical labour represented one of her most exacerbating challenges. We are not informed that she was exempted from bodily exertion any more than were other medieval recluses. Reading, meditation, and contemplation were common practices within anchoritic culture, but so too were more physically taxing labours. The manual tasks in which many anchorites engaged (for example, in needlework, weaving, or, if the anchorite was literate, in copying texts) would of course have been more challenging for some than for others. Moreover, the bowing

54 *LML*, 68.392; *VMC*, p. 97.

and genuflections that attended an anchoress's prayer life are described in detail in the thirteenth-century Middle English anchoritic text *Ancrene Wisse*.[55] It is entirely possible that Margaret's duties as an anchoress would likewise have been physically rigorous. At the same time, and in a procedure similar to that which guides the author's (and authors') distinction between *fragilitas* and *debilitas*, a terminological variation registers her physical labours (*labor*) as well as her spiritual work (*opus*). These terms, which often referred to the work performed through manual tasks and intellectual (or divine) activity respectively, also mark the transformation of her work over time as it becomes more authorial and less oriented around the body.

While bodily exertion also induced considerable suffering in Margaret, it does not follow that she remained inactive, or refrained from work entirely. On the contrary, her 'work' forms part of the same internalized and paradoxical development seen throughout the text. The *Life* is invested in the notion that it is neither Margaret nor God who performs her work; instead, the two in collaboration transform her external and bodily *labour* into inner and spiritual *opus*, though this occurs in ways that rework the structures of agency. Paradoxically, this collaboration establishes her as neither wholly passive nor active; it is a recurrent theme throughout the *Life*: in a way that pushes the limits of intelligibility, Margaret's experience merges active 'doing' and passive 'being-done-unto'. Due almost entirely to her disability, her relinquishment of personal agency has the effect of investing her with a more expansive and inner form of agency than she would have otherwise possessed without her limitations. As her passivity transmutes into a new form of activity, and as her relinquishment of power invests her with still greater power, the *Life* becomes an extended meditation on the inner mechanics of spiritual power and agency.

In one sense, Margaret's turn from external to internal work is not at all paradoxical; it is 'simply' a transition necessitated by her disability, which, as we have seen, prevented Margaret from performing most manual tasks. Her function as a charismatic counsellor to others, while also a strenuous form of work, was nonetheless precisely the kind of internal work that she requested from God. She specifically requests 'that God might give her to compensate on the inside for any physical work she could not do on the outside' (*ut Deus daret ei interius recuperare, quod non poterat exterius corporaliter laborare*).[56]

55 On the various manual tasks that marked the anchorite's life, see, for example, Doerr, *Das Institut*, pp. 55–57. For the descriptions of a physically demanding set of morning prayers in *Ancrene Wisse*, see pp. 7–8. See also *LML*, 3.314 and n. 5.

56 *LML*, 3.314; *VMC*, p. 4.

The spiritual instructions that she issued to her lay visitors and to her own confessor argue that Margaret's disability did not entirely impede her agency, and that she did indeed find herself inwardly compensated in this manner. On the other hand, even such work was onerous, and Margaret was at times deprived of the strength required to perform even the work of praising God, though this work was far less physically oriented than most other activities that she might have otherwise engaged in. In one of her conversations with Christ, the alternative form of agency to which her spiritual labours guide Margaret is treated through a discussion of prayer.

> Where does your prayer come from? When you can pray well and have more consolation than when you cannot pray, you are unfaithful by putting your consolation into your works [*operibus tuis*], for then you believe that you are heard through your travails and works [*tuos labores et opera*]. But if you put your prayers in my goodness, the less you do in yourself and the less consolation you have within yourself, the more you will find in me. For prayer is nothing else than trust in me. And because of a certain blindness, all human travails [*labor hominis*] are nothing else than that people do not trust me fully.[57]

Here she is guided to the logical consequences of performing spiritual work that, paradoxically, does not in fact originate with the performer. Christ instructs Margaret that *her* spiritual labours, or prayers, will bear fruit, though this will occur only insofar as she herself performs less rather than more labour. Her sense of powerlessness comes precisely from placing too much trust in her own power.

The point is repeated elsewhere and in connection with the physical weakness occasioned by Margaret's disability. Christ imposed a 'burden' (*onus*) upon her—the desire to praise God—though it was a burden that she need not carry, and which involved no effort on her part. This burden's entire purpose was to divest her of 'exterior effort' (*exteriori labore*) and strength so that all of her subsequent accomplishments would in fact come 'only through the grace of Jesus Christ' (*ex sola gratia Ihesu Christi*).

57 *LML*, 59.371; *VMC*, p. 72: 'Unde est oratio tua? Quando tu bene potes orare, si tunc plus habes consolationis quam, dum nichil potes orare, tunc tu es infidelis, quia solatium in operibus tuis ponis, quia tunc tibi videtur, quod propter tuos labores et opera exaudiris. Si autem in bonitate mea orationes tuas posuisses, quanto minus in te posses et quando minus solatii haberes in te, tanto in me amplius invenires. Quia oratio nichil aliud est nisi hoc, quod michil credatur. Et labor hominis propter aliud non est nisi propter quondam cecitatem, quod michi homines plene non confidunt'.

> For after this immeasurable desire to praise God had been poured into her, her body became so frail [*in corpore debilitata*] that it could no longer sustain any other work [*exteriora opera*]. Jesus Christ did so not because he was unable to strengthen her body, but only in order that she would always remain a poor little woman and would find consolation neither in her works [*in operibus*] nor in anyone else, for she was to have absolutely no consolation except him alone. Jesus Christ did not want her to serve him but wanted himself to serve her more, because all his work was accomplished [*omnia opera eius operatus*] in her. […] She desired greatly to lose all her vigour and bodily strength. Then God alone would be praised for his works [*operibus*], since she could not do anything out of her own strength but only through the grace of Jesus Christ.[58]

None of this implies that Margaret was completely without agency, only that her agency was not exclusively hers. Again, the paradox remains: through losing she receives more, and through weakness she finds her strength. In this way, agency appears in a form radically different from that which it is conventionally assumed to be. These points are reiterated at the very end of the *Life*, again by redirecting attention from the body and externals to the spirit and internal experience. John accordingly calls Margaret's experiences the 'inner miracles' (*interiora miracula*), by which God wishes to 'reveal his glory through wonders that he works on the inside' (*suam gloriam revelare per interiora mirabilia*).[59] In this final set of reflections on the divine 'work' that was performed through his saint, John redirects impairment to the spiritual level and directs it against his readers, who are 'blind' in spiritual matters. Because they are attuned to what they are already able to understand, such readers cannot 'see' the miracles that God works on the inside, where neither physical sight nor superficial understanding have any place. Here as on so many other occasions, we encounter the immense value of Margaret's own experience, for without the suffering induced by her lameness the teachings that she communicates to others, in part through the *Life* itself, would in fact be non-existent.

58 *LML*, 7.321; *VMC*, p. 11: 'Immenso enim desiderio laudis Dei sibi infuso ita in corpore debilitate fuit, quod non poterat exteriora opera plus portare. Non fecit hoc Ihesus Christus propter hoc, quin potens fuisset ipsam exterius confortare, sed ideo fecit, ut paupercula semper esset, ut nec in operibus, nec in aliquot alio solatium haberet, quia nullum penitus solatium habere debuit nisi ipsum solum. Noluit Ihesus Christus, quod ista serviret ei, sed voluit ipse potius servire isti, quia omnia opera eius operates est in ea. […] Magno desiderio desideravit hoc, ut omnem virtutem et fortitudinem amitteret corporalem, ut Deus solus, si qua essent in eius operibus, laudaretur, cum ex naturali virtute nichil posset, sed ex sola gratia Ihesu Christi'.
59 *LML*, 395 (epilogue); *VMC*, p. 101.

Few if any of Margaret's spiritual advances would have been possible without the disabilities she suffered at the level of the body. The point pertains as much to the *Life* as an expression of devotional labour as it does to Margaret as both its collaborating author and the instrument through which the work comes into being. One is reminded that the many psychological and physical challenges (and indeed disabilities) suffered by the fifteenth-century English mystic Margery Kempe became catalysts for the composition of her eponymous book, which repeatedly refers to the collaborative nature of its own composition.[60] Closer to home, Margaret's near contemporary Mechthild of Magdeburg succumbed to blindness during the twilight of her career and, while completing the final book of her mystical treatise, *Flowing Light of the Godhead* (*Das fließende Licht der Gottheit*), required the assistance of the nuns of Helfta.[61] This is, of course, not to say that impairments of any sort are absolute requisites for collaborative forms of authorial work. Yet it is critical to note the prosthetic element inherent in virtually all modes of collective expression. Disability marks the borderlines of our limitations. In this sense, John's literacy and rhetorical facility operate as the prostheses that allow Margaret to extend her textual and public presence. The amanuensis becomes a living mechanism even as the recluse herself becomes little more than an instrument through which the divine author expresses himself.

In other words, neither Margaret nor her text are anything—both are the 'nothing' that the *Life* repeatedly insists they are—though not because they are worthless, but because they are mere vehicles or channels through which God's work enters into the world. The vehicle is itself nothing in comparison to the divine work, which nonetheless cannot be accomplished without that same vehicle. But of course, Margaret's work of praise, prayers, counselling, and teaching resulted in yet a further work (*opus*)—namely, the text itself. In this regard, we witness an erasure of the boundaries separating her various identities as passive subject of the text, spiritual counsellor, and co-author with her confessor.[62] Her *laudes et orationes* become the very textual material (*librum*) of God's working within her. Thus, without the inner work to which Margaret was guided by her physical disability, the written text of the *Life*, which came about in collaboration with John, would not have been possible. In this sense disability becomes a determining

60 It is relevant to the present discussion that the disability (blindness) of her clerical scribe marked and somewhat impeded the beginnings of Margery's text; see Margery Kempe, *Book*, ll. 103–5.

61 Mechthild's blindness has been discussed on several occasions; see, for example, Newman, 'Mechthild of Magdeburg', pp. 383–84.

62 On this 'partnership', see Benedict, *Empowering Collaborations*.

factor both in the overall course of Margaret's life, and in the textual form in which that life ultimately appeared.

Conclusion

Margaret's embodied experiences become the site of an inner transfiguration wherein loss and suffering, while never simply eliminated, are reoriented around the dictates of the spirit. Although the ridicule that she faced prior to her enclosure also continued in some measure thereafter, the spiritual power that eventually expressed itself through her was facilitated by that reorientation. So too did the biological and material enclosures together shape the experience of disability, which became for her '*this* ability'—a specific power to re-establish, or reacquire, those forms of personal, spiritual, and even textual agency that her status otherwise inhibited. Thus, the disabled body becomes interwoven with forms of empowerment. Far from eliminating an active construction of her life and community, Margaret's physical suffering restructures and reorients her capacity for doing so. In a dialogic relationship, that experience interacts with those forms of agency that the enclosure facilitated and that actively transfigured her experience. Like other disabled saints, she challenges disabling assumptions about (physical) alterity and agency, particularly the ways in which we conceptualize the interactions between the inner life of the spirit and embodied experience.

The paradoxical expression of agency that comes through Margaret both necessitates and precludes her active participation. This dynamic is no less operative at the level of textual work. Whether embodied or textual, agency emerges here as neither strictly communal nor reducible to single individuals; Margaret performs spiritual and textual 'works' in part by surrendering rather than asserting her will. For this reason, it is finally difficult to identify the author of this text, or to stabilize its image of authorial work. This feature of the *Life* addresses the general absence of a 'stable position' or an 'effective praxis' for addressing disability.[63] Moreover, as extended meditations on the abundance acquired through lack, the power acquired through (physical) incapacitation, and the forms of agency made possible through disability, the images and discourse of disability are afforded their decisive function in transforming and being transformed by both her experience and her capacity for reimagining the 'limitations' imposed by the condition of physical impairment. Margaret's bodily limitations positively *enabled* her capacities

63 Stiker, *A History of Disability*, p. 87.

as a spiritual teacher, and were therefore seminal in the formation of her mystical teachings as recorded in the *Life*. In this way, experience becomes the lifeblood of instruction, both of which reinterpret the very notion of loss and privation. Thus, the *Life* prompts readers to ask not simply what Margaret lost through her disability, but also what she thereby gained. Her text also speaks to the need, in Julie Singer's formulation, to 'loosen Disability Studies' rigid discourse of marginalization'.[64] For in Margaret, the margin becomes centre, as was the case for many other medieval anchoresses. Privation and abundance, margin and centre, operate not as the opposites that they are conventionally assumed to be, but rather, and paradoxically, as interdependent aspects of a single life in thirteenth-century Magdeburg.

Abbreviations

LML	John of Magdeburg, 'The Life of Margaret the Lame, Anchoress of Magdeburg', trans. by Gertrud Jaron Lewis and Tilman Lewis, in *Living Saints of the Thirteenth Century: The Lives of Yvette, anchoress of Huy; Juliana of Cornillon, author of the Corpus Christi Feast; and Margaret the Lame, anchoress of Magdeburg*, ed. by Anneke B. Mulder-Bakker (Turnhout: Brepols, 2011), pp. 303–96
PL	*Patrologia Latina*, ed. by Jacques-Paul Migne, 217 vols (Paris: 1841–1864)
VMC	John of Magdeburg, *Die Vita der Margareta Contracta, einer Magdeburger Reklusedes 13. Jahrhunderts*, ed. by Paul Gerhard Schmidt (Leipzig: Benno, 1992)

Bibliography

Primary Sources

Ancrene Wisse: A Corrected Edition of the Text in Cambridge, Corpus Christi College, MS 402, with Variants from other Manuscripts, ed. by Bella Millett, EETS 325 (Oxford: Oxford University Press, 2005)

Bernard of Clairvaux, *S. Bernardi Opera*, ed. by Jean Leclercq, C. H. Talbot, and N. M. Rochais, 8 vols (Rome: Editiones Cistercienses, 1957–1977)

64 Singer, 'Toward a Transhuman', p. 175.

Gerald of Wales, *The History and Topography of Ireland*, trans. by John J. O'Meara (London: Penguin Books, 1982)

Hildegard of Bingen, *Scivias*, trans. by Mother Columba Hart and Jane Bishop (New York: Paulist Press, 1990); *Sanctae Hildegardis Scivias*, PL 197, cols 383–738

John of Magdeburg, 'The Life of Margaret the Lame, Anchoress of Magdeburg', trans. by Gertrud Jaron Lewis and Tilman Lewis, in *Living Saints of the Thirteenth Century: The Lives of Yvette, anchoress of Huy; Juliana of Cornillon, author of the Corpus Christi Feast; and Margaret the Lame, anchoress of Magdeburg*, ed. by Anneke B. Mulder-Bakker (Turnhout: Brepols, 2011), pp. 303–96

John of Magdeburg, *Die Vita der Margareta Contracta, einer Magdeburger Rekluse des 13. Jahrhunderts*, ed. by Paul Gerhard Schmidt (Leipzig: Benno, 1992)

Margery Kempe, *The Book of Margery Kempe*, ed. by Lynn Staley (Kalamazoo: Medieval Institute,1996)

Mechthild of Magdeburg, *The Flowing Light of the Godhead*, trans. by Frank Tobin (New York: Paulist Press, 1998)

Secondary Sources

Benedict, Kimberley M., *Empowering Collaborations: Writing Partnerships Between Religious Women and Scribes in the Middle Ages* (London: Routledge, 2004)

Bynum, Caroline Walker, *Fragmentation and Redemption: Essays on Gender and the Human Body in Medieval Religion* (New York: Zone Books, 1992)

Coakley, John W., *Women, Men, and Spiritual Power: Female Saints and Their Male Collaborators* (New York: Columbus University Press, 2006)

Davis, Lennard J., *Enforcing Normalcy: Disability, Deafness, and the Body* (London: Verso, 1995)

Doerr, Otmar, *Das Institut der Inclusen in Süddeutschland* (Münster: Aschendorff, 1934)

Eyler, Joshua R., ed., *Disability in the Middle Ages: Reconsiderations and Reverberations* (Burlington, VT: Ashgate, 2010)

Gilchrist, Roberta, 'Medieval Bodies in the Material World: Gender, Stigma and the Body', in *Framing Medieval Bodies*, ed. by Sarah Kay and Miri Rubin (Manchester: Manchester University Press, 1994), pp. 43–61

Griffiths, Fiona, and Julie Hotchin, eds, *Partners in Spirit: Women, Men, and Religious Life in Germany, 1100–1500* (Turnhout: Brepols, 2014)

Holloway, Anne, 'Performing Poverty: The Vices and Virtues of the Order of Preachers', in *Poverty and Devotion in Mendicant Cultures*, ed. by Constant J. Mews and Anna Welch (London: Routledge, 2016), pp. 151–63

Hollywood, Amy, 'Inside Out: Beatrice of Nazareth and Her Hagiographer', in *Gendered Voices: Medieval Saints and Their Interpreters*, ed. by Catherine M. Mooney (Philadelphia: University of Pennsylvania Press, 1999), pp. 78–98

Kestemont, Mike, Jeroen Deploigne, and Sara Moens, 'Collaborative Authorship in the Twelfth Century: A Stylometric Study of Hildegard of Bingen and Guibert of Gembloux', *Digital Scholarship in the Humanities*, 30.2 (2015), 199–224

Kieckhefer, Richard, *Unquiet Souls: Fourteenth-Century Saints and Their Religious Milieu* (Chicago: University of Chicago Press, 1984)

Kuuliala, Jenni, Katariina Mustakallio, and Christian Krötzl, 'Introduction: *Infirmitas* in Antiquity and the Middle Ages', in *Infirmity in Antiquity and the Middle Ages: Social and Cultural Approaches to Health, Weakness and Care*, ed. by Christian Krötzl, Katariina Mustakallio, and Jenni Kuuliala (Farnham, Surrey: Ashgate, 2015), pp. 1–11

Metzler, Irina, *Disability in Medieval Europe: Thinking about Physical Impairment during the High Middle Ages, c. 1100–1400* (New York: Routledge, 2006)

Metzler, Irina, 'Liminality and Disability: Spatial and Conceptual Aspects of Physical Impairment in Medieval Europe', in *Medicine and Space: Body, Surroundings and Borders in Antiquity and the Middle Ages*, ed. by Patricia A. Baker, Han Nijdam, and Karine van 't Land (Leiden: Brill, 2012), pp. 273–96

Metzler, Irina, *A Social History of Disability in the Middle Ages: Cultural Considerations of Physical Impairment* (New York: Routledge, 2013)

Mitchell, David T., and Sharon L. Snyder, *Narrative Prosthesis: Disability and the Dependencies of Discourse* (Ann Arbor: University of Michigan Press, 2000)

Morgan, Ben, 'The Spiritual Autobiographies of Visionary Nuns and Their Dominican Confessors in Fourteenth-Century Germany', in *Autobiography by Women in German*, ed. by Mererid Puw Davies, Beth V. Linklater, and Gisela Shaw (Oxford: Peter Lang, 2000), pp. 35–51

Mulder-Bakker, Anneke B., 'Lame Margaret of Magdeburg: The Social Function of a Medieval Recluse', *Journal of Medieval History*, 22 (1996), 155–69

Mulder-Bakker, Anneke B., *Lives of the Anchoresses: The Rise of the Urban Recluse in Medieval Europe*, trans. by Myra Heerspink Scholz (Philadelphia: University of Pennsylvania Press, 2005)

Newman, Barbara, 'Mechthild of Magdeburg at Helfta: A Study in Literary Influence', in *Women Intellectuals and Leaders in the Middle Ages*, ed. by Kathryn Kerby-Fulton, Katie Ann-Marie Bugyis, and John Van Engen (Cambridge: D. S. Brewer, 2020), pp. 383–95

Orlemanski, Julie, 'How to Kiss a Leper', *postmedieval: a journal of medieval and cultural studies*, 3.2 (2012), 142–57

Pearman, Tory Vandeventer, *Women and Disability in Medieval Literature* (New York: Palgrave, 2010)

Simons, Walter, *Cities of Ladies: Beguine Communities in the Medieval Low Countries, 1200–1565* (Philadelphia: University of Pennsylvania Press, 2010)

Singer, Julie, 'Disability and the Social Body', *postmedieval: a journal of medieval cultural studies* 3 (2012), 135–41

Singer, Julie, 'Toward a Transhuman Model of Medieval Disability', *postmedieval: a journal of medieval cultural studies*, 1 (2010), 173–79

Stiker, Henri-Jacques, *A History of Disability*, trans. by William Sayers (Ann Arbor: University of Michigan Press, 1999)

Thurber, Shari, 'Disability and Monstrosity: A Look at Literary Distortions of Handicapping Conditions', *Rehabilitation Literature*, 41 (1980), 12–15

Vauchez, André, *Sainthood in the Later Middle Ages*, trans. by Jean Birrell (Cambridge: Cambridge University Press, 1997)

Wells, Scott, 'The Exemplary Blindness of Francis of Assisi', in *Disability in the Middle Ages: Reconsiderations and Reverberations*, ed. by Joshua R. Eyler (Burlington, VT: Ashgate, 2010), pp. 67–80

Wendell, Susan, *The Rejected Body: Feminist Philosophical Reflections on Disability* (New York: Routledge, 1996)

Wendell, Susan, 'Toward a Feminist Theory of Disability', *Hypatia*, 4.2 (1989), 104–24

Wheatley, Edward, 'Monsters, Saints, and Sinners: Disability in Medieval Literature', in *The Cambridge Companion to Literature and Disability*, ed. by Clare Barker and Stuart Murray (Cambridge: Cambridge University Press, 2018), pp. 17–31

Wheatley, Edward, *Stumbling Blocks Before the Blind: Medieval Constructions of a Disability* (Ann Arbor: University of Michigan Press, 2010)

Williams, David, *Deformed Discourse: The Function of the Monster in Medieval Thought and Literature* (Exeter: University of Exeter Press, 1996)

Winzer, Margaret A., *The History of Special Education: From Isolation to Integration* (Washington, DC: Gallaudet University Press, 1993)

Wisbey, Roy A., 'Die Darstellung des Häßlichen im Hoch- und Spätmittelalter', in *Deutsche Literatur des späten Mittelalters: Hamburger Colloquium 1973*, ed. by Wolfgang Harms and L. Peter Johnson (Berlin: E. Schmidt, 1975), pp. 9–34

About the Author

Joshua S. Easterling competed his PhD at The Ohio State University in 2011 with emphasis on late medieval religious culture and texts. His work in this area was recently supported by a fellowship from the Alexander von Humboldt foundation. His chapter in this volume was in part made possible by that fellowship and research conducted in Berlin, Germany at the Freie Universität. His monograph, *Angels and Anchoritic Culture in Late*

Medieval England (Oxford, 2021), as well as several articles on thirteenth- and fourteenth-century admonitory, mystical, and visionary writings in England, were also generously supported by that fellowship. He currently researches, writes, and teaches in the Department of English and Philosophy at Murray State University (Kentucky).

3. Perspectives on Blindness, Deafness, and Muteness in the Chinese *Eminent Monks* Literature: The 'Eight Difficulties' in Context

Christopher Jensen

Abstract: Is there a 'Buddhist approach' to disability? This paper employs hagiographical materials from medieval China (up to the mid-seventh century) to problematize this question. Exploring the uses of terms translatable as 'blindness', 'deafness', and 'muteness' in the *Eminent Monks* and its sequel volume, it argues for the tradition's polyvocality, noting cases where disability discourses serve as metaphors for ignorance and others in which sensory impairments are explained away as karmic punishments. On the other hand, these traditions also include accounts of Buddhist thaumaturge monks as miraculous healers, and even a case of a deaf monk being accommodated by his community and thereby rising to prominence. This case study demonstrates the necessity of focusing on historical particulars, especially when dealing with a tradition as variegated as Buddhism.

Keywords: Chinese Buddhism, hagiography, blindness, deafness, disability studies

Many contemporary studies that explore disability in Asian religions do so in a somewhat reductive fashion, treating the cultural resources of these traditions as grist for the Western philosophical mill, instead of as aspects

I would like to thank James Benn, Ruifeng Chen, and Alice Zhao for their thoughtful comments on this chapter, and their assistance with some translation quandaries. All translations are mine unless otherwise noted, and any infelicities therein are mine as well. I would also like to thank the editors of this volume for their diligence and professionalism; this chapter has improved markedly thanks to their assistance. Finally, thank you to Emma Porter for her last minute review of the proofs. My sincere gratitude to all.

Grace-Petinos, Stephanie, Leah Pope Parker, and Alicia Spencer-Hall, eds. *Disability and Sanctity in the Middle Ages.* Taylor & Francis Group, 2025
DOI 10.5117/9789463724333_CH03

of living traditions that have guided the lives of (and were in turn been shaped by) innumerable individuals over the course of millennia.[1] As such, rather than attempting to offer a definitive picture of 'disability' in Chinese Buddhism, my goal in the present chapter is narrower, but resultantly more achievable: namely, to identify a 'local' Chinese category (or categories) roughly analogous to the English-language notion of 'disability' and to trace this category through a corpus of historically situated Chinese Buddhist literature. Chinese hagiographical stories provide a perfect source for such an investigation, as they were simultaneously the literary productions of elite monks, while also being written and compiled to promote and disseminate Buddhist ideals to a wide audience. That said, they also—by their very genre commitments—focus on human exemplarity, which is often symbolically represented in bodily terms. This means that any discussion of impaired or non-normative bodies was likely to be ideologically freighted, with descriptions of such bodies tending to serve as 'narrative prostheses'.[2]

I focus on two hagiographical collections: the *Biographies of Eminent Monks* (*Gaoseng zhuan* 高僧傳, composed in approximately 530 CE; hereafter *GSZ*), compiled by Huijiao (慧皎, 497–554 CE), and the *Continued Biographies of Eminent Monks* (*Xu gaoseng zhuan* 續高僧傳, composed in approximately 645 CE; hereafter *XGSZ*), compiled by Daoxuan (道宣, 596–667 CE).[3] Existing at the intersection between popular and elite

1 For instance, see Benjamin Lukey's 'Confucianism and Disability', which focuses almost entirely on the perspective(s) outlined in the *Analects* of Confucius, and Andrew Lambert's 'Daoism and Disability' (in the same volume), which situates its discussion in the *Daodejing* and the *Zhuangzi*. Deriding such approaches, Miles, in 'Disability', suggests that 'it would be merely reciprocal politeness to contemplate some of the Asian heritage, without a utilitarian yardstick in hand' (p. 104). While I certainly appreciate any attempt to extend the boundaries of the philosophical canon beyond Euro-American sources, it is also the case that neither of these living traditions is adequately represented by one or two texts associated with them. In the present volume, see the chapter by Vargas-O'Bryan for a case study of disability in the Indian Buddhist tradition, focusing on the nun Gelongma Palmo (pp. 115–46); and Edwards's discussion of the Buddhist Empress Kōmyō of Japan (pp. 248–50).

2 On the comparative utility of hagiographical materials, see Rondolino, 'Case for Hagiography'. On these collections as proselytic tools, see Kieschnick, *The Eminent Monk*. On narrative prosthesis, see Mitchell and Snyder's book of the same name. They concisely define this notion as follows: '*narrative prosthesis* is meant to indicate that disability has been used throughout history as a crutch upon which literary narratives lean for their representative power, disruptive potentiality, and analytical insight. Bodies show up in stories as dynamic entities that resist or refuse the cultural scripts assigned to them' (p. 49, emphasis in original).

3 See the list at the end of this chapter for all abbreviations employed herein. Also, while I would have liked more 'gender parity' in this analysis, there were no comparable accounts in the contemporaneous *Biographies of Nuns* (T. 2063). On the composition and key themes of these texts, see Kieschnick, *The Eminent Monk*. For more general bibliographical info, as well as

religion, these texts were composite productions, combining the literary prose and organizational impulses of their erudite compilers with material sourced from epitaphs and popular story traditions. By narrating the lives of monastic heroes, they offered both practical religious instruction and escapism, and in so doing, they became widely popular with both monastic and lay Buddhist audiences, eventually being copied and circulated not only in China but also throughout East Asia.[4] Moreover, given that they are collections of previously extant narrative materials, they also provide insights into the goals, biases, commitments, and assumptions of the early medieval Chinese Buddhist 'discourse community' (in Robert Campany's sense of the term): the uncountable, unnamed Buddhists who effortfully told, retold, hand-copied, and circulated these accounts before their eventual compilation.[5] In addition to assembling a composite picture of the various, often messy and non-systematic ways that non-normative bodies were discussed and imagined by sixth- and seventh-century Chinese Buddhists, looking at these two collections in tandem also allows us to consider some ways that these ideas might have changed diachronically, given that the texts were compiled within approximately 150 years of each another. That said, given the paucity of data points from the first collection, any such conclusions are provisional.

In order to pursue a local Chinese-language term to compare with the English-language notion of 'disability', this chapter explores concepts tied to the karmic framework, which was often used aetiologically in both Indic and Chinese Buddhism to explore a variety of life outcomes. As such, I am focusing on the Buddhist doctrine of the 'Eight Difficulties' (*banan* 八難), which was already ubiquitous by the time that the hagiographical collections under discussion were compiled, and which refers to eight rebirths that imperil one's ability to adopt the Buddhist path and/or achieve liberation.[6] Huiyuan's (慧遠, 523–592 CE) influential sixth-century encyclopaedia,

a discussion of their respective compilations, see Kieschnick, 'Gaoseng zhuan' (p. 76), and 'Xu gaoseng zhuan'. In the case of the second text, while the preface lists a concluding date of 645 CE, material compiled by Daoxuan after its completion was incorporated into the text after his death, meaning that *XGSZ* includes accounts ranging to 665 CE; Kieschnick, 'Xu gaoseng zhuan', p. 430. Material in *GSZ* has been cross-referenced with Yoshikawa and Funayama's translation of *Gaoseng zhuan* 高僧傳.

4 For a helpful overview of the sources and contents of these texts, as well as their influence throughout East Asia, see Kieschnick, 'Gaoseng zhuan' and 'Xu gaoseng zhuan'.

5 For several excellent examples of this 'discourse communities' approach to medieval Chinese materials, see Campany, *Making Transcendents*, and *Signs*.

6 For a helpful introduction to the textual history of this term and its usage(s) in the medieval Chinese context, see Nicol, 'Outsiders', especially pp. 34–40.

entitled *Essay on the System of Mahāyāna* (*Dasheng yi zhang* 大乘義章), includes the following items within the list of eight:

1. [Being born in] an earth-prison [i.e., a hell];
2. Being born as an animal;
3. [Being born as] a hungry ghost;
4. Being blind, deaf, or mute;
5. Being a worldly philosopher;
6. [Being born] prior to or after a Buddha;
7. [Being born in] the country of Uttarakuru [i.e., a land of worldly pleasures];[7]
8. [Being born as] a long-lived deity.[8]

While this list represents an influential sixth-century articulation of the 'Eight Difficulties', Janine Nicol notes that there are a variety of different versions, with the majority referencing 'incomplete sense faculties or some other physical factor', including the earliest attested usage, which can be dated to the later Han dynasty, c. 150–170 CE.[9] In order to trace the perspectives on non-normative bodies presented in our hagiographical sources,

7 DDB (鬱單越).

8 言八難者。一是地獄。二是畜生。三是餓鬼。四盲聾瘖瘂五世智辯聰。六佛前佛後。七鬱單越國。八長壽天。(T. 1851: 628c23–25).

9 Nicol, 'Outsiders', p. 35. An important feature of this list of 'difficulties' is its focus on the epistemological conditions of various births/lives: for instance, a reader unfamiliar with Buddhist doctrine/soteriology might be perplexed by the overt linkage here between being born into a land of worldly pleasures, as a longevous god, or even as a worldly philosopher, and being born blind, as an animal, or as a hungry ghost. Here is essentially what is being proposed: in the early Buddhist context, it was assumed that one must undergo specific experiences in order to become committed to the Buddhist path; namely, one must jointly experience the unsatisfactoriness (Sanskrit: *dukkha*) of embodied existence, and also encounter (and have the capacity to internalize/enact) Buddhist teaching and Buddhist practice. The first creates the impetus to seek liberation, the second provides the necessary tools to achieve it. As such, these 'Eight Difficulties' are 'disabling' for different reasons: an animal (in general) is not thought to be able to comprehend Buddhist doctrine or to be able to engage in Buddhist practice. (For a discussion including some counterexamples, see Ohnuma, *Unfortunate Destiny*, pp. 5–23 and throughout.) A god in a paradisical realm or a dweller in a mythic land of plenty, by contrast, lacks the experiential preconditions to recognize the suffering endemic to embodied life, and will thus fail to seek liberation for that reason. (For an introductory overview of Buddhist cosmology, including the karmic episteme, see Strong, *Buddhisms*.) Clearly, being born 'blind, deaf, or mute' is a problem of the first kind, in that it is assumed to prevent either engaging with Buddhist ideas (inability to read sutras or hear teachings) or Buddhist practice (inability to chant Buddhist texts or hymns). Given that the conditions of one's current life are, according to Buddhist cosmology, determined by karma amassed in previous births, it was common for

I have searched through the digital editions of both *GSZ* and *XGSZ*, and will discuss *all* instances of the terms blind (*mang* 盲), deaf (*long* 聾), and mute (*yinya* 瘖瘂) (using the terms in Huiyuan's definition of the 'Eight Difficulties'), with the goal of allowing a composite picture to emerge.[10]

In general, the usages of these 'disability' terms can be divided into two categories: rhetorical and narrative. These will be considered in sequence below. To foreshadow my conclusions, the majority of accounts that reference these terms for non-normative bodies do so from the standpoint of the 'medical' model of disability, focusing on such somatic conditions as sources of suffering and incapacity, situating them squarely in the bodies of those thus 'afflicted', and positing that they can only be ameliorated (if at all) through magico-medical intervention.[11] Moreover, one of the most common usages of all such terms is as a generalized metaphor for the inability to access the Buddha's salvific teaching (the Dharma): a metaphorical 'crutch' supporting the texts' construal of normative bodies and their sensory modalities.[12] That said, a few rare cases also provide evidence of a 'social' approach to such conditions, whereby a bodily incapacity is *not* seen as debilitating, specifically because sensory impairment is reimagined more positively or, in one case, because a given monk's social circumstances allowed his full

these specific disabilities to be characterized as a form of punishment for prior misdeeds (as we will see below).

One of the primary strengths of a comparative volume like this one is that it provides its authors and readers with an opportunity to (re)consider the assumptions and logics of second-order categories like 'disability'. (On this process of 'rectification and theory formation' in the context of comparative analysis, see Freiberger, *Considering Comparison*, pp. 104–09, 158–60.) My decision to focus on the 'blindness, deafness, and muteness' subset of the Eight Difficulties is tied to this goal: these are categories that seem readily mappable onto intuitive English-language notions of disability. The particulars of this mapping are considered throughout the present chapter. That said, the *epistemic* basis of the Buddhist approach to disability (at least in philosophical/doctrinal texts) is a potential point of discontinuity, as we see when we consider the Eight Difficulties in sum. These are issues that deserve further investigation, though doing so is beyond the scope of the current chapter.

10 On the importance of assessing whole textual corpora to avoid cherry-picking data in studies like this one, see Slingerland, *Mind and Body*, pp. 14, 143–46. While working on this study, I also came across seven uses of a synonym for blindness (*gu* 瞽) in *XGSZ* (which is absent from *GSZ*). That said, all but one were already covered in the accounts treated below. The one that was not is a rhetorical use of the compound *menggu* 蒙瞽 as a reference to ignorance (which is another potential meaning of 瞽 as a monad). As such, I have not included it. See T. 2060: 528c9. One account that will not be considered is a story about a monk's adoption of a deaf dog (T. 2060: 588b–c), as any ideological assumptions concerning the animal's deafness would surely be dwarfed by those tied to animal birth in general (as discussed in Ohnuma, *Unfortunate Destiny*).

11 On the 'medical model', see Siebers, *Disability Theory*, pp. 3, 24.

12 As per Mitchell and Snyder, *Narrative Prosthesis*, p. 49.

participation in the community regardless of his sensory impairment.[13] On the issue of diachronic change, it appears that Huijiao was more circumspect about discussing the seemingly negative traits of 'blindness, deafness or muteness', perhaps indicating discomfiture about the prospect of associating such notions with monastic exemplars. Daoxuan's collection, in contrast, includes a broader range of responses and assessments (both positive and negative), which is perhaps congruent with the greater social prominence and prestige of Buddhism in the early Tang dynasty (mid-seventh century).[14] Before we can get to these conclusions, however, we must first consider why 'blindness, deafness, and muteness' were associated with karma in the first place.

Karma and Bodies in Indian and Chinese Buddhism

Buddhism, which developed in centuries prior to the Common Era among other South Asian renunciant religions (such as Jainism and the religion of the Upanishads), shared many cosmological assumptions with them, including the notion of *karma*: an impersonal force that causes moral behaviour (defined broadly) to yield positive consequences, and immoral behaviour to yield the opposite. Importantly, these consequences were not exclusively experienced in one's current life, but rather informed one's future births as well. This theory provides an internally consistent response to the twinned problems of evil and suffering: namely, that hardships (including sensory impairment, as per the 'Eight Difficulties') are the unfortunate result of immoral activity, either in this birth or a previous one. In any case, delving further into the doctrinal particulars of the Buddhist notion of karma would take us too far afield, given that the Chinese narratives under consideration do not hinge on any terms or concepts related to them.[15]

13 On the 'social model', see Siebers, *Disability Theory*, pp. 3, 72–75.

14 While the imperial court's support for Buddhism varied throughout the Tang era, it should also be noted that the period between the compilation of these two texts also saw the reunification of the Chinese state under the banner of the short-lived but self-consciously Buddhist Sui dynasty (581–618 CE), as well as the development of novel, distinctively Chinese Buddhist traditions (such as the Tiantai Buddhism of Zhiyi). See Weinstein, *Buddhism*.

15 For a concise introduction to these issues, with particular attention paid to their relevance to the field of disability studies, see Harris, 'Buddhism and Disability'. For a detailed exploration of the philological, philosophical, and sociological issues related to the development of the doctrine of karma in the South Asian context, see Doniger O'Flaherty, *Karma*. See also the relevant material in Vargas-O'Bryan's chapter in the present volume, pp. 115–46.

Instructively, in light of the notion of the 'eight difficulties', this karmic framework posits a direct correlation between the qualities of an individual's current body and their moral conduct in prior births, with the Buddha himself serving as the preeminent example of earned bodily excellence.[16] In particular, the canonical lists of the 'thirty-two great marks' and 'eighty lesser marks' of a great man—physiognomic signs that a Buddha's body will manifest—include 'clear and pure sight', 'unimpaired hearing', and the 'voice of a roaring elephant', highlighting the fact that these sensory and communicative modalities were classed as necessary features of a perfected body.[17] While such a birth was necessary to 'turn the wheel of Dharma' (to rediscover Buddhist truths anew and to teach them to others, i.e., the job of a Buddha), the ultimate goal of liberation was obviously open to those without Buddha bodies. Even for early Buddhist monks and nuns, however, liberation (*nirvana*) was understood epistemologically, in that it was tied to the complete and accurate perception of the true nature of reality, achieved after engaging with a Buddha's liberative teaching.[18] It is perhaps for these reasons that individuals with non-normative bodies (including those who were blind or deaf) were to be denied ordination, at least according to many traditions of *Vinaya* (Buddhist law), though the degree of adherence to this rule varied over time.[19]

When itinerant monks and traders began to transport Buddhist texts, artwork, and practices from India into China in the early centuries of the Common Era, they brought the system of karmic causality discussed above, and its associated understanding of bodies, with them. Summarizing the

16 See Mrozik, *Virtuous Bodies*, p. 62. On Buddhist physiognomy and the thirty-two marks, see Strong, *A Bull of a Man*; Guang, *The Concept of the Buddha*.

17 See the DDB entry for the 'eighty [lesser] marks' (*bashi zhong hao* 八十種好), which draws them from *The Sutra of the Collection of the Past Activities of the Buddha* (佛本行集經 [T. 190]). Also see Guang, *The Concept of the Buddha*, pp. 29–31.

18 Harris, 'Buddhism and Disability', p. 36. Likewise, in his conclusion, Harris notes that 'Buddhist texts also emphasize the limited access people with intellectual disabilities and sensory impairments have to Buddhist teachings' (p. 43).

19 On monastic rules seemingly forbidding the ordination of individuals with non-normative bodies/minds, see Mrozik, *Virtuous Bodies*, p. 72. That said, the Vinaya scholarship of Gregory Schopen and Shayne Clarke (among others) has compellingly demonstrated that the formulation of many such rules was motivated by the desire to avoid social censure of (and encourage continued donations from) mainstream brahminical society, and that their application was much less cut-and-dried than a simple list of the rules themselves might suggest. For one example, Clarke's *Family Matters* offers a detailed overview of the rules intended to both police and protect nuns who maintained contact with their natal/conjugal families after renouncing, who continued to nurse babies while serving as nuns, and even those who found themselves pregnant.

received scriptural position, the famed Chinese exegete Huiyuan (慧遠, 334–416 CE) stated:

> the sutra says that there are three types of karmic response: (1) in this life; (2) in the next life; (3) in one of the following lives. They are explained as follows: good deeds are rewarded and bad deeds are punished.[20]

As an explanatory framework, these Buddhist theories found themselves in active competition with (at least) three pre-existing Chinese aetiologies for the same phenomena: (1) correlative cosmology; (2) 'extrahuman' assault; and (3) fate and the 'allotted lifespan'.[21] In the first case, impairment of any sensory modality could be explained as the result of either the repletion or depletion of material energy (*qi*) in specific bodily systems, or an imbalance in the types of *qi* present.[22] While this understanding of the body was central to the hybrid Chinese/Buddhist medical discourse that was developing at the time (see below for examples), it is not referenced in any of the *GSZ* or *XGSZ* accounts related to blindness, deafness, or muteness, so it need not concern us further.[23] The second traditional aetiology for all manner of adverse bodily effects was the malefic influence of various types of ghosts, spirits, and aggrieved underworld bureaucrats.[24] Since the appeal of Buddhism to the Chinese public was due in part to the perceived exorcistic power of many early monks, it is perhaps unsurprising that some of the *XGSZ* accounts considered below describe blindness, deafness, and muteness as conditions caused by spirits, rendering them curable by such wonder-workers.[25] Finally, the notion that every individual was allotted a specific lifespan at birth, and that various other positive and negative life outcomes could be foretold (and were thus to some extent fated), was a cultural commonplace in early China,

20 As translated in Yün-hua Jan, 'The Chinese Understanding', p. 148.

21 Poo Muzhou has argued that the term 'extrahuman' is more apt in the early Chinese context than either 'supernatural' or 'superhuman', because many such beings were understood to be part of the natural order, and to have some capacities and vulnerabilities that were comparable to those of humans (*Personal Welfare*, p. 6). This 'allotted lifespan' is Robert Ford Campany's translation of *ming* (命): *To Live as Long*, p. 47.

22 The role of the correlative cosmology in Chinese medical thought is summarized well in Unschuld, *Medicine in China*, pp. 51–100.

23 On the historical development of a hybrid Chinese/Buddhist medical tradition, see Salguero, *Translating Buddhist Medicine*.

24 As described in Poo, *Personal Welfare*, pp. 69–102, 123–78.

25 On exorcism in medieval Chinese Buddhism, see Mollier, *Buddhism and Taoism*, pp. 55–99 and passim. See also the discussion of monastic thaumaturgy in Kieschnick, *The Eminent Monk*, pp. 67–111, and particularly pp. 82–87.

long pre-dating the arrival of Buddhism.[26] As such, it is often not possible to determine whether the proper explanatory framework for a particular case of blindness, deafness, or muteness found in our hagiographical sources was being attributed to 'karma' or to the more traditional Chinese notion of 'destiny', which speaks to the sort of hybrid discourse environment in which Chinese Buddhism developed.

Rhetorical Uses

All uses of the terms 'blind' (*mang* 盲) and 'deaf' (*long* 聾) in Huijiao's early sixth-century *Eminent Monks* collection are dialogical, with monastic speakers using them rhetorically to describe an extreme impediment to engaging with the Buddha's teachings.[27] The terms are depersonalized: instead of describing specific historical individuals, they merely signify a generalized imaginary of incapacity—David T. Mitchell and Sharon L. Snyder's metaphorical crutch that prosthetically supports an ideology of 'normalcy'. The first two such examples can be seen in the biography of Zhu Shixing (朱士行), a mid-third-century Chinese monk famed for being the first to trek along the Silk Road to retrieve Buddhist scriptures from the Western Regions.[28] According to his *GSZ* biography, when he attempted to leave Khotan with a Mahayana text, local monks—who rejected the Mahayanist doctrinal position outlined therein—interceded with a local ruler to prevent his departure. Addressing the king, they outlined their objections:

> This *śramaṇa* from the land of Han wants to use this *brahmin* book to confuse [people about] the true scriptures. Since you, O King, are the master of this land, if you do not prohibit this, and it then causes the destruction of the Great Dharma, deafening and blinding the ruler of the Han territories, it will be your fault.[29]

26 On issues related to destined lifespans, see Jan, 'The Chinese Understanding', pp. 146–48; Campany, *To Live as Long*, pp. 47–52; on fate more broadly, and the technologies used to prognosticate about such issues, see Poo, *Personal Welfare*, pp. 73–74; Von Glahn, *The Sinister Way*, pp. 4–5, 15.

27 The terms for muteness mentioned above do not occur in T. 2059.

28 See Tsukamoto, *A History*, pp. 138–39; Zürcher, *The Buddhist Conquest*, pp. 62–63.

29 未發之頃于闐諸小乘學眾遂以白王云：「漢地沙門欲以婆羅門書惑亂正典。王為地主。若不禁之將斷大法聾盲漢地王之咎也。」(T. 2059: 346b21–24, following Yoshikawa and Funayama's Japanese translation [vol. 2, p. 26]).

While the historicity of this account has been called into question, it nonetheless allows us to make two clear observations.[30] First, this usage suggests that blindness and deafness were so strongly associated with rendering the Dharma (i.e., the Buddha's teaching) inaccessible that these terms could be employed as metaphors for life in a country whose local form of Buddhism had been thrown into disarray by incorrect doctrines. Second, whether or not such an appeal was actually made by the Khotanese monks in question, the unquestioned inclusion of this statement in Zhu Shixing's biography suggests that such a claim would have been seen as so unequivocally understandable to a Buddhist discourse community as to require no explanation or justification, even when placed in the mouths of non-Chinese monks.[31]

Kang Senghui's (康僧會) biography contains the only other use of these terms in *GSZ*, and it follows the same general logic.[32] In this account, the King of Wu sends one of his wisest officials (Zhang Yu 張昱), to interrogate the monk on his understanding of Buddhism. After successfully answering all of his interlocutor's questions, Kang Senghui led his visitor to the door, where they happened to find some adherents of a licentious cult right beside the temple. This piqued his visitor's curiosity:

> Yu said: 'If the profound teaching [of the Buddha] is definitely trustworthy, how can these fellows be so close [to it] without being affected?' Senghui replied: 'When thunder and lightning smash a mountain, a deaf person does not hear it, but not because the sound is too minute. If one penetrates this Principle, one could comply with it even at a vast distance. If one's [ears] are obstructed and closed off [to it], then [even things as close together as the] liver and gallbladder [might as well be as distant as] the kingdoms of Chu and Yue.'[33]

After hearing Kang's reply, Zhang returns to the capital and eulogizes the monk's brilliance to his ruler. Once again, Kang's statement relies on

30 Tsukamoto, *A History*, p. 139; Zürcher, *The Buddhist Conquest*, p. 63.

31 This interpretation represents an instance of the 'principle of irrelevance', drawn from Biblical Studies and employed to great effect in the Buddhist Studies context by Jan Nattier in *A Few Good Men*, pp. 66–67.

32 See Tsukamoto, *A History*, pp. 151–63; Zürcher, *The Buddhist Conquest*, pp. 51–55.

33 時寺側有淫祀者。昱曰：「玄化既孚此輩何故近而不革。」會曰：「雷霆破山聾者不聞。非音之細。苟在理通。則萬里懸應。如其阻塞則肝膽楚越。」(T. 2059: 325c14–17). For a French rendering of this entire biography, see *Biographies des moines*, pp. 25–26. On the unsignalled *Zhuangzi* reference here, see *The Complete Works*, p. 34.

the assumption that deafness represents an impediment to receiving the Buddhist message. Moreover, and even more overtly than in the previous example, the blame for such a situation is squarely placed upon the individual, rather than on any failing of the Dharma itself: a seeming allusion to the karmic understanding of disability.

While the uses of the terms *mang* (blind 盲), *long* (deaf 聾), *yin* and *ya* (both meaning 'mute' 瘖瘂) in Daoxuan's collection are considerably more varied than the few examples seen in Huijiao's text, as reviewed above, a reasonable percentage of them (ten out of twenty-two, or 45%) are also employed rhetorically, albeit in a wider variety of situations and with a wider variety of aims than seen in the earlier collection. This disparity suggests the intriguing possibility that by the early Tang dynasty the seemingly ineluctable link between such conditions and a (karmically foreordained) difficulty in accessing the Dharma was in the process of being questioned. The magnitude of such developments should not be overstated, as many of the rhetorical uses of these disability terms in *XGSZ* continue to be predicated on the assumption that sensory impairment is equivalent to (or indicative of) an inability to access the teachings of the Buddha. For instance, the monk Huijing, in a debate with a Daoist (the organized religion with which Tang Buddhists were most often competing for patronage and donations), argues that his rival's teaching is like delusion or drunkenness, which (symbolically) renders its hearers blind and deaf.[34] Similar language is employed by the monastic translator and pilgrim Xuanzang in a missive attempting to convince the emperor to write a foreword to the record of his travels, as well as by Daoxuan in the commentary to his chapter on reciters, wherein he likens ignorance and improper religious practice to blindness and deafness.[35]

In contrast to these unilaterally negative usages (which match those we saw above in *GSZ*), several of the rhetorical uses in *XGSZ* also suggest a slightly more nuanced perspective. For instance, an edict by the Sui emperor Wen, attempting to convince the monk Lingyu (靈裕, 518–605 CE) to enter the public service, suggests that his teaching can 'lead the deaf and blind'.[36] In a similar fashion, Chen Ziliang, in his preface to the early Tang apologetic text 'Discerning the Correct' (*Bianzheng lun* 辯正論), argues that court Daoists had slandered the True Dharma, leading to

34 T. 2060: 444a.

35 T. 2060: 455c. This entreaty is included verbatim in Huili and Yancong's biography of Xuanzang (T. 2053: 254c). Daoxuan's commentary on the 'Reciters' chapter can be found at T. 2060: 690c.

36 開導聾瞽。(T. 2060: 496b12).

a rise in mistaken beliefs among the general populace. Chen then describes the text's monastic author's motives (Falin 法琳) as follows: 'The Dharma Teacher [i.e., Falin] was sympathetic to their blind ignorance and so has proceeded to compose this discourse'.[37] For our purposes, we must note that, in both of these cases, even though 'blindness' and 'deafness' were still being employed as signs of ignorance and spiritual incapacity, both usages assume that individuals with such conditions can, and indeed should, be taught. This, in turn, suggests that such forms of impairment were not necessarily seen as permanent or insurmountable issues.

Indeed, the remaining rhetorical use implicitly assumes that conditions like blindness and deafness were not intractable impediments, as we have seen in an argument made by the monk Zhiyi (智顗, 538–597 CE): one of the most singular figures in the development of a distinct Chinese form of Buddhism, due to his innovative reading and systematizing of the enormous corpus of translated Buddhist texts, as well as his painstaking development of a detailed programme of meditation practice.[38] Near the end of his *XGSZ* biography, in a section including summaries of a variety of his teachings, the following exchange is recorded:

> When someone asked him about his conditions of enlightenment [wei 位], Zhiyi replied: 'You all are lazy [when it comes to] planting good roots, so when you ask someone else about their merits, it is like a blind person asking about [the colour of] milk or a stumbling person [asking about] the road. If I had not focused on regulating the [members of the] assembly, I would have purified my six sense faculties, but I neglected myself for the sake of others, and have only reached the fifth rank [those who hear and rejoice in the Lotus Sutra] and no more.'[39]

This approach to blindness was a common rhetorical device for Zhiyi. For example, his *magnum opus*, *The Great Calming and Contemplation* (Mohe

37 法師愍其盲瞽遂著斯論 (T. 2060: 638a11–12).

38 For Zhiyi's life and contributions to Chinese Buddhism, see Hurvitz, *Chih-i*. For the social context and proselytic aims of the composition of Zhiyi's biography, from which Daoxuan drew much of his material for the present account, see Shinohara, 'Guanding's Biography of Zhiyi'.

39 有問其位者，答曰：「汝等嬾種善根。問他功德，如盲問乳蹶者訪路。云云。吾不領眾，必淨六根，為他損己，只是五品內位耳。」 (T. 2060: 567b16–19, punctuated as per *XGSZ* [2014], pp. 632–33). On the term *wupin* (五品), I am following DDB: 'A division of the disciples, in the Lotus Sutra, into five grades—those who hear and rejoice; read and repeat; preach; observe and meditate; and transform self and others'. My thanks to James Benn and Ruifeng Chen for helpful feedback on this passage.

zhiguan 摩訶止觀), uses the term 'blind' (*mang* 盲) sixty times, the majority of which hew closely to the generally denigratory rhetorical pattern described above.[40] That said, in his exhaustively annotated translation of this text, Paul Swanson makes a rather intriguing observation: when Zhiyi employs the image of attempting to instruct a blind person about the colour of milk, he is implicitly citing the Mahayana *Mahāparinirvāṇa sūtra*, though his interpretation of the text is quite idiosyncratic. Specifically, and in contrast to his scriptural source, Zhiyi does *not* assume that such individuals are, by dint of their perceptual disabilities, irrevocably unable to receive Buddhist instruction; instead, he reinterprets this metaphor as referring to the necessity of such individuals finding enlightened teachers.[41] While this rhetorical usage is still ableist by modern standards (in that the monastic teacher is criticizing his presumably sighted disciples by referring to them as 'blind'), Zhiyi's conviction that such aspirants can and should still be taught suggests that the karmic difficulty (*nan* 難) of blindness is perhaps more surmountable than some previous sources would have had us believe.

Finally, we must turn our attention to the most provocative rhetorical usage of the terms 'blind' and 'deaf' in *XGSZ*, as recorded in a short, poetic text entitled the 'The Precious Man's Inscription' (*Baoren ming* 寶人銘), written by the monk Wangming (亡名, sixth century).[42] Therein, as part of a discourse on meditation, the monk states: 'barring one's seven apertures, shutting one's six sense [organs], one must not look at colours, one must not listen to sounds, one sounds will deafen [*long* 聾] the ears, colours will blind [*mang* 盲] the eyes'.[43] While these instructions clearly refer to the utility of *temporarily* blocking one's sensory inputs, it nonetheless alludes to an intriguing possibility considered by Stephen Harris: '[r]ather than being seen as intrinsically negative, disability could be considered an advanced training for those dedicated toward progressing quickly toward enlightenment'.[44]

40 I arrived at this number through a full-text search of T. 1912. For Swanson's edition, see *T'ien-t'ai Chih-i's Mo-ho Chih-kuan*.

41 For instance, in a section on 'Contemplating the Sense Fields', Zhiyi states that a blind student who receives this analogical teaching will 'reach [a certain] understanding of milk' (*T'ien-t'ai Chih-i's Mo-ho Chih-kuan*, p. 829). Commenting on this passage, Swanson notes that, 'contrary to the interpretation given by [Zhiyi], the *sūtra* says that no matter how many examples are given (a shell, rice powder, snow, and a white crane), a blind person cannot know the true meaning of "white"' (ibid.).

42 For a brief biographical sketch of this monk, see Knechtges, 'Shi Wangming', pp. 934–35.

43 關爾七竅閉爾六情。莫視於色莫聽於聲。聞聲者聾。見色者盲。(T. 2060: 482a20–22). CJKV (七竅): 'Seven apertures; seven orifices; seven holes. The seven apertures of the head: two eyes, two ears, two nostrils, and the mouth'.

44 Harris, 'Buddhism and Disability', p. 39. While the selected passage is from a section in Harris's argument concerned with general Buddhist perspectives (as opposed to his subsequent

In any case, arguing that the sights and sounds of the world are themselves inherently 'blinding' and 'deafening' (from the standpoint of the quest for enlightenment) certainly normalizes these conditions; likewise, in making the suggestion that practitioners should intentionally close themselves off to such inputs, Wangming's claim provocatively reimagines the logic of including sensory impairments among the 'Eight Difficulties', given that it essentially argues that such conditions could—at least theoretically—*enhance* one's ability to engage with Buddhist practice.

Narrative Uses

Highlighting the diversity of seventh-century opinions on the topic, the narratives collected by Daoxuan that contain references to the Chinese terms for blindness, deafness, and muteness range widely, in terms of both their affective valences and their symbolic resonances.

For an example of sensory impairment cast in a purely negative light, we can turn to the biography of the monk Puming (普明, 550–650 CE), a monk from Mount Tiantai and a disciple of Zhiyi, who was overseeing the casting of a great bell. When a blind man stops by to check on their progress, Puming worries that it is a bad omen and, indeed, when the mould is opened, the bell shatters.[45] This narrative represents a clear instance of the medieval Chinese *stimulus/response* (*ganying* 感應) cosmology, wherein actions within the human realm were understood to be capable of inducing corresponding reactions from the natural world.[46] More specifically, it suggests that—at least in certain contexts—the mere appearance of an individual with a non-normative body could be parsed as an adverse omen, in much the same way that an eclipse, an earthquake, or a multiheaded animal prodigy might. This brief episode sheds a grim light on the discrimination faced by such individuals.

In contrast, *XGSZ* also includes several tales of exemplary monks using some combination of thaumaturgical ability and spirituo-moral suasion to cure blindness, deafness, and muteness.[47] The biography of the monk

discussion of Mahayana views), it is nonetheless relevant, as the linkage between suffering and unsatisfactoriness, and the desire to renounce the secular life and seek liberation, remains relatively constant across historical Buddhisms.

45 T. 2060: 586a–b.

46 On the Chinese Buddhist reception of this cosmological principle, see Sharf, *Coming to Terms*. For *ganying* in Chinese Buddhist narrative traditions, see Campany, *Strange Writing*, pp. 321–34; Campany, *Signs*, pp. 43–48, 49 and passim.

47 Kieschnick, *The Eminent Monk*, pp. 67–111.

Fashun (法順, 558–641 CE) provides a clear introduction to this narrative trope, as it directly invokes the *ganying* framework as an explanation for the monk's curative prowess.

> At this time, Fashun contracted [*huan* 患] a swelling that festered and leaked pus. Among the people, there were some who revered him and sucked it out, and others who used a silk cloth to wipe it up. Immediately, it was cured, and the remaining pus emitted a [marvellous] fragrance whose flowing *qi* was incomparable. Nowadays, the wiping cloth is still there, and the marvellous aroma has not ceased.[48]
> In Sanyuan County, there was a person named Tian Saduo who had contracted [*huan* 患] deafness from birth. There was also a person named Zhang Su, who had contracted [*huan* 患] muteness from birth.[49] Fashun heard about their fates and came. He then spoke with them, and they were, always and forever after, completely cured. There was a monk from Wugong Prefecture who had been bewitched by a poisonous dragon, causing the assembly to send him out [to see Fashun]. Fashun began by clasping his hands and sitting across from him, when the dragon who had possessed the sick monk spoke to him, saying: 'The meditation master has now come, so it is appropriate [for me] not to stay for a long time. [I'm] agonized by having troubled you.' Soon thereafter, the monk's [infirmity] dissipated.
>
> For this reason, when there were people near or far who were vexed by disease, there were none who did not visit Fashun and find succour with him. He did not [take] charitable contributions or employ other techniques, but instead he would only sit and face a person. Those who know say that there is a [numinous] stimulus [*gan*] from his hidden virtue, which is the reason that the spirits of the dead were inclined to honour [him] and bring about [such results].[50]

48 On the image of sucking pus as a cultural signifier of devotion, see Knapp, *Selfless Offspring*, pp. 121–22.

49 As per DDB (患): highlighting the polyvocality of this term, it should be noted that can be used to describe a variety of misfortunes, from being afflicted with anxiety, to contracting an illness, and even being subject to calamity or evil.

50 順時患腫，膿潰外流，人有敬而㖒者，或有以帛拭者，尋即差愈　餘膿發香，流氣難比，拭帛猶在，香氣不歇。三原縣民田薩埵者生來患聾，又張蘇者亦患生瘂，順聞命來，與共言議，遂如常日，永即痊復。武功縣僧，毒龍所魅，眾以投之。順端拱對坐，龍遂託病僧言曰：「禪師既來，義無久住，極相勞嬈。」尋即釋然。故使遠近瘴癘淫邪所惱者無不投造，順不施餘術，但坐而對之，識者謂有陰德所感，故幽靈偏敬致 (T. 2060: 653c6–16). My thanks to Ruifeng Chen for some helpful comments on my translation of this passage.

The monk's ability to cure named individuals of their lifelong deafness and muteness, as well as his exorcism of a possessed monk, are clearly posited here as analogous acts, and each of them is explained—through explicit reference to the *ganying* (stimulus/response) framework—as resulting from the monk's 'hidden virtue'. Moreover, the author's specific reference to Fashun's avoidance of 'other techniques', and his simple reliance upon his own spiritual potency, emphasizes the competitive nature of the 'religio-medical marketplace' in medieval China, in which an individual struck by an acute or chronic condition could avail themselves of a local doctor, Daoist, spirit medium, *or* Buddhist monk for treatment.[51]

By describing Buddhist religious professionals treating such conditions, accounts like this one promote the this-worldly power and efficacy of Buddhism, while also seemingly challenging the karmic view of disability.[52] Finally, despite Fashun's exemplarity, this episode begins with a depiction of his transient, acute affliction with some sort of pustulous disease. Instead of viewing this illness as the result of a moral failing, however, this account treats it as a simple given in the monk's life. The narrative then uses the actions of those who opted to nurse him back to health as positive stimuli (*gan*) prompting twinned miraculous responses (*ying*): his recovery and the production of an otherworldly fragrance. This suggests that, for Daoxuan's discourse community, any given adverse health condition (such as disability and/or disease) was something of an open signifier, to which a variety of values could be ascribed depending on context and rhetorical agenda.

While the previous account offers a medicalized understanding of sensory impairment as a curable condition, neither the monk's methods nor the details provided about his patients yield any clues about how a medieval Chinese reader would have understood the cause(s) of their conditions.[53] Fortunately, several other relevant healing narratives from *XGSZ* allow us to shed additional light on this question. First, the biography of the Silla monk Jajang (慈藏, dates unknown) includes a number of miraculous responses in its description of his travels to China, including his use of a confession ritual to cure an individual who had 'suffered from blindness since birth'.[54]

51 See Salguero, *Translating Buddhist Medicine*, pp. 60–66.

52 Campany, *Strange Writing*, p. 323.

53 While I have invoked the contemporary categorization of 'medicalized' views of disability here (as per Sieber), I use it while recognizing that the 'medical' realm in medieval China also included spirit possession as a disease aetiology (see Unschuld, *Medicine in China*, pp. 29–50; Strickmann, *Chinese Magical Medicine*, pp. 58–88).

54 T. 2060: 639b. For an overview of contemporaneous Buddhist confession rituals, see Kuo Li-ying, *Confession et Contrition*.

This healing account provides a salient example of the fact that Daoxuan's discourse community must have found the karmic aetiology for bodily impairment, which linked such conditions to prior moral failings, plausible and intuitive. Otherwise, more ink would have been spilled explaining the connection between confession and healing. Also, and in keeping with the healing accounts treated above, it provides another example of an efficacious ritual or officiant seeming to short-circuit this karmic logic of bodily impairment as punishment.

These same dynamics are reflected in an episode from the biography of the Sui monk Zhiyin (智隱), which includes a list of miraculous responses to Buddhist relics. Included among this list of prodigies, we find the following:

> There were blind people who came and confessed, and suddenly their eyes recovered, [allowing them to] throw away their walking sticks and return home. Wind [illnesses], handicapped legs, and other such ailments were also [cured] in just this manner.[55]

This episode parallels Jajang's, with the inclusion of healings in a longer catalogue of miraculous episodes, the role of confession as a precursor to healing, and the necessary involvement of a Buddhist source of miraculous efficacy.[56] In addition, this account seems to posit a causal framework in which blindness, mobility problems, wind illnesses (a host of bodily conditions presumed to be caused by malign interactions between bodily and environmental energies), and other unnamed conditions are all receptive to the healing power of Buddhist relics and/or Buddhist ritual confession: a far cry from seeing such conditions as ineluctable fruits of karma.

In contrast, the *XGSZ* biography of the monk Zhikuang (智曠, 526–600 CE) includes another healing narrative, albeit one that posits a radically different aetiological framework:

> In Jiangling, there was [a person by the name of] Zhang Quan who was second-generation blind. Zhikuang said: 'A coffin inside your family's tomb was placed on top of an old well. If you move the grave and uncover the well, this will certainly allow you to banish [this misfortune]'. As a

55 盲者來懺欸獲雙目。捨杖而歸。風躄等病其例皆爾。」(CBETA, T50, no. 2060, p. 668b3–4). On 'wind illness', see Chen, 'Wind Malady'; and Kuriyama, *Expressiveness of the Body*, pp. 223–70.
56 Similarly, *XGSZ* includes an account of a layman named Qin Juhai (禽巨海) whose muteness spontaneously vanishes after he encounters some Buddhist relics (T. 2060: 673c).

> result of following the monk's words, the blind man came to see the Path, and he thereupon requested ordination.[57]

In this case, the unequivocal cause of Zhikuang's patient's blindness is a sepulchral plaint. As described in archeologically recovered tomb texts, the medieval Chinese were convinced that improper burial could aggrieve the denizens of the underworld and impel them to submit a legal case to the officers of the chthonic bureaucracy, which could result in any number of this-worldly consequences, from illness and premature death, to the loss of social station and penury.[58] From the Sinological standpoint, this miraculous cure is of note because the rituals for dealing with such plaints were much more typically associated with institutional Daoism, whereas here we see a Buddhist monk characterized as possessing the wherewithal to diagnose the ultimate (chthonic) causes for his parishioner's blindness.[59] Further, the success of this ritual cure inspires the patient to take ordination himself, dramatically enacting the linkage between vision, knowledge, and access to the Buddhist teaching.

The foregoing accounts can be usefully compared with Indian Buddhist healing narratives. Phyllis Granoff notes that comparable Indian tales are characterized by a general discomfiture with miraculous healing, as such cures could be seen as contraventions of the principle of karmic recompense.[60] In contrast, most of the Chinese healing narratives discussed above seem content to flout these concerns, especially when the patients were explicitly described as 'suffering' or 'being afflicted' (*huan* 患) with congenital conditions. In the cases of individuals *born with* sensory impairments, the karmic aetiology would have seemed especially apposite in this cultural context, given that such individuals could not yet have committed acts that would justify such 'punishments' in their current births. For this reason, and in contrast to the South Asian examples studied by Granoff, the healing narratives found in the hagiographical *Eminent Monks* literature suggest that demonstrating the numinous power of great Buddhist renunciants was a greater rhetorical concern than preserving the integrity of impersonal

57 江陵張詮者，二世眼盲，曠曰：「爾家塚内棺枕古井，移墳開甃，必獲禳焉。」因即隨言，瞽者見道，請求剃落。(T. 2060: 658c13–16).

58 See Hansen, *Negotiating Daily Life*, pp. 149–88; Davis, 'Texts for Stabilizing Tombs', pp. 592–612.

59 For a relevant section of a contemporaneous Daoist ritual text, see 'The Great Petition', p. 261.

60 Granoff, 'Cures and Karma', p. 286. The only exception she notes is in the case of plagues, whose indiscriminateness is incompatible with a karmic aetiology (pp. 300–01).

karmic justice, or—at the very least—that encountering the miraculous power of a healing monk could itself be attributed to one's karma.[61]

In an intriguing logical extension of the previous accounts, in which we saw spiritually potent Buddhist monks curing sensory impairments, *XGSZ* also includes several explicit references to the obverse process: namely, impious individuals being miraculously afflicted with such conditions. For an illustrative example, we turn to the biography of the sixth-century monastic exorcist Senglang (僧朗). Therein, we encounter a description of a nun who becomes possessed by a ghost. This spirit's malign influence gives her the ability to offer impressively erudite, but mystifying, lectures on Buddhist scriptures, thus earning her a considerable following in her home region. Hearing about the situation, Senglang recognizes it as a case of possession, visits her temple, and exorcizes the spirit, leaving her 'like one who was deaf and simple' (*longchi* 聾癡) until she recovers a hundred days later.[62] In addition to lauding its protagonist's exorcistic acumen, this account also includes a tangential reference to one of the causal frameworks for disability discussed above: namely, encounters with malign spirits as aetiologies for blindness, deafness, or muteness. More specifically, this story highlights the ideological linkage between ignorance, impairment, and punishment in a rather graphic way. First, the nun earns herself a sizeable following of adoring fans by offering complex and mystifying disquisitions on Buddhist scriptures through the power of this spirit. Once the monastic exorcist expels the malign force from her body, the nun finds herself uncommunicative for more than three months, as if an explicit punishment for having misled or confused the public about the Buddha's teachings. This is, of course, reminiscent of the various rhetorical uses discussed above, wherein such impairments were employed as metaphors for ignorance of and/or inability to access the Dharma. On a similar note, *XGSZ* also includes two accounts of officials and their servitors becoming immediately mute after they engage in campaigns to destroy Buddhist statues. As in the case of the unnamed nun, these anti-Buddhist actors become miraculously impaired, seemingly as a direct result of denying others access to Buddhist religious goods.[63] As such, we can see how accounts like these allow Daoxuan (and the original teller(s) of these tales) to radically foreshorten the karmic comeuppance of the malefactors described therein.

61 In his review of the common tropes featured in this literature, Kieschnick dedicates a lengthy chapter to 'monastic thaumaturges': see *The Eminent Monk*, pp. 67–111.

62 奄若聾癡 (T. 2060: 650c29).

63 T. 2060: 693a; 693b–c.

This is reminiscent of M. Miles's observation that many Indian Buddhist narrative sources approach karma as an 'educational force', allowing the Buddha (by virtue of his miraculous ability to perceive prior lives) to explain how an individual's current sensory impairments were a direct result of prior moral failings.[64] In these three examples, in contrast, the pedagogical role of bodily impairment (whether permanent or temporary) is cast into the present, such that one need not possess the miraculous vision of a Buddha in order to correctly parse the causal forces at work.

To round out our survey of these accounts, we now turn our attention to the *XGSZ* biography of the monk Daobian (道辯, 446–561 CE), as the description of its eponymous protagonist stands in stark contrast to the examples considered above.

> The monk Daobian was from the Tian clan and was a person of Fanyang. There is an *Additional Record* that says: 'Wearing a robe and clutching a monk's staff, thus he entered into her womb, and on account of that was born'. His heaven-endowed nature was surpassingly pure, and his genius and technical skill were widely renowned. Although he was said to be deaf, he eventually met Emperor Xiaowen [r. 471–499 CE] and never failed to meet the emperor's decrees. Thanks to his lofty reputation and illustrious appearance, people both near and far revered him. His specialties were clearly differentiating between good and evil, and providing clarification and interpretation of [challenging points] that impeded and obstructed [understanding].[65]

As the account continues, Daobian is seen playing an important role in preventing the dissemination of forged scriptures, as well as writing expansive and useful commentaries on a variety of Buddhist texts. It concludes with a short subsidiary biography of one of his disciples.[66]

The discrepancies between this account and those considered previously are striking. First and foremost, in contrast with the vast majority of the foregoing accounts, here we see a monk whose deafness presents no obstacle to a full and significant life as a contributing member of the monastic community. This is nowhere more clearly suggested than in the first several

64 Miles, 'Disability', pp. 98–99.

65 釋道辯、姓田氏、范陽人。有別記云: 著納擎錫入於母胎、因而生焉。天性踈朗、才術高世。雖曰耳聾、及對孝文、不爽帝旨。由是榮觀顯美、遠近欽茲。剖定邪正、開釋封滯、是所長也。(T. 2060: 471c1–c5).

66 T. 2060: 471c.

lines of the biography, which clearly invoke the 'exemplary child' trope to describe his birth and early years: a ubiquitous rhetorical signifier of sanctity that would have seemed utterly incongruous to a contemporary reader if deafness were seen as an insurmountable barrier to a meaningful Buddhist life.[67] Though a slight discomfiture with this situation is implied through the use of an explicit contrastive phrase to introduce the monk's condition ('Although he was said to be deaf', 雖曰耳聾), both the circumstances of his miraculous birth and his preternatural morality offer countervailing evidence. Moreover, the specific content of his mother's prenatal dream/vision (i.e., a monk entering her womb) suggests that her future child was destined for the monastic life: a fact that could be read as a rhetorical attempt to head off potential criticism over the ordination of an individual with a non-normative body.[68] Finally, and most significantly, this account presents us with circumstances that gesture to the social model of disability, in which 'impairment' only becomes 'disability' due to failures of accommodation. Rather than focusing on any instances where Daobian's deafness presented a challenge or impediment to living a full and meaningful monastic life, we instead see an individual who was able to make significant contributions to his religious order in ways that were compatible with his capacities: namely, by directing his considerable intellect towards the textual tasks of writing commentaries and scriptural exegeses.[69]

Conclusion

Some of the accounts considered above reinforce stereotypes about the premodern past, emphasizing the fact that individuals with sensory impairments like blindness, deafness, and muteness were often stigmatized and sidelined. In addition, the ways that texts circulated within specific religious communities created and reinforced these types of stigmatizing discourses. Many of these accounts treat the non-normative body as a 'narrative prosthesis', in Mitchell and Snyder's terminology: 'a destabilizing

67 See Kinney, 'The Theme of the Precocious Child'; Levering, 'The Precocious Child'; Jensen, 'Exemplary Child Trope'.

68 For a discussion of the historical context and rhetorical functions of such prenatal visions in the context of the medieval Chinese Buddhist hagiography, see Jensen, 'Dreaming Betwixt and Between'.

69 Though he is not mentioned in the *XGSZ*, as he was active slightly later than its compilation, the same case could be made for the monk Jianzhen (688–763), as briefly described in Chen, 'Brilliant Blind Monk', pp. 130–33.

sign of cultural prescriptions about the body and a deterministic vehicle of characterization for characters constructed as disabled'.[70] In so doing, most of these accounts also employ the 'medical model' of disability, approaching such conditions through the lens of lack, incapacity, and—in the best-case scenario—magico-medical treatment. That said, these materials—when considered as a whole—paint a much more multifaceted picture. While Huijiao's (admittedly limited) use of these terms was entirely commensurate with the logic of the 'Eight Difficulties', Daoxuan's usages were much more multifarious, with some rhetorical uses hewing closely to the inherited karmic logic of Buddhism. However, others raise the possibility that such conditions were not inherent, impassable barriers to enlightenment. Moreover, the narrative materials contained in Daoxuan's later collection demonstrate the hybrid nature of the cultural resources available to early medieval Chinese Buddhists, raising the possibility that the power of Buddhist actors (whether living monks or the numinous relics of them) could trump the logic of karma. The later collection even includes one example of a deaf monk being revered for his contributions to the Buddhist community, in which his sensory impairment was clearly a non-issue. This final example in particular demonstrates that a 'social model' of disability was also a living option to this discourse community, if perhaps an inchoate one. If nothing else, these observations highlight the inherently flawed nature of any attempt to define a singular 'Buddhist' perspective on disability, especially by focusing on doctrinal materials, as these doctrines were always being understood, interpreted, and occasionally flouted by specific named individuals, in response to the myriad political, cultural, economic, and ethical issues facing them at any given historical moment. Approaching such issues through the study of historical narratives is one corrective to this essentializing tendency.

Abbreviations

CJKV	*CJKV-English Dictionary of Confucian, Daoist, and Intellectual Historical Terms*, ed. by Charles A. Muller <http://www.buddhism-dict.net/dealt/>
DDB	*Digital Dictionary of Buddhism*, ed. by Charles A. Muller <http://www.buddhism-dict.net/ddb/>

70 Mitchell and Snyder, *Narrative Prosthesis*, p. 50.

GSZ *Biographies of Eminent Monks* (*Gaoseng zhuan* 高僧傳 [T. 2059])
T. *Taishō Tripitaka* [CBETA version] 《大正新脩大藏經》與《卍新纂續藏經》的資料引用是出自「中華電子佛典協會」(Chinese Buddhist Electronic Text Association, 簡稱 CBETA 的電子佛典系列光碟, 2016) <http://www.cbeta.org/>
XGSZ *Continued Biographies of Eminent Monks* (*Xu gaoseng zhuan* 續高僧傳 [T. 2060])

Bibliography

Primary Sources

Biographies de moines éminents (*Kao Seng Tchouan*) *de Houei-Kiao*, trans. by Robert Shih (Louvain: Bibliothèque du Muséon, 1968)

Biographies of Eminent Monks (*Gaoseng zhuan* 高僧傳 [T. 2059])

The Complete Works of Zhuangzi, trans. by Burton Watson (New York: Columbia University Press, 2013)

Continued Biographies of Eminent Monks (*Xu gaoseng zhuan* 續高僧傳 [T. 2060])

Daoxuan (道宣), *Xu gaoseng zhuan* 續高僧傳 [*Continued Biographies of Eminent Monks*] [T. 2060], collated and punctuated by Guo Shaolin 郭紹林 (Beijing: Zhonghua shuju, 2014)

'The Great Petition for Sepulchral Plaints', trans. by Peter Nickerson, in *Early Daoist Scriptures*, ed. by Stephen Bokenkamp (Berkeley: University of California Press, 1997), pp. 230–74

Gaoseng zhuan 高僧傳, trans by. Yoshikawa Tadao and Funayama Tōru 吉川忠夫, 船山徹 (Tokyo: Iwanami Shoten, 2009–2010)

Huijiao (慧皎), *Gaoseng zhuan* 高僧傳 [*Biographies of Eminent Monks*] [T. 2059], ed. and punctuated by Tang Yongtong 湯用彤 (Beijing: Zhonghua shuju, 1992; repr. 2007)

Huiyuan (慧遠), *Dasheng yi zhang* 大乘義章 [*Essay on the System of Mahāyāna* (T. 1851)]

Taishō Tripitaka [CBETA version] 《大正新脩大藏經》與《卍新纂續藏經》的資料引用是出自「中華電子佛典協會」(Chinese Buddhist Electronic Text Association, 簡稱 CBETA) 的電子佛典系列光碟 (2016) http://www.cbeta.org/

T'ien-t'ai Chih-i's Mo-ho Chih-kuan: Clear Serenity, Quiet Insight, trans. by Paul Swanson (Honolulu: University of Hawai'i Press, 2018)

Secondary Sources

Campany, Robert Ford, *Making Transcendents: Ascetics and Social Memory in Early Medieval China* (Honolulu: University of Hawai'i Press, 2009)

Campany, Robert Ford, *Signs from the Unseen Realm: Buddhist Miracle Tales from Early Medieval China—A Study and Translation* (Honolulu: University of Hawai'i Press, 2012)

Campany, Robert Ford, *Strange Writing: Anomaly Accounts in Early Medieval China* (Albany: State University of New York Press, 1996)

Campany, Robert Ford, *To Live as Long as Heaven and Earth: A Study and Translation of Ge Hong's 'Traditions of Divine Transcendents'* (Berkeley: University of California Press, 2002)

Chen Hsiu-fen, 'Wind Malady as Madness in Medieval China: Some Threads from the Dunhuang Medical Manuscripts', in *Medieval Chinese Medicine: The Dunhuang Medical Manuscripts*, ed. by Christopher Cullen and Vivienne Lo (Abingdon: Routledge Curzon, 2005), pp. 345–62

Chen Yaozhen, 'The Courageous and Brilliant Blind Monk Jianzhen', *Chinese Medical Journal*, 93 (1980), 130–33

CJKV-English Dictionary of Confucian, Daoist, and Intellectual Historical Terms, ed. by Charles A. Muller <http://www.buddhism-dict.net/dealt/>

Clarke, Shayne, *Family Matters in Indian Buddhist Monasticisms* (Honolulu: University of Hawai'i Press, 2013)

Davis, Timothy M., 'Texts for Stabilizing Tombs', in *Early Medieval China: A Sourcebook*, ed. by Wendy Swartz, Robert Ford Campany, Yang Lu, and Jessey J. C. Choo (New York: Columbia University Press, 2014), pp. 592–612

Digital Dictionary of Buddhism, ed. by Charles A. Muller <http://www.buddhism-dict.net/ddb/>

Doniger O'Flaherty, Wendy, ed., *Karma and Rebirth in Classical Indian Traditions* (Berkeley: University of California Press, 1980)

Freiberger, Oliver. *Considering Comparison: A Method for Religious Studies* (New York, Oxford University Press, 2019)

Granoff, Phyllis, 'Cures and Karma II: Some Miraculous Healings in the Indian Buddhist Story Tradition', *Bulletin de l'Ecole française d'Extrême-Orient*, 85 (1998), 285–304

Guang Xing, *The Concept of the Buddha: Its Evolution from Early Buddhism to the Trikāya Theory* (London: Routledge Curzon, 2005)

Hansen, Valerie, *Negotiating Daily Life in Traditional China: How Ordinary People Used Contracts, 600–1400* (New Haven, CT: Yale University Press, 1995)

Harris, Stephen E., 'Buddhism and Disability', in *Disability and World Religions: An Introduction*, ed. by Darla Y. Schumm and Michael Stoltfus (Waco: Baylor University Press, 2016), pp. 25–46

Hurvitz, Leon, *Chih-i (538–597): An Introduction to the Life and Ideas of a Chinese Buddhist Monk* (Bruges: Institut Belge des Hautes Écoles Chinoises, 1963)

Jan, Yün-hua, 'The Chinese Understanding and Assimilation of the Karma Doctrine', in *Karma and Rebirth: Post Classical Developments*, ed. by Ronald W. Neufeldt (Albany: State University of New York Press, 1986), pp. 145–68

Jensen, Christopher, 'Dreaming Betwixt and Between: Oneiric Narratives in Huijiao and Daoxuan's *Biographies of Eminent Monks*' (unpublished doctoral dissertation, McMaster University, 2018)

Jensen, Christopher, 'Rhetorical Uses of the Exemplary Child Trope in the *Biographies of Eminent Monks* and *Biographies of Nuns*', *Studies in Chinese Religions*, 7 (2021), 63–111

Kieschnick, John, *The Eminent Monk: Buddhist Ideals in Medieval Chinese Hagiography* (Honolulu: University of Hawai'i Press, 1997)

Kieschnick, John, 'Gaoseng zhuan', in *Early Medieval Chinese Texts: A Bibliographical Guide*, ed. by Cynthia Chennault, Keith N. Knapp, Alan J. Berkowitz, Albert E. Dien, (Berkeley, CA: Institute of East Asian Studies, 2015), pp. 76–80

Kieschnick, John, 'Xu gaoseng zhuan', in *Early Medieval Chinese Texts: A Bibliographical Guide*, ed. by Cynthia Chennault, Keith N. Knapp, Alan J. Berkowitz, Albert E. Dien (Berkeley, CA: Institute of East Asian Studies, 2015), pp. 428–31

Kinney, Anne Behnke, 'The Theme of the Precocious Child in Early Chinese Literature', *T'oung Pao*, second series, 81.1/3 (1995), 1–24

Knapp, Keith Nathaniel, *Selfless Offspring: Filial Children and Social Order in Medieval China* (Honolulu: University of Hawai'i Press, 2005)

Knechtges, David R., 'Shi Wangming', in *Ancient and Early Medieval Chinese Literature: A Reference Guide (Part Two)*, ed. by David R. Knechtges and Taiping Chang (Leiden: Brill, 2013), pp. 934–35

Kuo Li-ying, *Confession et contrition dans le bouddhisme chinois du Ve au Xe siècle* (Paris: EFEO, 1994)

Kuriyama, Shigehisa, *The Expressiveness of the Body and the Divergence of Greek and Chinese Medicine* (New York: Zone Books, 2002)

Lambert, Andrew, 'Daoism and Disability', in *Disability and World Religions: An Introduction*, ed. by Darla Y. Schumm and Michael Stoltfus (Waco: Baylor University Press, 2016), pp. 71–92

Lukey, Benjamin, 'Confucianism and Disability', in *Disability and World Religions: An Introduction*, ed. by Darla Y. Schumm and Michael Stoltfus (Waco: Baylor University Press, 2016), pp. 47–70

Levering, Miriam, 'The Precocious Child in Chinese Buddhism', in *Little Buddhas: Children and Childhoods in Buddhist Texts and Traditions*, ed. by Vanessa R. Sasson (Oxford: Oxford University Press, 2012), pp. 124–56

Miles, M., 'Buddhism and Responses to Disability, Mental Disorders and Deafness in Asia', *Center for International Rehabilitation Research Information and Exchange* (CIRRIE), November 2013, <https://www.independentliving.org/files/buddhism-disability-bibliography-m-miles201311.pdf> [accessed March 24, 2023]

Miles, M., 'Disability on a Different Model', *Journal of Religion, Disability & Health*, 6 (2002), 89–108

Mitchell, David T., and Sharon L. Snyder, *Narrative Prosthesis: Disability and the Dependencies of Discourse* (Ann Arbor: University of Michigan Press 2000)

Mollier, Christine, *Buddhism and Taoism Face to Face: Scripture, Ritual and Iconographic Exchange in Medieval China* (Honolulu: University of Hawai'i Press, 2008)

Mrozik, Susanne, *Virtuous Bodies: The Physical Dimensions of Morality in Buddhist Ethics* (Oxford: Oxford University Press, 2007)

Nattier, Jan, *A Few Good Men: The Bodhisattva Path According to the Inquiry of Ugra* (*Ugraparipṛcchā*) (Honolulu: University of Hawai'i Press, 2003)

Nicol, Janine, 'Outsiders: Medieval Chinese Buddhists and the "Borderland Complex", An Exploration of the Eight Difficulties', *SOAS Journal of Postgraduate Research*, 6 (2014), 27–48

Ohnuma, Reiko, *Unfortunate Destiny: Animals in the Indian Buddhist Imagination* (New York and Oxford: Oxford University Press, 2017)

Poo, Muzhou, *In Search of Personal Welfare: A View of Ancient Chinese Religion* (Albany: State University of New York Press, 1998)

Rondolino, Massimo A., 'Some Foundational Considerations on Taxonomy: A Case for Hagiography', *Religions*, 10 (2019), 1–9

Salguero, C. Pierce, *Translating Buddhist Medicine in Medieval China* (Philadelphia: University of Pennsylvania Press, 2014)

Siebers, Tobin, *Disability Theory* (Ann Arbor: University of Michigan Press, 2008)

Sharf, Robert H., *Coming to Terms with Chinese Buddhism: A Reading of the Treasure Store Treatise* (Honolulu: University of Hawai'i Press, 2002)

Shinohara, Koichi, 'Guanding's Biography of Zhiyi, the Fourth Patriarch of the Tiantai Tradition', in *Speaking of Monks: Religious Biography in India and China*, ed. by Phyllis Granoff and Koichi Shinohara (Oakville, Ontario: Mosaic Press, 1992), pp. 97–232

Slingerland, Edward, *Mind and Body in Early China: Beyond Orientalism and the Myth of Holism* (Oxford: Oxford University Press, 2019)

Strickmann, Michel, *Chinese Magical Medicine*, ed. by Bernard Faure (Stanford, CA: Stanford University Press, 2002)

Strong, John, *A Bull of a Man: Images of Masculinity, Sex, and the Body in Indian Buddhism* (Cambridge: Harvard University Press, 2009)

Strong, John, *Buddhisms: An Introduction*, (London: OneWorld, 2015)

Tsukamoto, Zenryū, *A History of Early Chinese Buddhism: From Its Introduction to the Death of Hui-yüan*, trans. by Leon Hurvitz (Tokyo: Kodansha International, 1985)

Unschuld, Paul U., *Medicine in China: A History of Ideas* (Berkeley: University of California Press, 1985)

von Glahn, Richard, *The Sinister Way: The Divine and Demonic in Chinese Religious Culture* (Berkeley: University of California Press, 2004)

Weinstein, Stanley, *Buddhism under the T'ang* (Cambridge: Cambridge University Press, 1987)

Zürcher, Erik, *The Buddhist Conquest of China: The Spread and Adaptation of Buddhism in Early Medieval China*, 3rd edn (Leiden: Brill, 1959; repr. 2007)

About the Author

Christopher Jensen is an Assistant Professor in the Religion Program (College of Humanities) at Carleton University in Ottawa. His ongoing research interests include dreams and dreaming, Chinese Buddhist hagiography, Religious Studies pedagogy, and the theory and practice of comparison in twenty-first-century Religious Studies. The present project represents one facet of his broader attempt to attend to the lived experience of medieval Chinese Buddhists, using narrative sources to explore aspects of religious life that are often elided in other forms of literature (e.g., disability, dream-related practices, and the experiences of children). He is grateful to have been given the opportunity to present an early version of this research and to meet the editors of this volume at the International Congress on Medieval Studies, and to have subsequently been included in this collection.

4. Perfect Disabled Embodiment: Gelongma Palmo in the Tibetan Buddhist Hagiographies

Ivette Vargas-O'Bryan

Abstract: The hagiographies of Gelongma Palmo (*Dge slong ma Dpal mo*, 'Lustrous Nun' in Tibetan) contain the story of an early tenth-century Indian Buddhist nun and former leper, whose life story and fasting ritual formed the foundation for one of the most popular legacies in Tibetan Buddhist history and contemporary Tibetan communities throughout Asia. This study explores the intersectionality between disability and gender in the Gelongma Palmo legacy of life stories uncovering relations of power by contrasting social-institutional (monastic) norms of ableism with more inclusive Buddhist tantric theories of spiritual development and embodiment. The select hagiographies in this study draw attention to tantric Buddhist notions of embodiment in contrast to Indian and Tibetan Buddhist societal and medical norms.

Keywords: Tibetan Buddhism, disability studies, feminist studies, Gelongma Palmo, gender, monasticism, Tibetan medicine

The story begins with a familiar tale of a beautiful young princess during the reign of a powerful medieval kingdom. This maiden defies the wishes of her royal family by choosing to follow a religious vocation instead of succumbing to a political marriage arranged for her by her family. Her chosen path—to become a celibate nun—is difficult for a woman in a patriarchal society. In several retellings, she is described as an erudite abbess of an all-male monastery, rare for her time and context. However, she finds that the religious path is not an end in itself, but just the beginning of a series of internal and external struggles. After a few years, the scholarly monastic

Grace-Petinos, Stephanie, Leah Pope Parker, and Alicia Spencer-Hall, eds. *Disability and Sanctity in the Middle Ages.* Taylor & Francis Group, 2025
DOI 10.5117/9789463724333_CH04

contracts a disfiguring skin disease. Thereafter, she is stripped of her position in the monastery and wanders, homeless due to her illness. She then realizes that her greater purpose is to embrace her illness as instrumental for the salvation of all beings. Depending on the account, she is transformed in a spiritual union with the divine, or is revealed as a divine figure herself, who then founds a fasting healing practice for communities of followers.

This is not the story of a medieval European Christian female saint, who came from a noble background, suffered stigmatized illness, and became a founder of a religious community. This is the story of an early tenth-century Indian Buddhist nun and former leper, Gelongma Palmo (*Dge slong ma Dpal mo*, 'Lustrous Nun' in Tibetan) whose life story and fasting ritual formed the foundation for one of the most popular legacies in Tibetan Buddhist history and contemporary society.[1]

This chapter focuses on how female-gendered, stigmatized illness, seen through a tantric Buddhist lens, is not a problem to be cured but instead serves as a valuable site of resistance to normative, ableist Buddhist monastic (and by extension, societal) notions of perfection as a criterion for enlightenment.[2] Perfection is, therefore, problematized since the religious ideal of a 'fluid' Buddha (enlightened being) is itself a perfect being who utilizes the body as a skillful method of compassion for others' enlightenment, while the monastic, and by extension, patriarchal society's understanding of higher spiritual development and embodiment is undergirded by norms of ableism, a perspective of marginalization based on bodily difference. This study explores the intersectionality between disability and gender in the Gelongma Palmo legacy of life stories, uncovering forms of meaning in relations of power by contrasting social institutional (that is, monastic) norms of ableism with more inclusive Buddhist tantric theories of spiritual development and embodiment. The select hagiographies in this study draw attention to tantric

1 In contemporary Tibetan Buddhism, this nun's legacy is commemorated in annual fasting practices. Tibetan nuns embrace her legacy as a model for Tibetan Buddhist women's struggle for rights to access full monastic ordination and education at a time without fully ordained Tibetan or Indian nuns (Sanskrit: *bhikṣuṇī*; Tibetan: *dge slong ma*) as well as a model of female enlightened embodiment. The first English-language novel in Bhutan, written in 2004 by a female Bhutanese novelist and well known among school-age children, memorializes Gelongma Palmo as a healer and protector of humans and mangy stray dogs. Pilgrimage sites related to Gelongma Palmo's legacy in Bhutan and Nepal reflect the cultural memory of her as a kind of St Francis of Assisi. See Choden, *Dawa*. On St Francis, see the chapter by Trembinski in this volume, pp. 39–62.

2 On this, see also Edwards's chapter in the present volume, analysing the signification of leprosy in the life of Buddhist Empress Kōmyō of Japan (d. 760) (pp. 248–50); and Jensen's study of disability in the Chinese Buddhist context of the *Eminent Monk* biographies (pp. 87–113).

Buddhist notions of embodiment as equanimity and fluidity that go beyond more conservative Indian and Tibetan Buddhist monastic, societal, and even medical norms. Unlike the binary (and ambivalent) representations often encountered in other non-tantric Buddhist scriptures and monastic rules—such as female/male, sick/well, nun/monk, and others—here, a reframing of enlightened embodied experience enable us to explore it in terms that reverse stigma and recast it as a virtue. Exposing the socially constructed and, therefore, contingent status of categories like the body, and identities such as *leper* and *woman*, opens up the possibility for more empowering interpretations of Buddhist literature. Critical disability and feminist theories provide fresh theoretical lenses through which to view this legacy of Tibetan hagiographies of a medieval Indian Buddhist nun, which were transmitted by mostly male Tibetan Buddhist monastics. Furthermore, my work on disease spirits and the intersections of Buddhist scripture and the Tibetan medical tradition (the latter being heavily indebted to Indian Āyurvedic medical views) point to an underlying medicalization of the leper body that potentially inform the Gelongma Palmo hagiographies. This brief study will draw on two of the earliest Tibetan Buddhist texts (dating from the fourteenth century) and a modern version, as well as contemporary ethnographic studies in Tibetan communities in Asia, which offer consistent examples of the nature of these perspectives across time and region.[3]

The Gelongma Palmo Legacy and Buddhist Doctrine

Gelongma Palmo's life story was transmitted over several centuries from the eleventh century to the present day as indicated in the scholarly literary collections of Tibetan Buddhist monastic libraries, popular literature, and oral legends in South Asia and Tibetan areas of East Asia.[4] My research

3 The two fourteenth-century texts are Jo gdan Bsod nams bzang po's *Smyung gnas bla ma brgyud pa 'i rnam thar*, and 'Od dpag rdo rje's *Thugs rje chen po bcu gcig zhal gyi bla ma brgyud pa 'i rnam thar nor bu 'i phreng ba*. *Dge slong ma dpal mo'i rnam thar nges 'byung rgyud la skye ba 'i chos gtam* is the anonymous modern work printed at the request of a Bhutanese monastic leper. I have conducted archival, field- and ethnographic work over the past twenty years in India, Nepal, and Tibet. For ethnographic studies on these and related texts, see Vargas-O'Bryan, 'Disease, the Demons and the Buddhas', pp. 81–99.

4 Most attention in Western scholarship has been given to the fasting ritual rather than to the hagiographies: see Zivkovic, 'Embodying the Past', pp. 45–63. There are currently about 168 texts on the Gelongma Palmo (Tibetan: *dpal mo lugs*) legacy dated from the eleventh century to the present day as evident in the Buddhist Digital Archives and local communities. See also my forthcoming book: Vargas-O'Bryan, *Historical Study*.

links her appearance and the early transmission of her teachings with the reintroduction of Buddhism (and re-introduction of the tantric strand) into Tibet and with the flourishing of monasticism into Tibetan areas from the Indian subcontinent in the late ninth or early tenth centuries, after a brief hiatus of Buddhist transmission due to civil unrest and suppression of Buddhism in Tibet.[5]

According to the hagiographies, Gelongma Palmo became the head of a male monastic order in India, a rare occurrence in her time period, and the founder of what became a popular fasting ritual (*smyung gnas*) in Tibetan Buddhist culture, revealed to her by the renowned bodhisattva of compassion, Avalokiteśvara (Tibetan: Chenrezig). In Buddhism, a bodhisattva is believed to be an enlightened being who appears in bodily form out of compassion in order to help others develop their spiritual states. Gelongma Palmo revealed herself as a bodhisattva in a spiritual journey. As a Buddhist tale, suffering or dissatisfaction (*duḥkha*) is a central concern in the Gelongma Palmo life stories. Briefly, according to Buddhist doctrine, sentient beings are caught in an endless cycle of rebirth due to their attachment to selfish desires and a lack of understanding that everything is impermanent, including one's identity (self). It is only when sentient beings realize this transitory nature of existence, act non-dualistically (without preference for one perspective), and direct their energies intentionally towards the betterment of others through compassion that they are released from the cycle of rebirth and realize their Buddhanature (the potential to be enlightened, a 'Buddha').[6] A Buddha is a figure who realizes the nature of reality and has detached herself from personal perspectives and desires (and is released from the cycle of rebirth); she has instead dedicated her existence to helping others get out of the same cycle. In the Buddhist tradition of the Mahāyāna, achieving the quality of the Buddha as a compassionate being—becoming a bodhisattva—is the most critical state of enlightenment, and it is through intentional re-embodiment that the Buddha-bodhisattva helps others. An enlightened being must act skilfully (the doctrine of skillful means), in other words, use different methods to help other sentient beings achieve enlightenment based on others' capacity to understand and *karma* (the fruit of their own past actions).

5 Davidson, *Tibetan Renaissance*.

6 A Buddha has achieved the highest level of certain virtues, 'perfections', including generosity, morality, patience, energy, meditation, and wisdom. A Buddha is perfect, that is, fully enlightened, in that he is omniscient, altruistic, and non-detached.

In the Buddhist philosophical context, illness, along with old age and death, are interpreted as transitory states that all beings share in existence. The realization of these states played a major role in transforming what became known as the historical Buddha, Śākyamuni, to an enlightened being in about the fourth century BCE in South Asia; he established the monastic institution in order to help others achieve this Buddha state.[7] According to the framing narrative in the historical Buddha's biographies, it was not until he (Gautama) as an Indian prince or tribal chieftain's son saw illness, old age, and death in others during three of his royal excursions that he was able to embark on a spiritual journey that led to his understanding about the nature of existence, and find a way to alleviate this 'suffering' (an attachment to the transitory) in his own realization as a Buddha. His founding of a monastic institution (*sangha*) served as a training centre for 'future bodhisattvas' and as a learning centre for the laity. Throughout the centuries, Indian Buddhist monastics, the early healers and founders of the Indian medical traditions along with their Hindu counterparts, often treated (with teachings and rituals) people's bodies and minds.[8] In a predominantly patriarchal society, Buddhist monastics—mostly male monastics—made it their purpose to act as male nurses to treat patients (the world of suffering beings) with the medicine of the Buddha-physician's *Dharma* (literally, Buddhist teachings). Modern Tibetan medical institutions are based on these earlier Buddhist ideas of healing through the Dharma.

The Gelongma Palmo stories in particular represent the tantric strand of Buddhism, a new, often antinomian approach to Buddhism transmitted in India from around the third to the sixth centuries and embraced in Tibetan areas around the ninth century. Tantra seeks to harness experiences and mental and physical energies through ritual practices (in the case of the hagiographies, it was fasting) to help realize the true nature of existence and enable a rapid transformation (enlightenment) in one's current body.[9] One of the unique characteristics of tantric texts, besides having elaborate rituals and more female enlightened beings than any other Buddhist tradition, is that they fervently represent the body as fluid and changing, a stance that

7 By founding a new religion that, among other things, transgressed his contemporary pre-Hindu tradition's caste system—utilized as a means to achieve higher rebirths, reach 'God', or attain a permanent higher reality—the historical Buddha, by contrast, created a model monastic society meant to uphold ethical values and seek higher spiritual aspirations for all sentient beings through their own efforts. The collection of monastic rules (*Vinaya*) contained his experiments in narrative form and guidelines during his lifetime. See Hanh, *The Heart*.

8 See Zysk, *Asceticism*.

9 Davidson, *Tibetan Renaissance*, pp. 34–44.

is meant to challenge normative notions of permanence and identity.[10] As tantras, these texts are meant to be read on two levels: on one level, from the perspective of an ordinary person undergoing hardships in order to achieve a spiritual experience, and on the other level, as a magical illusion or ploy used by a Buddha-bodhisattva to help others achieve enlightenment.[11]

Tibetan Hagiography's Spectacle and Enigmatic Enlightened Embodiment

In a Mahāyāna tantric Buddhist story, the Buddha-bodhisattva appears physically human; however, she is ultimately (albeit covertly) at a spiritually divine level. In other words, she is an enlightened being disguised as a human. The Buddha-bodhisattva can appear in different embodiments, a kind of shape-shifter who is in control, balanced, and skillful, and able to transform based on what is needed by others. At the beginning of the corpus of hagiographies, Gelongma Palmo is identified as an enlightened being worthy of being the subject of Tibetan Buddhist tantric biographical literature:

> Homage to the bodily constituents of the Illustrious Palmo,
> a *yoginī* who came as a luster of the world in this degenerate time,
> subsumed into one the Buddha activity of all the conquerors of the three times.
> Such a *yoginī* like that is Rdo rje Phag mo, the supreme mother of the conquerors of the three times [...]
> she has [voluntarily] miraculously re-embodied into the body of a female for the sake of sentient beings.
> It will be shown on the basis of the constellation,
> just a part of the sun and the moon of what is inconceivable and inexpressible.[12]

10 The Gelongma Palmo legacy texts do not contain higher-level tantric esoteric teachings that explicitly transgress social norms concerning bodily fluids, alcohol, and sexual acts (deemed against monastic rules).

11 Tibetan tantric biographical literature is interpreted as generally following a triadic structure (outer, inner, and secret) signifying different levels of spiritual development. Most of the Gelongma Palmo narratives represent the outer structure of tantra, much more exoteric and accessible to the general public.

12 *Dge slong ma dpal mo*, 1.1–1.7: dus gsum rgyal ba kun gyi 'phrin las pa// gcig tu sdud cing snyigs ma'i dus 'di ru // 'gro ba'i dpal tu byon pa'i mal 'byor ma/ dpal ldan dpal mo'i tshogs la

> Now, what master composed this means for the spiritual realization [*sādhanā*] of the holy Eleven-faced One? Having heard it, Nun Palmo listened directly to the holy one and composed it with ease.[13]

These descriptions from two different texts reflect common openings in Tibetan Buddhist tantric biographies, known in Tibetan as *rnam par thar par* ('namthar'), literally meaning 'full liberation'. These texts are the Tibetan version of Western Christian hagiographies.[14] Like Western hagiographic literature, Tibetan hagiographic literature provides records for those on a spiritual quest that are often transmitted by a male monastic official or mentor who serves as a scribe or later 'historian' of a saint figure's spiritual journey. However, it is to be understood in the Tibetan Buddhist case that the saintly figure's human body, through which her experiences are described, is later revealed in the writings as a ruse or spectacle for her true 'hidden' nature. The central figure is first presented in the narratives with saintly titles and suprahuman qualities, that is, with physical manifestations typical of a divine being or Buddha. In these texts, Gelongma Palmo is identified as a Buddha figure with different titles such as a *lob dpon* (spiritual master or scholar), *yoginī* (female master of yoga), *sku sprul* (pronounced 'tulku', reincarnated body), *ḍākinī* (female embodiment of enlightened energy), and *bodhisattva* (an embodied and reincarnated enlightened being with compassionate qualities).[15] As a *ḍākinī*, she is a special female form that

phyag 'tshal lo// de lta bu'i mal 'byor ma de nyid dus gsum rgyal ba'i yum mchog rdo rje phag mo 'gro ba bud med kyi lu su skur sprul nas sems can gyi don la bsam gyis mi khyab cing brzod kyi mi lang shing rgyu skar nas nyi zla'i zur tsam ston pa la/

13 The Sanskrit term *sādhanā* means 'accomplishing a realization connected with a Buddha figure', which generally entails ritually evoking a divinity, and eventually identifying with and absorbing that figure. See Jo gdan, *Smyung gnas*, fols 2a.l–4: de yang 'phags pa zhal bcu gcig pa'i sgrub thabs 'di slob dpon gang gis mdzad na / dge slong ma dpal mos 'phags pa la dngo[s] su gsan nas /des bde blag tu mdzad do//

14 These 'saints' that exhibit qualities of an enlightened being under various titles in Tibetan Buddhism are not officially canonized, as in the Catholic tradition. However, they are recognized and commemorated for their special spiritual qualities by Tibetan Buddhist monastics and local communities throughout the centuries.

15 Generally, terms such as Buddha (a fully enlightened being), *bodhisattva* (a compassionate enlightened being on his way to becoming fully enlightened), *tulku* (emanation body referring to a reincarnated body), *Dharmakāya* (the body of the Buddhist teachings, not necessarily a physical body), and the others mentioned above, including material objects, refer to different aspects of enlightened experience that are not often mutually exclusive. Bodies that appear in sentient existence or in the world of *saṃsāra* (rebirth) are considered temporary receptacles. A Buddha body is a sign of perfection that is irreversible and therefore expresses a complete detachment from anything transitory.

shows her detachment literally by severing her head.[16] As a bodhisattva, her method is to intentionally choose a body that is useful for particular sentient beings. As she listened to another bodhisattva's teaching (who is later revealed to have 'healed' her by teaching her fasting), she 'composed' the story, also reflecting her agency in this tale.

Related to the notion of intentionality, Tibetan tantric biographies are meant to be read (understood) by its (monastic) readers and transmitted to its (lay) audience on two levels at once, according to the doctrine of the two levels of reality: that is, relative or conventional truths and ultimate truths. In other words, on one level, these texts present a struggling human being, who through a spiritual journey eventually achieves a spiritual awakening and liberation. On the ultimate level, there is in actuality no struggle, since this is a Buddha-bodhisattva in disguise using the story for didactic purposes. As these stories develop, they reveal that Gelongma Palmo appears to undergo obstacles (experiences pertaining to impermanence) in relation to a body that is in reality an ingenious construct that allows others to learn from experience and attain spiritual elevation. Gelongma Palmo uses the tool of the sick and female body in her narratives in order to reveal the enlightenment experience so that others may also achieve it.

The Power Dynamics of Ableism versus Perfection

One of the ways to better understand the power relations underlying the Gelongma Palmo hagiographies is to first situate them within the interpretive framework of ableist social institutional (that is, Buddhist monastic) norms regarding health and related 'normalcy' standards, as well as illness and perspectives on disability, and gender. Critical to several religious traditions is the view that the sick body is a powerful image doctrinally, and in both Hinduism and Buddhism, it relates to the fruits of one's actions, *karma*.[17] In the Buddhist context, karma is a moral doctrine based on one's attachment or desires; the strongest attachment is to the body (and the need for self-preservation). A sick body reflects a state of imperfection, a lack of cognitive understanding (ignorance) of the true nature of reality,

16 Here she is a special type of Buddha, often also seen as a manifestation of other Buddha figures that commit self-mutilation by beheading, thus representing her severance of attachment to contingent existence and appearances. See Benard, *Chinnamasta*.
17 Leslie, 'Implications', pp. 23–45.

which is applied to the physical body. In contrast, ultimate health is the permanent body of the Buddha, who is omniscient, lacks attachment to any one perspective normally based on selfish desires, and is thus free of any karmic residue. As a stable experience, the enlightened being acts (and exists) completely altruistically. Her body and mind do not exhibit pain; the physical body is anatomically intact (a mark of 'health'), although it does not necessarily take what we may define as a human form.[18]

In the case of Gelongma Palmo, as a bodhisattva she intentionally chooses a body that is marked historically by marginalization and stigma: a sick, leprous, female body. The two biographies both describe her bodily condition in detail:

> About three months passed,
> the ten toes of the lama's feet fell off.
> Then five months later,
> the ten fingers of her hands fell off.[19]
> Despite [the fact] that this nun was knowledgeable
> in the five domains of knowledge [*rig pa 'i gnas lnga*]
> and also instructions and vows were present [in her] in a very noble way,
> leprosy arose due to the force of previous karma. [...]
> Even though knowledgeable in the five domains of knowledge,
> by being afflicted with a virulent illness,
> there arose immeasurable suffering settling in her mind as if without recourse.
> Attendants carried her into an isolated thatched hut where she stayed crying.[20]

18 The body of a Buddha has been discussed extensively in different Buddhist texts; for example, a large head and a third eye signal his omniscience and insight, and covered genitalia signify detachment. See Powers, 'Body'.

19 *Dge slong ma dpal mo*, 7.19–8.4: zla ba gsum tsam lon pa dang bla ma'i zhabs kyi sor mdzub bcu chad/ de nas zla lnga long pa dang phyag mdzub bcu chad / de tshe dpon g.yog gnyis po thugs la sdug bsngal drag po byung bas/ bsam 'phel mas bla ma la yul bas skor te / sku lus gzhan gyis mi mjal ba ltar bzhugs pa'i dus 'dir / kun gyis mag khrag tshor nas skabs 'dir lo rdzogs pa dang phyi la ston byung /

20 Jo gdan, *Smyung gnas*, fol. 2b.3–6, 3a.3–5: dge slong ma 'di ni rig pa'i gnas lnga la mkhas shing / bslab sdom mams kyang shin tu btsun par bzhugs pa las / sngon gyi las dbang gis mdze byung ste / phyag g.yas pa'i 'khrigs ma nas chad / zhal gyi gdong la yang khro gzer btab pa bzhin du gyur /sha mdog ni ston ka'i me tog la ba mos phog pa bzhin du gyur / bza' btung byed pa yang phyag gis bsnyod mi shes par dud 'gro rtsa za ba bzhin du gyur /rig pa'i gnas lnga la mkhas kyang / nad drag pos btab pas sdug bsngal sems la bzhag thabs med pa lta bu dpag tu med pa byung ste / 'khor rnams kyis logs shig tu rtsa'i spyil bu cig tu bskyal nas der bshum gyin bzhugs

Despite the monastics' training in perceiving an inclusive Buddha-bodhisattva ideal with the endorsement of a powerful Dharmic 'medicine' to overturn the effects of karma, underlying these quotes are more conservative notions of health and illness intertwined with the Buddhist doctrine of suffering and karma. Historically, the belief in karma has led to the marginalization of certain segments of the population in Indian society. Monastics' interpretation of physical and cognitive impairments or disability of any sort were infused with karmic understanding; therefore, they were viewed as impediments to the 'purity' of the religious order and final realization of enlightenment (a permanent elevation to ultimate health).

Ironically, the way that monastic officials were trained about karmic fruits and the Dharma's power to overturn them counteracted the actual 'treatments' that they provided to potential human monastic candidates to the order. In other words, any karmic impairment on a physical (and even mental) level barred entry into the model monastic "society", even though the teachings of the Buddha had the 'power' to neutralize karmic fruit (the potential for Buddhanature to take fruition). Driven by moral preoccupations within an ableist monastic institution, different monastic (*Vinaya*) rules delineated 'normalcy standards' for monastic entry requirements and for continued service to the monastic order with detailed anatomical gender specifications, health symptomatology, and instructions about sexual behaviours. Monastics required 'suitable bodies', normative bodies, with particular attention to body parts being in appropriate places for each gender and with detailed descriptions of what marked healthy mental and physical conditions (and behaviour). Only those with specific sex characteristics that clearly marked them as males and females were accepted. For example, individuals with missing or additional body parts, such as those who were intersex, as well as those considered to have some form of deficiency in male sexual reproductive capacity, or those who experienced excessive sexual desire, were kept out of the institution, although there were rules in place to discipline those already in it. According to various Vinaya commentaries, the five groups of people considered to have sexual 'disabilities' that barred them from ordination were: (1) those who were intersex (Sanskrit: *paṇḍaka*; Tibetan: *pho mo ma ning*); (2) people with diseased genitals or venereal disease (Tibetan: *mtshan dug*), or physical deformities (Tibetan: *mdze*); (3) people without genitals; (4) people who had changed sexes three or more times;

pa na / *'Rig pa 'i gnas lnga* refers to linguistics, medicine, technology, logic and epistemology, and inner science (Buddhism).

and (5) eunuchs or impotent men (Sanskrit: *ṣaṇḍha*; Tibetan: *za ma*).[21] This monastic rule model of Buddhism fits well with the medical and moral models of disability.[22] People were judged based on physical and mental limitations (in this case, however, extended to the spiritual level) and based on a person's inner character or karma that needed to be overcome in order to train for or achieve liberation. By extension, following the religious model of disability, disease is an impairment due to sin or moral failing.

Moreover, societal stigma towards certain diseases that exhibit physical impairments, such as leprosy, the loss of a limb, or the existence of what was considered uncommon anatomical parts, crept into Buddhist doctrine and monastic rules since such impairments were perceived as being connected with karma. These 'impairments' impacted suitability requirements for entry into the Buddhist monastic community—a community meant to serve as a model of 'perfection' for lay society on a moral level as they strove for perfection as a Buddha. However, monastic ableist responses to disease in religious training run sharply athwart to the underlying premise of spiritual development, particularly Buddhism's doctrinal inclusiveness with regard to everyone's equal capacity for salvation (Buddhanature) and tantric Buddhism's notion of embodiment.

Leprosy: A Stigma or an Opportunity?

As her narrative unfolds further, it becomes clear that it was not just any common kind of karmic disease that Gelongma Palmo exhibited: she showed signs of a condition that was powerful enough to merit expulsion from the monastic order, despite her initial qualifications to enter and lead a religious community:

> When the nun was afflicted and consumed with severe leprosy, because of this, suffering arose like an arrow struck into the mind of that very servant Sampelma. Although she offered whatever services were possible [to Nun Palmo], it had no effect. About three months passed, the ten toes of the lama's feet fell off. Then five months later, the ten fingers of her hands fell off. At that time, severe suffering arose in the minds of both the master and the servant. Sampelma enclosed the lama with a curtain. During this time, it was as if her body was not seen by anyone […] After

21 See Cabezón, *Sexuality*, pp. 381–84.

22 See Yuill, Crinson, and Duncan, 'The Social and Medical Models'.

all [in the temple] noticed the pus and blood, [Nun Palmo and Sampelma] were thrown out after the end [of the] year.[23]

Responses to skin conditions like leprosy have been shown to be one of the most powerful examples of marginalization based on morality in Indian society and by extension, by the ableist structure of the monastic order as described earlier.[24] Leprosy was alterity par excellence. While the exact reasons behind the expulsion are unclear, the servant's concealment of Gelongma Palmo strongly implies that there was a stigma associated with her condition. Although it is difficult to definitively confirm a disease as leprosy in different cultures, leprosy's widespread impact in the history of medieval and modern Indian and Tibetan cultures correlated well with the Buddhist theory of karma and the Indian Buddhist monastic anxiety and exclusiveness based on restricted notions of the body.[25] Leprosy (Sanskrit: *galitakuṣṭham*; Tibetan: *mdze, mdze nad*) was well known historically as a disease of one's internal moral state, linked with karma in medical, religious, and later legal texts in Indian Hindu and Buddhist traditions.[26] According to Indian Āyurvedic medical traditions based on Hindu and Buddhist teachings, as well as Tibetan Buddhist medical sources, leprosy has multiple causes—moral, non-human, and supernatural.[27] Leprosy's physical manifestations—detached limbs, shedding of fluids like blood, and neuropathy—provided Buddhists with proof of its karmatic aetiology and even dehumanizing effects, paralleling certain European and Chinese medieval societies' preoccupation with internal morality, social and sacred purity boundaries, and the female gender.[28]

23 *Dge slong ma dpal mo*, 7.16–8.4: dge slong ma mdze snyung drag po zhig gis zin te bzhugs pa'i tshe / g.yog mo bsam 'phel ma de nyid sems la mda' phog pa lta bu'i sdug bsngal byung bas i zhabs tog gang cir byed kyang mi phan par/ zla ba gsum tsam lon pa dang bla ma'i zhabs kyi sor mdzub bcu chad/ de nas zla lnga long pa dang phyag mdzub bcu chad / de tshe dpon g.yog gnyis po thugs la sdug bsngal drag po byung bas/ bsam 'phel mas bla ma la yul bas skor te / sku lus gzhan gyis mi mjal ba ltar bzhugs pa'i dus 'dir / kun gyis mag khrag tshor nas skabs 'dir lo rdzogs pa dang phyi la ston byung.

24 De Bruin, *Leprosy*. On leprosy in the present volume, see the chapters by Edwards (pp. 235–63) and Escobedo (pp. 207–34, esp. 220–23) in this volume.

25 Ibid.

26 See Leslie, 'Implications', pp. 23–45; and Jacob, 'Stigmatization'. Western medical perspectives on leprosy (Hansen's disease) also became common in India.

27 Indian and Tibetan medical theories traditionally ascribed leprosy to a large category of causes typically translated as 'demons' (*gdon*) when they are offended by an action. G.yu thog Yon tan mgon po, *Bdud rtsi snying po yan lag brgyad pa gsang ba man ngag gi rgyud*, pp. 392–400.

28 Cross-cultural studies include: Allen, *Wages of Sin*; de Bruin, *Leprosy*; Brody, *Disease of the Soul*; and Ki Che Leung, *Leprosy in China*.

In the history of conditions like leprosy in a caste-conscious Indian society that established strict rules of purity and pollution, the transgression of boundaries was a serious issue.[29] Although Buddhism attempted to liberate itself from its neighbouring religion's premises, notably Hinduism's concerns over caste-based social differentiation and ritual purity, it still needed to maintain the support of the laity by respecting social concerns.[30] As both Mary Douglas and Patrick Olivelle have argued elsewhere, the 'protection of the boundaries' has strong moral implications in religious traditions and is directly related to power in society.[31] Olivelle leverages Douglas's notion of 'dirt out of place' with regard to the relationship of the body to boundaries in order to understand Indian religious traditions:

> If [...] we define dirt as matter out of place, then it seems that, at least as far as the social perception of the human body is concerned, dirt gathers predominantly on its margins and in a special way at the openings that lets the inside of the body meet the outside both by letting bodily excreta and fluids flow out and permitting outside elements—especially food and water—to come inside, the protection of the boundaries has been a major preoccupation of most traditional religions.[32]

Therefore, these excrescences (pus and blood) not only mark a 'sick' body, but also represent a crossing of social purity borders between polluted and sacred space, and ideological biases against access by the body.[33] As the Buddhist monastic community depended on the support of the laity and even royal patronage, leprosy violated the sacred–secular boundaries set by Indian Buddhist and Hindu traditions and for societal order.[34] With the barring of leprosy's seeping of bodily fluids (blood, pus) from sacred spaces (monasteries and temples), the response to a disabling condition like leprosy reflected a preoccupation with keeping sacred spaces pure in a caste-conscious society

29 From antiquity to modernity, Indian society treated leprosy singularly (and akin diseases) with respect to custom and law, a response shaped by both scientific knowledge and cultural attitudes. See Jacob, 'Stigmatization'.

30 Both Buddhism and Hinduism were affected by traditional views of purity and pollution in terms of caste, food, marriage, gender, and sacred spaces. Polluting substances were often identified as blood and pus.

31 Olivelle, 'Deconstruction', p. 189; Douglas, *Purity and Danger*.

32 Ibid.

33 Blood is also a mark of female gender, another sign of marginalized identity in the Buddhist tradition.

34 For the Buddhist monastic order to maintain support and even patronage by the laity, it must reflect a moral society and not simply be equipped to teach the Dharma.

and the protection of a model moral monastic community. Furthermore, as in the case of Gelongma Palmo, the leprous body was pathologized as a condition of alterity through the support of Indian and Tibetan medical texts that were exclusively authorized by a predominantly male monastic institution for many centuries. Julie Avril Minich's definition of critical disability theory is helpful in understanding what happens with leprosy in these texts, and the Gelongma Palmo hagiographies in particular; this theory 'scrutiniz[es] not bodily or mental impairments but the social norms that define particular attributes as impairments, as well as the social conditions that concentrate stigmatized attributes in particular populations'.[35] Leprosy therefore provides a perfect case study of medieval Indian and Tibetan Buddhist conceptions of disability that crosses the boundary of what may be considered simply sickness. This relates to what Julie Orlemanski states in her study of the leper's kiss in medieval saints' stories: 'To my mind, the exemplary status of leprosy in representing physical infirmity and institutionalizing practices of care in the Middle Ages demands the pathology's inclusion within "medieval disability".'[36]

Moreover, since the monastics, as the healers and doctors of Indian and Tibetan societies, set the parameters for health and disease, it is not surprising that the monastic authors of the hagiographies were aware (as they undoubtedly were) of the dehumanizing effects of leprosy and the impact of their storytelling. In one of the hagiographies, Gelongma Palmo declares:

> I am not a person,
> I am a leprous corpse.[37]

Here Gelongma Palmo's identification within the liminal space of the diseased and deceased, a hybrid form of disability, has a two-pronged effect: it disempowers her in society and also affects her legitimacy as a monastic figure. Research into Indian and Tibetan medical literature's treatment of leprosy as a spirit-inflicted disease illuminates another layer of interpretation in this passage and the understanding of stigma in the Gelongma Palmo hagiographies.[38] For example, according to a tenth-century Tibetan medical text, the *Rgyud Bzhi* (closely connected to other Indian medical texts that pre-date it), composed around the time of Gelongma Palmo's life,

35 Minich, 'Enabling Whom?'.

36 Orlemanski, 'How to Kiss a Leper', p. 144.

37 *Dge slong ma dpal mo*, 11.16–17: nga ni mi min mdze ma'i ro yin no//

38 See my work on the intersection of Tibetan religions and Indian and Tibetan medicine, Vargas-O'Bryan, 'Falling Rain', pp. 99–114.

leprosy was interpreted as not only morally caused, but also as having been inflicted by a race of spirits with animal features (snakes) known as *nāgas*, or non-human spirits (*mi min*), implying that Gelongma Palmo was affected (or 'possessed') by them.[39] Therefore, the dehumanizing effect of leprosy in this genre extends our analysis of disability. In other words, in addition to the religious model of disability that is evident in these stories, there is an underlying medicalization of the leper body, or a medical model of disability, within Buddhist scriptures/hagiographies. Moreover, the disease-afflicted being must be 'medically treated', which in the Indian and Tibetan medical contexts includes ritual control and transformation, reminiscent of the medicalization of disability coupled with the religious model.[40] Furthermore, Gelongma Palmo's identification as non-human is in direct violation of the monastic code, which bars 'certain magical animals'—for example, *nāgas*—or a 'nonhuman spirit' (*mi min*) that are believed to 'temporarily take on a human form' and often trick monastic authorities in order to gain entry into the Order.[41] The Gelongma Palmo hagiographies therefore pathologized leprosy not just as an immoral condition, a violation of monastic norms, but also as a deviant condition outside the societal constructions of normalcy owing to its non-humanness (animal and/or demonic origins). In other words, monastics must be human! This extends the disability model even further, implying that to be disabled with leprosy in this context is to be deviant, different, and no longer entirely human.[42]

The notion of the inhuman is further problematized by the fact that the main character of the hagiographies is embodied in a female form. As is evident already, the diseased body and enlightened body, in conjunction with gender, complicate the disability models. Therefore, these bodies do not take on their full transgressive value in these hagiographies without reference to the significance accorded to gender.

39 Well known in Indian and Tibetan societies, *nāgas* are theriomorphic beings described and depicted as half-human and half-serpent (or half-reptilian). Connected to the natural environment in Indian and Tibetan Buddhist scriptural and medical literatures, they are described as inflicting diseases like leprosy (and others that cause mental instability) through possession when they are offended by humans. See ethnographic studies on these texts in Asia, in Vargas-O'Bryan, 'Falling Rain'. It is interesting to note the correlations to European fears of demonic possession, saints' powers, and antinomian saint behavior. For a study of saint zombification and possession, see Spencer-Hall, 'The Horror of Orthodoxy'.

40 The medicalization of disability regards disability as an individual misfortune, and people with disabilities are assumed to suffer primarily from physical and/or cognitive differences that medicine can and should treat, cure, or at least prevent. See Oliver, *Politics of Disablement*.

41 Cabezón, *Sexuality*, p. 381.

42 Vargas-O'Bryan, 'Disease', pp. 81–99.

Gender and Disability

Observers of Buddhism are often struck by the contradictory representations and apparent ambivalence towards women and the feminine that one finds in Buddhist texts, where women are described as temptresses, nurturing mothers, and enlightened figures; their bodies must either undergo transformation into a male form or remain as female to show that they are capable of enlightenment. There is also the perspective that gender does not matter in terms of final enlightenment. The androcentric and gynocentric perspectives sometimes inhabit single texts, while other writings highlight one view over the other.[43] The Gelongma Palmo hagiographies inhabit this middle ground of perspectives.

Although diverse Buddhist perspectives on gender are certainly present in the Gelongma Palmo hagiographies, the common societal attitude displayed towards the leprous female who prays in a temple draws attention to underlying gender biases:

> [The custodian of the temple said:]
> 'On top of being of low birth [*skye dman*],
> you are a leprous woman.
> Stay behind the door and make your request.'[44]

> 'You beggar woman, who are a leprous beggar, came inside my temple. I myself cannot make offerings of incense to the deities and ablutions in the temple. If the crops fail, hail strikes and so forth, it is certain that [all] will come to my head.'
> With the key handle, he beat her from the crown of her head to the soles of her feet. Having pulled the nun from her feet, he brought her to the back of the temple. In Nun Palmo's mind, she generated an enlightened attitude [and thought], 'Sentient beings' minds are obscured by ignorance.'[45]

43 Alan Sponberg identified four distinct attitudes in Buddhist texts: soteriological inclusiveness, institutional androcentrism, ascetic misogyny, and soteriological androgyny; see 'Attitudes', pp. 3–36. On leprosy and gender in the Western Christian context, see also the chapter by Edwards in the present volume, pp. 235–63.

44 'Od dpag rdo rje, *Thugs rje chen po*, 23.1–2: dkon gnyer na re khyod skye ba dman pa 'i thog du mdze mar 'dug pa sgo rgyab tu 'dug la gsol ba thob cig gsungs/

45 *Dge slong ma dpal mo*, 16.7–17.3: mdze sbrang gi sbrang mo khyod nged gyi lha khang nang 'ongs pa dang / nged rang ni lha khang nang Iha bsangs khrus gsol byas mi tshugs pas / lo thag nyes pa dang ser bas rdung pa la sogs pa byung na nged rang gi mgor 'ong nges yin zer nas / lde mig gi thag pa des spyi gtsugs nas rkang thil yan chad du brdungs shing / dge slong ma'i shabs

There are several examples in these passages that point to the marginalization of women. First, the use of the common derogatory Tibetan term for 'woman' (*'skye dman*, literally meaning 'low birth') indicates the view of gender hierarchy in Indian culture.[46] This term in the hagiographies objectifies and demeans the female in contrast to the male gender. There is not only a local bias towards women in a sacred space, but implicitly, this also reflects Buddhist philosophical and monastic views about a suitable body for enlightenment and underlying assumptions that women have insatiable desires (or function solely as sex objects for men).

Secondly, as indicated earlier, in addition to her gender, the leprous Gelongma Palmo is seen as a polluting entity in a sacred space. Not only is she sick, but she also secretes polluting substances like pus and blood. In Indian society at the time, and even to this day, the secretion of blood is reminiscent of female menstruation and childbearing, and is closely connected to death; blood is a substance considered impure for entry into temples or monastic spaces. During menstruation, women were advised for centuries not to 'enter temple, work in kitchen, wear flowers, have sex, touch other males or females, or come in contact with any creative energies to ensure free flow of *Apana*', admonitions that also reveal an underlying sexist medical model of disability.[47] Menstruation was seen as a period of purification, and women were often separated from places of worship or any object pertaining to it for the length of their period because of the potentially polluting and dangerous substances that were excreted from the body. Furthermore, women in medieval Indian society often died during childbirth and there was much apprehension about miscarriage. Procedures on how to abort a fetus, including their potential dangers, were also readily available in Indian medical texts; the presence of blood was therefore of major concern due to its various implications. Closely related to these ideas, the detail about the presence of blood in the episode of Gelongma Palmo's expulsion has led to all types of oral interpretations among the laity in local modern Sherpa communities in Nepal—from accusations of pregnancy to contraction of venereal disease— which again reinforce the sexist interpretations prevalent in

nas 'then te lha khang gi rgyab la bskal bas/ dge slong ma'i thugs dgongs la sems can gyi blo ma rig pas sgrib pa yin snyam byang chub tu thugs bskyed de /

46 See Gyatso and Havnevik, *Women in Tibet*, p. 78.

47 *Apana* refers to downward wind in the Indian Āyurvedic medical tradition; see Bhartiya, 'Menstruation', pp. 523–27. In Hindu and Buddhist upper-level tantric rituals, disciplining the mind to restrict the shedding of bodily fluids like semen and blood marks a high-level practitioner.

society and also the sexual connotations that were historically often ascribed to leprosy.[48]

In addition, the fact that the custodian attempts to beat Gelongma Palmo into submission reflects how her body is treated as if it were that of an animal, that is, a dehumanization of her body; it also indicates treatment of non-submissive women, supplying another example of demarcation of boundaries against and societal alienation of a body that does not fit into an ableist society or institution.[49] As Gelongma Palmo's previous assertion that she is a non-human corpse implies, women have also often been symbols of death or rebirth in Buddhist texts. From the time of the historical Buddha, women's bodies were seen by male monastics as ideal objects for meditation in cremation grounds in order to combat desire and achieve a deeper understanding of impermanence.[50] In terms of attaining the highest Buddhist goal—to leave the cycle of rebirth (*saṃsāra*) and achieve enlightenment—the fact that women menstruate, thereby marking their fertility, puts them at a disadvantage. Menstruation indicates that her body propagates *saṃsāra* and this body is a potential barrier to higher spiritual states. In addition, certain monastic rules that listed other diseased or unsuitable bodies were biased against women and were meant to control their bodies (regulation of the feminine body) to bar women from entering the order, receiving higher ordination, and continuing service.[51] Against this background, Gelongma Palmo's leprous female embodiment represents her multilayered disability, a marginalized, outcast identity reinforced by the hierarchical power structure of an ableist, patriarchal society and monastic institution. This adds nuance to Iris Marion Young's contention that '[w]

48 Ortner, *High Religion*, p. 181; March, *Intermediacy of Women*, p. 277. See also de Bruin, *Leprosy*. The sexual connotation is in reference to the widespread belief that the blood shed during leprosy may indicate a hidden pregnancy or abortion by a monastic, thus transgressing prescribed moral behaviour. Indian Buddhist monastics are supposed to be celibate and/or have renounced sexual behaviour and their families before entering the order.

49 Hinduism developed alongside Buddhism so both had major societal impacts. The Hindu law book, *Dharmaśāstra* [*Laws of Manu*] states, 'A wife, a son, a slave, a pupil, and a (younger) brother of the full blood, who have committed faults, may be beaten with a rope or a split bamboo' (*Laws of Manu*, ch. 7, para. 299).

50 Wilson, *Charming Cadavers*.

51 Among the questions posed to female candidates interested in being ordained into the Buddhist monastic order, particularly those related to the sick body include: 'Have you any of the following diseases; scabies, malaria, carbuncles, hemorrhoids, uncontrollable bowl movements, yellow fever and ague, coughing, tuberculosis, epilepsy, fever, swelling due to gas, welling [... or swelling?] due to water, swelling in the stomach, or any other illnesses?' See Guṇaprabha, *Ekottarakarmaśataka*, 117b–118a.

omen in a sexist society are physically handicapped'.[52] However, if we take this as fitting into a particular 'domain of abjected bodies', Judith Butler asks:

> How does that materialization of the norm in bodily formation produce a domain of abjected bodies, a field of deformation, which in failing to qualify as the fully human, fortifies these regulatory norms? What challenge does that excluded and abjected realm produce to a symbolic hegemony [...] ?[53]

Gelongma Palmo's stories bring to the foreground the cultural norms at work underlying a number of Mahāyāna Buddhist texts that profess that female embodiment is a disadvantage and must instead transform into a more suitable 'gender' or 'spiritual' state in order to be elevated; that is, in order to be accepted in an androcentric/misogynist society and achieve a higher spiritual state.[54] Despite the fact that an able-bodied woman like Gelongma Palmo attained a high level of intellectual religious training and status in a male monastic order, which was rare in this period, the contraction of such an 'inflammatory' disease as leprosy (steeped in a history of stigma that signals the transgression of norms of morality and purity/pollution boundaries), and the fact that her female and diseased body signals transgression of monastic ideals and moral monastic norms, accentuate the underlying power structures within highly androcentric and sexist Indian and Tibetan societies. Gelongma Palmo's leprous female embodiment, with its excrescences and perceived moral turpitude, is a disabling condition in itself, reinforced in Indian society and promoted to a Tibetan audience. In this framework, both gender and disability function, as Ellen Samuels notes, 'to materialize norms and their constitutive others', though it should be kept in mind that the two categories cannot be uncritically substituted for one another.[55]

On the other hand, although figures like Gelongma Palmo were trapped in societally constructed, binary spaces—the pure and sacred versus the polluted Others, lepers, and women—and subjected to exclusionary measures and institutional barriers that either directly state or imply the barring from higher spiritual elevation, such discourses of exclusion and contestation do not tell the whole story. Buddhism, like other religious traditions, is often a

52 Young, *Throwing Like a Girl*, p. 153.
53 Butler, *Excitable Speech*, p. 15.
54 Paul, *Women in Buddhism*, pp. 166–216.
55 Samuels, 'Critical Divides', p. 65.

site of reflection upon and contestation of societal norms despite the impact of these norms within the religion itself.

The Leprous Female Bodhisattva Body: La Pièce de Résistance

In contrast, although the ableist patriarchal monastic (including medical and societal) framework, with its representation of a sick female disabled monastic identity, undergirds the Gelongma Palmo hagiographies, it is certainly superseded by tantric Buddhist resistance in an ultimate spiritual sense. Further exploration of the narrative reveals tantric Buddhist notions of bodies and embodiment that go beyond what critical disability theorists David T. Mitchell and Sharon L. Snyder call 'narrative prosthesis', in which narrative uses the representation of disability as a device of characterization or metaphor.[56]

After the custodian throws Gelongma Palmo out of the temple and calls her a 'leprous woman', she insists on remaining nearby.[57] Settling herself outside at the back of the temple, she prays to the statue of her bodhisattva (her personal Buddha figure she prayed to for guidance) housed in the inner sanctum of the temple. Suddenly, a miraculous event occurs: 'And [...] the faces of the images of 'Bigs Srī Temple turned in the direction of where Nun Palmo was and remained [that way].'[58] Besides the implicit message that enlightened beings inhabit even statues as their bodies, the behaviour of the animated images shows that the leprous woman's prayers are worthy despite societal restrictions and monastic violations.[59] It is also at this point that the animated image of the bodhisattva imparts his fasting practice that Gelongma Palmo later transmits to others as a practice for achieving enlightenment. Shortly thereafter, Gelongma Palmo claims that her embodiment as a leper-woman has a higher purpose—to liberate others:

56 Disabled characters act as a 'crutch upon which literary narratives lean for their representational power, disruptive potentiality, and analytical insight'; Mitchell and Snyder, *Narrative Prosthesis*, p. 49. See also Corker, 'Differences', pp. 627–42.

57 'Od dpag rdo rje, *Thugs rje chen po*, 23.1–2.

58 *Dge slong ma dpal mo*, 9.15: 'bigs srī lha khang gi bris sku rnams kyang zhal dge slong ma bzhugs pa'i phyogs la skor te bzhugs so //

59 Animation of images is a common occurrence in both Hindu and Buddhist traditions; see Reinders and Rambelli, *Buddhism and Iconoclasm*, pp. 16–28. The 'dynamic presence' of icons is evident in other medieval stories; see Spencer-Hall, *Medieval Saints*, pp. 243–53. I am also inspired by Alfred Gell's notion of 'object agency' to understand the images as having agency beyond societal and even ritual structures; see Gell, *Art and Agency*.

> [Gelongma Palmo] said to Sampelma [her servant], 'I am sick for the sake of sentient beings who are as vast as the sky.'[60]

On the level of Tibetan tantric Buddhist practice, these scenes are pivotal points in the narrative. Gelongma Palmo receives a ritual empowerment from a higher being and attains a realization about her mission as a Buddha figure, whose intrinsic nature is that of a compassionate and skillful bodhisattva. She attains the empowerment through her meditative fasting practice and as a result, she removes non-human entities out of specific body parts and intentionally 'transforms' (or 'forces') them to vow to protect the teachings transmitted to her earlier:

> When she stayed there five days, in an experiential vision in which sleep and light were mixed, she saw many tadpoles, fish, frogs, snakes, and so forth come out of her vagina and anus and glide into the earth while she recited the six-syllable mantra without distraction.[61]

> By having bound them to an oath, they pledged to be the Dharma protectors of the practice of the Great Compassionate One, and in particular, the eight great *nāgas* pledged to be the Dharma Protectors of the Eleven-faced One.[62]

In contrast to assumptions of weakness in previous descriptions of a sick female, Gelongma Palmo here displays incredible agency as she binds 'non-human' entities, the 'pathogens' of her disease, and transforms them as protectors. In time, her discovery as a bodhisattva reveals her ability to shape-shift, which empowers her even more, especially when the community critiques her based on societal biases. The fourteenth-century hagiography states:

60 *Dge slong ma dpal mo*, 7.12–13: bsam 'phel ma la gsungs pa / nam mkha' dang mnyam pa'i sems can gyi don la na ba yin gsungs / For a comparison of a leper saint and her commitment to the instrumentality of her leprosy, see Spencer-Hall, 'Christ's Suppurating Wounds', pp. 389–415.

61 *Dge slong ma dpal mo*, 13.14–14.6: 'der zhag po lnga lon pa dang/ mnal dang 'ad zer 'dres pa'i nyams snang zhig la/ sku smad kyi shang lam chu lam nas mar lcong nya sbal sbrul la sags pa mang po than te zhal nas yi ge drug pa yengs med kyi nang nas gnang/ sa 'ag la 'dzul ba'i mnal lam gzigs te/ de nas dgung zhag nyer gcig song ba'i dus na/ mo rang gi mdun gyi nam mkha' la lo brgyad gnyis bcu drug Ion pa'i lang tsho dang ldan pa zhig gis/ phyag g.yas pas shel gyi 'phreng ba brgya rtsa brgyad bsnams/ g.yon pas chu skyes kyi sdong bu 'dzin pa zhig gis /

62 Jo gdan, *Smyung gnas*, 6a.3–6: khyad par du klu chen brgyad kyis zhal bcu gcig pa'i sgos kyi chos skyong du khas blangs/

When she went to Magadha,
people said,
'Since the cause for this nun's illness subsided,
she became lax in her instructions and vows. How is it?'
In order to reverse their disbelief,
at a congregation for a worship service for Khasarpaṇa.
[Nun Palmo] cut off her own head.
Since she placed it on her monastic staff [*mkhar bsil*] and danced,
now the people,
in realizing that she was one who attained spiritual realization,
all requested a blessing and obtained a realization as well.[63]

Here she reveals herself (as often seen in iconography) as a *ḍākinī*, a female enlightened being who typically appears in tantric texts to enforce the Dharma with the *khatvãnga* staff, the implement of an enlightened female *ḍākinī* who goes beyond the restrictions of monasticism and is now in command of all means to enlightenment. This passage points to her embodied resistance to normativity, the critiques of the community, through her revelation as an enlightened being. The act of self-mutilation by utilizing her 'weapon' signifies an act of intentional severance of limitations set by society, freeing others in the process. Paradoxically, the act of her dancing (which is against monastic rules and seen as an act of sensual pleasure) signifies her bliss as an enlightened being. Her embodiment as a female enlightened being (bodhisattva and *ḍākinī*) may lead to the conclusion that Sarah McNamer came to in her book, *Affective Meditations and the Invention of Medieval Compassion*: that women were linked by their male biographers with affective, compassionate tendencies.[64] It is interesting to note, however, that in this context, these hagiographies align with the tantric strand of Buddhism, which has a more inclusive body image than other Buddhist traditions owing to the presence of many more female Buddhas and bodhisattvas (or both) embodiments.[65] Moreover in this context, the

63 Jo gdan, *Smyung gnas*, 7a.3–5- 7a.6.

64 McNamer, *Affective Meditation*. It is interesting to note that the male bodhisattva who taught Gelongma Palmo the fasting ritual is known as female (Guanyin) in the Chinese Buddhist context because Chinese culture could not conceive of compassion as a male quality embodied by a male Buddha. See Yü, *Kuan-yin*.

65 It is beyond the scope of this chapter to bring to light the different Tibetan biographies of female Buddhas in the Tibetan Buddhist tradition; many biographies have not been translated into English or other Western languages. However, suffering, androcentric views, misogyny, and sexism in the lives of female enlightened teachers are common features. The Tibetan saint

powerful purpose of Gelongma Palmo's act of severance is connected with her embrace of her body as a tool to be used by an enlightened being, who is in command of the mission she undertakes for the sake of others.

Paradox, Intentionality, and Fluid States in Buddhist Tantra

One possible problematic area in the above-mentioned scene is the incidence of transcendence. How do we understand Gelongma Palmo as an affirmative symbol of leprous womanhood when her disability (leprosy) is ultimately fixed and removed? Through her agency, Gelongma Palmo disengages with her disintegrating, corpse-like body and emerges not as a leprous woman, but as a healed divine woman. In some scholarship on Western feminism, feminist disability studies and feminist theology, transcending the body may be seen as problematic, with such research often drawing from Christian writings that devalue the body (especially women's bodies) and bodily experience.[66]

It is critical to note that in the tantric context all of Gelongma Palmo's embodiments are tools that she intentionally takes up on behalf of others' spiritual development. Two popular Mahāyana Buddhist scriptures express the nature of non-dualism and emptiness (impermanence) in which these hagiographies operate philosophically:

> Form is emptiness, emptiness is form
> Emptiness is not separate from form, form is not separate from emptiness
> Whatever is form is emptiness, whatever is emptiness is form.[67]

> There exists the imagination of the unreal, there is no duality, but there is emptiness, even in this there is that.[68]

The implicit meaning in these rather paradoxical passages is that categories are not fixed. According to the critical Buddhist doctrine of identity known as non-self (*anātman*), our desire for a fixed 'whole' identity is connected to

Yeshe Tsogyal, in the process of being raped, transformed her abusers into her spiritual followers. See Kunga, *The Life and Visions of Yeshe Tsogyal*.

66 Wendell, *Rejected Body*. See also Erevelles, *Embodied Rhetoric*, pp. 92–111; and Shoop, 'Body Wise', pp. 240–55.

67 Rupan śūnyatā śūnyatāiva rupan. Rupan na prithak śūnyatā śūnyatā na prithag rupan. Yad rupan sa śūnyatā ya śūnyatā tad rupan. *The Heart Sutra*.

68 Cited in King, 'Early Yogācāra', p. 665; Nagao, *Madhyāntavibhāga*, 1.1.

the origin of suffering (that is, attachment or desire) and rebirth as things that are ultimately transient. From a Buddhist perspective, a being's identity is composed of an amalgamation of five aspects (form, perceptions, feelings/ sensations, volition, and consciousness), which come together to form a person or self. When one is suffering, bodily constituents are perceived as if 'whole' and fixed. With powerful meditative ritual techniques, a perceptual deconstruction takes place and the self is ultimately (and perceptually) understood not as a fixed entity, but as parts that are fluid and changing. This was a turning point for the historical Buddha under the tree of enlightenment in the fourth century BCE; after coming to this realization, he became known as a Buddha. In the role of a Buddha-bodhisattva, categories are contingent, and as such, so is identity. Difference in terms of embodiment is relative and contingent, and therefore not based on hierarchy or binaries but, rather, represents a tool for enlightenment.

In addition, the fact that the enlightened being appears as a female in these narratives has a very specific intentional tone regarding the nature of female religiosity in this society. From Caroline Walker Bynum's essays in *Fragmentation and Redemption*, we appreciate the relations of parts to wholes, gender among fragmented bodies, and the significance of the patterns of practices that are gendered. Bynum discovers that there is an ordinariness, continuity, and physical foundation to women's lives, and to the ways in which women in the Christian tradition embraced their femaleness to get closer to God's redemption. She notes that there is an a-institutional nature to female piety as reflected in ascetic practices (for example, fasting), an interesting correlation with what occurs in Indian and Tibetan medieval practices,

> not by reversing what they were but by sinking more fully into it. In fact and in image suffering (both self-inflicted and involuntary) and food (both eucharist and fasting) were women's most common ways of attaining God.[69]

Therefore, in a sense, Gelongma Palmo shows in her embodiments and sickness the ideal of a bodhisattva—that is, the ability to delve into humanness. Gelongma Palmo appears as a leper-woman (bodily form) that gains authority because of, rather than despite, her embodied condition and her relationship to others. Transcendence is revealed through the experiences

69 Bynum, *Fragmentation*, p. 172; see also p. 89 on her discussion of female redemption. No extensive historical studies have been done on the role of fasting by women in Buddhist traditions. See Sanyal and Kumar, *Food, Faith and Gender.*

of impermanence that permeate the texts, the nun's intercession on behalf of others as a female leper, bodily performance of fasting (including ecstatic visionary experiences), and female re-embodiment as a divine being. Here Gelongma Palmo shows that she is an autonomous embodiment that is not contingently vulnerable; as a bodhisattva; she intentionally takes on the mission to help others reach enlightenment.[70] As tantric Buddhist hagiographies show, the outer reality was a tool; she was never disabled on an intrinsic level, at least not disabled by social constructions. Through the lens of Tibetan tantric Buddhism, Buddhist notions of embodiment are reframed to show that a body—any body—is a tool for liberation of static notions of identity, and not a barrier. Even the image of dehumanization and inferred de-gendering are empowering in that they refer to her higher spiritual state being defined ultimately beyond the human (or not confined by humanness) since she is divine.[71] As James I. Porter notes:

> [W]riting the disabled body will mean that our most basic conceptions of the body will need to be rewritten [...] Like the normative ideologies of the body to which they often stand opposed, theoretical discourses of the body already contain within themselves a series of unacknowledged and/or disavowed assumptions and theories about disability.[72]

The work of feminist disability theorists such as Rosemarie Garland-Thomson is helpful here. She states that:

> A feminist disability theory introduced what Eve Sedwick has called a 'universalizing view' of disability that will replace an often persisting 'minoritizing view.' [...] In other words, understanding how disability operates as an identity category and cultural concept will enhance how we understand what it is to be human, our relationships with one another, and the experiences of embodiment.[73]

70 Relational views of human life affect models of autonomy. See Scully, 'Disability and Vulnerability', pp. 204–21. See also Spencer-Hall, 'Chronic Pain and Illness'.

71 This has striking parallels with Alicia Spencer-Hall's analysis of Alice the Leper in 'Christ's Suppurating Wounds' and her description of the thirteenth-century 'holy zombification' of Christina Mirabilis in 'The Horror of Orthodoxy'. As in this case, the *vita* of Christina Mirabilis is a 'vehicle for educating the audience about religious truths' and 'reveals the divine order that orients all earthly things' (Spencer-Hall, 'The Horror of Orthodoxy', p. 358).

72 Porter, 'Foreword', p. xiv.

73 Garland-Thomson, 'Integrating Disability', p. 5.

Rather than limiting Gelongma Palmo's experience with her body (and thus the message to her readers about embodiment) to a constructed marginalized status based on ableist binary norms, the female-diseased body is an empowering embodiment within the Buddhist context. In keeping with Buddhist teachings, Gelongma Palmo's performative materialization as a leper-woman may instead be taken in a positive light. Unlike some feminist theorists, such as Butler, who take 'metaphors of illness' as being negative, in this corpus of materials, illness and its so-called disabling effects alongside gender are necessary for embodied spiritual elevation and revelation. The dismemberment, leaking fluids, and bodily differences do not need to be read as limitations and moral fragmentation based on karmic causation that require purificatory rituals or to be cast out. The body is, in reality, not a boundary because it is porous; it has the ability to transform, therefore transgressing and transcending restrictive interpretations. The gendered, decomposing, perfect able embodied subject is an alternative corporeality, a tool that has agency to liberate all bodies from oppressive attitudes about the body.[74] A Buddha-bodhisattva's responsibility in her multiple manifestations as an enlightened being is to help others realize that ultimately the body can never lack; it is the tool to overcome any preconceived notions about limitations or societal biases. Gelongma Palmo's embodiment as a divine being not only transforms at will: she is also in command of her environment.

Concluding Aspirations

Overall, the Gelongma Palmo hagiographies are an inclusive space for thinking about disability and gender that remind us that the body is a useful site of conflict.[75] Buddhist notions of transcendence or liberation from limited thinking reinforce the necessity of bodily engagement and not a resistance to it. Susan Stocker makes us aware in her work on disability and embodiment that there is the possibility of what she calls 'mutuality' in our 'biological vulnerability' that enables empathic connections.[76] This is affirmed in the Mahāyana Buddhist philosophical position of

74 See McRuer, 'Composing Bodies', pp. 48–78.

75 The work of Nancy Mairs is helpful in understanding that the body is a site of conflicts of power: see Mintz, *Unruly Bodies*, p. 26; Mairs, *Literary Nonfiction*.

76 Stocker, 'Problems', pp. 48–49. Stocker's utilization of postmodern queer theorist Judith Butler and paleoanthropologist Maxine Sheets-Johnstone includes both genetically and genealogical approaches in order to better understand mutuality in response to embodiment and disability.

universal re-embodiment and Buddhahood. Gelongma Palmo's revelation as a Buddha figure therefore indicates a transcendence of herself as a dualistic body, not one inscribed with binary characteristics carrying moral connotations. Gelongma Palmo was able to transform both within *saṃsāra* (the cycle of life and death) and outside of it, depending on what was needed. This is a critical issue to understand. This type of embodied experience challenged the static (and linear) androcentric views of access to enlightenment and the regimented monastic views of the gendered body and disease. It calls into question any embodied identity as static, liberating all bodies from fixed categories. This is especially clear in the way Gelongma Palmo's lineage of hagiographies and practices are commemorated throughout the ages. To this day in Asia and in the West in Tibetan communities, Gelongma Palmo is not depicted as a leper nun or even with lepers, but most often as a nun or as a *ḍākinī* keeping to the revelation of the Buddhist notion of embodied enlightenment. She is most remembered for her suffering and her illness as instrumental to her mission as a bodhisattva. She empowers others (male and female monastics) to act through the transmission of her texts and the performance of her rituals, which I have had the privilege to view and undertake throughout South Asia and Tibet.[77]

As is often the case, there are sites of resistance in any religious tradition. The Gelongma Palmo hagiographies remind the reader that our shared humanity and innate empowerment in all its diversity have the capacity for greatness, despite obstacles framed by ableist institutional structures and societal assumptions. This legacy provides another lens through which to view the Asian Buddhist context in order to understand alternative religious meaning about the body, health, and gender.

See also Foucault, *Discipline and Punish*; and Schriempf, '(Re)fusing the Amputated Body', pp. 53–79.

77 As is common in Tibetan cultural areas, nuns and monks today in India, Nepal, and Tibet orally recite the Gelongma Palmo hagiographies and perform extensive fasting annually during the most sacred Tibetan Buddhist holiday, *Sagadawa*, commemorating the enlightenment of the historical Buddha. At Dolma Ling Nunnery in particular, located in Dharamsala, India, the nunnery's male abbot directly promotes the figure of Gelongma Palmo as a model for Tibetan renunciant women by hanging *thangkas* (Buddhist cloth paintings) depicting her image and the words of her hagiographies at the main prayer hall. In addition, Gelongma Palmo's fasting ritual is promoted in the nunnery in order to support the nuns' aspirations for higher levels of monastic status and to reach spiritual advancement. This is also a rare site among Tibetan nunneries where nuns can undertake higher Buddhist monastic training and attain academic degrees traditionally restricted to male monastics.

Bibliography

Primary Sources

Dge slong ma dpal mo 'i rnam thar nges 'byung rgyud la skye ba 'i chos gtam [English title: *The Biography of Kamala Bhikshuni, Princess of King Dharma Pal, an Ancient King of Kashmir, India*], trans. by Bla ma Rab brtan (Kalimpong: Tibet Mirror Press, 1953; repr. 1963)

Guṇaprabha, *Ekottarakarmaśataka, Las brgya rtsa gcig pa*. Sde dge bstan 'gyur. Toh 4118, 'dul ba wu (n.d.), 100b–259a

G.yu thog Yon tan mgon po, *Bdud rtsi snying po yan lag brgyad pa gsang ba man ngag gi rgyud* (Lhasa: Bod ljongs mi dmangs dpe skrun khang, 1993)

The Heart Sutra: Prajna Paramita Hrdaya Sutra, Buddhanet.net <https://www.buddhanet.net/e-learning/heartstr.htm> [accessed 4 February 2020]

Jo gdan Bsod nams bzang po, *Smyung gnas bla ma brgyud pa 'i rnam thar* (Lhasa: Dpal ldan Par khang, n.d.), fols 1–107 [blockprint]

The Laws of Manu, trans. by George Bühler, in *Internet Indian History Sourcebook*, Fordham University, <https://sourcebooks.fordham.edu/india/manu-full.asp> [accessed 26 March 2023]

Nagao, G., *Madhyatavibhaga* (Tokyo: Japan: Suzuki Research Foundation, 1972)

'Od dpag rdo rje, *Thugs rje chen po bcu gcig zhal gyi bla ma brgyud pa 'i rnam thar nor bu 'i phreng ba'*, in *Instructions for the Practice of the Gso Sbyong and Smyung gnas Focusing Upon the Invocation of Avalokitesvara in the Eleven Faced Form* (Thimphu: Dorji Namgyal, 1985), fols 1–233

Secondary Sources

Allen, Peter Lewis, *The Wages of Sin: Sex and Disease, Past and Present* (Chicago: University of Chicago Press, 2000)

Benard, Elisabeth Anne, *Chinnamasta: The Aweful Buddhist and Hindu Tantric Goddess* (Delhi: Motilal Barnarsidass, 2010)

Bhartiya, Aru, 'Menstruation, Religion and Society', *International Journal of Social Science and Humanity*, 3.6 (November 2013), 523–27

Brody, Saul Nathaniel, *The Disease of the Soul: Leprosy in Medieval Literature* (Ithaca, NY: Cornell University Press, 1974).

Buddhist Digital Archives, The Buddhist Digital Resource Center <https://library.bdrc.io/>

Butler, Judith, *Excitable Speech: A Politics of the Performative* (New York: Routledge, 1997)

Bynum, Caroline Walker, *Fragmentation and Redemption: Essays on Gender and the Human Body in Medieval Religion* (Cambridge, MA: MIT Press, 1992)

Cabezón, José Ignacio, *Sexuality in Classical South Asian Buddhism* (Somerville, MA: Wisdom Publications, 2017)

Choden, Kunzang, *Dawa: The Story of a Stray Dog in Bhutan* (Thimphu, Bhutan: Riyang Books, 2014)

Corker, Mairian, 'Differences, Conflations and Foundations: The Limits to "Accurate" Theoretical Representation of Disabled People's Experience?', *Disability and Society*, 14.5 (1999), 627–42

Davidson, Ronald M., *Tibetan Renaissance: Tantric Buddhism in the Rebirth of Tibetan Culture* (New York: Columbia University Press, 2005)

De Bruin, Hanne M., *Leprosy in South India: Stigma and Strategies of Coping* (Pondicherry: Institut Français de Pondichéry, 1998)

Douglas, Mary, *Purity and Danger: An Analysis of the Concepts of Pollution and Taboo* (London: Ark, 1984)

Erevelles, Nirmala, 'In Search of the Disabled Subject', in *Embodied Rhetoric: Disability in Language and Culture*, ed. by James C. Wilson and Cynthia Lewiecki-Wilson, (Carbondale: Southern Illinois University Press, 2001), pp. 92–111

Federman, Asaf, 'Literal Means and Hidden Meanings: A New Analysis of Skillful Means', *Philosophy East and West*, 59.2 (2009), 125–41

Foucault, Michel, *Discipline and Punish: The Birth of the Prison* (New York: Pantheon, 1997)

Garland-Thomson, Rosemarie, 'Integrating Disability, Transforming Feminist Theory', *NWSA Journal*, 14.3 (2002), 1–32

Gell, Alfred, *Art and Agency: An Anthropological Theory* (Oxford: Clarendon Press, 1993)

Gyatso, Janet, and Hanna Havnevik, *Women in Tibet* (New York: Columbia University Press, 2006)

Hanh, Thich Nhat, *The Heart of the Buddha's Teaching: Transforming Suffering into Peace, Joy, and Liberation* (Pittsburgh: Harmony, 1999)

Jacob, Jesse, and C. Franco-Paredes, 'The Stigmatization of Leprosy in India and its Impact on Future Approaches to Elimination and Control', *PLOS Neglected Tropical Diseases*, 2.1 (January 2008), e113, 1–3 <https://doi.org/10.1371/journal.pntd.0000113>

Ki Che Leung, Angela, *Leprosy in China: A History* (New York: Columbia University Press, 2009)

King, Richard, 'Early Yogācāra and its Relationship with the Madhyamaka School', *Philosophy East and West*, 44.4 (October 1994), 659–83

Kumarajiva, Tripitaka Master, trans., *The Diamond of Perfect Wisdom Sutra*, Chung Tai Translation Committee (New York: Simon & Schuster, 2009)

Kunga, Drime, *The Life and Visions of Yeshe Tsogyal: The Autobiography of the Great Wisdom Queen* (New York: Snow Lion, 2017)

Leslie, Julia, 'The Implications of the Physical Body: Health, Suffering and Karma in Hindu Thought', in *Religion, Health and Suffering*, ed. by John R. Hinnells and Roy Porter (London: Kegan Paul, 1999), pp. 23–45

March, Kathryn, 'The Intermediacy of Women: Female Gender Symbolism and the Social Position of Women Among Tamangs and Sherpas of Highland Nepal' (unpublished doctoral dissertation, Cornell University, 1979 [1986])

Mairs, Nancy, *On the Literary Nonfiction of Nancy Mairs: A Critical Anthology*, ed. by Merri Lisa Johnson and Susannah B. Mintz (London: Palgrave, 2011)

McNamer, Sarah, *Affective Meditation and the Invention of Medieval Compassion* (Philadelphia: University of Pennsylvania Press, 2010)

McRuer, Robert, 'Composing Bodies; or, De-Composition: Queer Theory, Disability Studies, and Alternative Corporealities', *JAC*, 24.1 (2004), 48–78

Minich, Julie Avril, 'Enabling Whom? Critical Disability Studies Now', *Lateral*, 5.1 (2016) <https://doi.org/10.25158/L5.1.9>

Mintz, Susannah B., *Unruly Bodies: Life Writing by Women with Disabilities* (Chapel Hill: University of North Carolina Press, 2007)

Mitchell, David T., and Sharon L. Snyder, *Narrative Prosthesis: Disability and the Dependencies of Discourse* (Ann Arbor: University of Michigan Press, 2000)

Olivelle, Patrick, 'Deconstruction of the Body in Indian Asceticism', in *Asceticism*, ed. by Vincent L. Wimbush and Richard Valantasis (Oxford: Oxford University Press, 1998), pp. 188–210

Oliver, Michael, *The Politics of Disablement* (London: Palgrave, 1990)

Orlemanski, Julie, 'How to Kiss a Leper', *postmedieval: a journal of medieval and cultural studies*, 3.2 (2012), 142–57

Ortner, Sherry, *High Religion: A Cultural and Political History of Sherpa Buddhism* (Princeton, NJ: Princeton University Press, 1989)

Paul, Diana, *Women in Buddhism: Images of the Feminine in the Mahayana Tradition* (Berkeley: University of California Press, 1985)

Porter, James I., 'Foreword', in *The Body and Physical Difference: Discourses of Disability in the Humanities,* ed. by David T. Mitchell and Sharon L. Snyder (Ann Arbor: University of Michigan Press, 1997), pp. xiii–xiv

Powers, John, 'The Body of the Buddha', in *Oxford Research Encyclopedia of Religion* (Oxford: Oxford University Press, 2021), <https://doi.org/10.1093/acrefore/9780199340378.013.745> [accessed 26 March 2023]

Reinders, Eric, and Fabio Rambelli, *Buddhism and Iconoclasm in East Asia: A History* (London: Bloomsbury, 2012)

Samuels, Ellen, 'Critical Divides: Judith Butler's Body Theory and the Question of Disability', *NWSA Journal*, 14.3 (Autumn 2002), 58–76

Sanyal, Usha, and Nita Kumar, eds, *Food, Faith and Gender in South Asia: The Cultural Politics of Women's Food Practices* (New York and London: Bloomsbury Academic, 2020)

Schriempf, Alexa, '(Re)fusing the Amputated Body: An Interactionist Bridge for Feminism and Disability', *Hypatia*, 16.4 (Fall 2001), 53–79

Scully, Jackie Leach, 'Disability and Vulnerability: On Bodies, Dependence, and Power', in *Vulnerability: New Essays in Ethics and Feminist Philosophy*, ed. by Catriona Mackenzie, Wendy Rogers, and Susan Dodds (London: Oxford University Press, 2014), pp. 204–21

Shoop, Marcia Mount, 'Body-Wise: Re-Fleshing Christian Spiritual Practice in Trauma's Wake', in *Trauma and Transcendence: Suffering and the Limits of Theory*, ed. by Eric Boyton (New York: Fordham University Press, 2018), pp. 240–55

Spencer-Hall, Alicia, 'Christ's Suppurating Wounds: Leprosy in the Vita of Alice of Schaerbeek (†1250)', in *Wounds and Wound Repair in Medieval Culture*, ed. by Larissa Tracy and Kelly DeVries (Leiden: Brill, 2015), pp. 389–416

Spencer-Hall, Alicia, 'Chronic Pain and Illness: Reinstating Crip-Chronic Histories to Forge Affirmative Disability Futures', in *A Cultural History of Disability in the Middle Ages*, ed. by Jonathan Hsy, Tory V. Pearman, and Joshua R. Eyler (London: Bloomsbury, 2020), pp. 51–66

Spencer-Hall, Alicia, 'The Horror of Orthodoxy: Christina Mirabilis, Thirteenth-Century "Zombie" Saint', *postmedieval: a journal of medieval and cultural studies*, 8.3 (2017), 352–75

Spencer-Hall, Alicia, *Medieval Saints and Modern Screens: Divine Visions as Cinematic Experience*, Knowledge Communities (Amsterdam: Amsterdam University Press, 2018)

Sponberg, Alan, 'Attitudes toward Women and the Feminine in Early Buddhism', in *Buddhism, Sexuality and Gender*, ed. by José Ignacio Cabezón (Albany: State University of New York Press, 1992), pp. 3–36

Stocker, Susan, 'Problems of Embodiment and Problematic Embodiment', *Hypatia*, 16.3 (2001), 48–59

Vargas-O'Bryan, Ivette, 'Disease, the Demons and the Buddhas: A Study of Tibetan Conceptions of Disease and Religious Practice', in *Health and Religious Rituals in South Asia: Disease, Possession and Healing*, ed. by Fabrizio M. Ferrari (New York: Routledge, 2010), pp. 81–99

———, 'Falling Rain, Reigning Power in Reptilian Affairs: The Balancing of Buddhism and the Environment', in *Charming Beauties and Frightful Beasts. Non-Human Animals in South Asian Myth, Ritual and Folklore*, ed. by Fabrizio M. Ferrari and Thomas Dahnhardt (New York: Equinox Publications, 2013), pp. 99–114

———, *Historical Study of the Gelongma Palmo Legacy* (forthcoming 2026)

Wendell, Susan, *The Rejected Body: Feminist Philosophical Reflections on Disability* (New York: Routledge, 1996)

Wilson, Liz, *Charming Cadavers: Horrific Figurations of the Feminine in Indian Buddhist Hagiographic Literature* (Chicago: University of Chicago Press, 1996)

Young, Iris Marion, *Throwing Like a Girl and Other Essays in Feminist Philosophy and Social Theory* (Bloomington: Indiana University Press, 1990)

Yü, Chün-fang, *Kuan-yin: The Chinese Transformation of Avalokiteshvara* (New York: Columbia University Press, 2001)

Yuill, Chris, Iain Crinson, and Eilidh Duncan, 'The Social and Medical Models of Disability', in *Key Concepts in Health Studies*, ed. by Chris Yuill, Iain Crinson, and Eilidh Duncan (Newbury Park, CA: SAGE, 2010) <https://doi.org/10.4135/9781446251676>

Zivkovic, Tanya, 'Embodying the Past: Gelongma Palmo and the Tibetan Nyungne Rituals', *Journal of Ritual Studies*, 27.2 (2013), 45–63

Zysk, Kenneth G., *Asceticism and Healing in Ancient India: Medicine in the Buddhist Monastery* (Delhi: Motilal Banarsidass, 1998

About the Author

Ivette Vargas-O'Bryan is a Professor of Asian Religions and Chair of the Department of Religious Studies at Austin College in Sherman, Texas. She is a specialist in Indian and Tibetan Buddhist traditions. Her special interest is on the intersection between Asian religions and medical traditions. In addition to having been President of the Southwest Commission on Religious Studies and resident scholar at humanities and medical research institutes in Asia, Vargas-O'Bryan has also been the recipient of prestigious awards and grants including the Fulbright Scholar Program, Andrew W. Mellon Foundation, American Council of Learned Societies Project Development Grant, and numerous teaching and scholarship awards.

5. Writing Sanctity Upon the Body: The Healed Wounds of St Æthelthryth and St Edmund

Aidan Holtan

Abstract: In Ælfric of Eynsham's tenth-century Old English homilies, 'Natale Sancte Æðeldryðe Virginis' and 'Passio Sancti Eadmundi Regis Et Martyris', St Æthelthryth and St Edmund are described as incorrupt when they are translated; however, their notionally incorrupt bodies are also marked by scars that appear during the post-mortem healing process. In this paper, I analyse the expressive and transmissive mediality of the holy saints' bodies and contend that the scars add to the saints'—and their bodies'—narratives, indicating identity, preserving important moments in their vitae, and ultimately confirming their sanctity.

Keywords: mediality, scar, St Æthelthryth, St Edmund, Ælfric of Eynsham

In *Why Can the Dead Do Such Great Things*, Robert Bartlett describes a saint as 'not a person of a particular type but a person who was treated in a particular way'.[1] While this description applies to the human treatment of those identified as saints (for example, the creation of relics, hagiographies, and other accoutrements of a saint's cult), it also applies to the heavenly treatment of saints described in their *vitae*. One particularly noteworthy indicator of sainthood is the incorruption of their corpse: rather than decaying after death, a saint may appear to be merely sleeping and, in some cases, return to a premortem, uninjured state of being.[2] However, not all incorrupt saints' bodies are preserved in a state of perfection. Most notably, St Æthelthryth

1 Bartlett, *Why Can the Dead*, p. 95.
2 Tomaini, *Corpse as Text*, p. 5.

Grace-Petinos, Stephanie, Leah Pope Parker, and Alicia Spencer-Hall, eds. *Disability and Sanctity in the Middle Ages.* Taylor & Francis Group, 2025
DOI 10.5117/9789463724333_CH05

and St Edmund are both described in their *vitae* as incorrupt, but both of their hagiographies focus on healed wounds that serve as reminders of premortem injuries. While it is possible to read these as 'disfigurements', I suggest that these healed wounds also serve an important function within the hagiographical texts.[3] Instead of simply disfiguring the saints, these markers inscribe the narrative journey from human to saint, (re)creating the saint's body as a text that can be read by its Christian audience both viewing the physical body and reading the hagiography.[4]

In this essay, I will be exploring the scarred incorruption of St Æthelthryth and St Edmund. Although there are several hagiographical texts for both saints, I will be referencing their *vitae* in the *Lives of Saints*, Ælfric of Eynsham's collection of hagiographic homilies composed c. 994–998. While there are other notable hagiographers for these saints, using Ælfric allows me to focus on a single hagiographical text and explore how these saints are discussed in the vernacular.[5] The first hagiographical text I will address concerns St Æthelthryth (d. 679). Over the course of her *vita*, St Æthelthryth assumes a wide variety of roles. She is a wife, both to the ealdorman Tondberht and, after his death, to King Ecgfrith, then a nun in Coldingham and an abbess in Ely; finally, after her death, Æthelthryth becomes a saint. As I will discuss, Æthelthryth's sanctity is largely tied to her status as a virgin, which is maintained through both her marriages, and is reflected in the incorruption of her body upon translation by her sister, Seaxburh.[6] The second saint I will consider here is the martyr-king of East

3 Patricia Skinner discusses disfigurement in much greater detail in her monograph *Living with Disfigurement*. While such disfigurement is, as Skinner notes, 'highly gendered' and varies depending on other contextual factors, it does impact the individual's perception by society (p. 17). For example, Skinner states 'there is plenty of evidence for damaged faces being "read" by contemporaries, and appearance being associated with honor or a lack of it' (p. 8). One exception here is the case of female saints, many of whom deliberately seek facial disfigurement to maintain their virginity (p. 17). For more on female disfigurement, see also Skinner, *Living with Disfigurement*, pp. 133–58.

4 Bartlett, *Relics and Writing*, p. 20.

5 For example, St Æthelthryth's *vita* is recorded by Bede in his *Ecclesiastical History of the English People* (completed in 731), and St Edmund's *vita* is recorded in Abbo of Fleury's *Passio Sancti Eadmundi* (c. 986).

6 For a diachronic analysis of St Æthelthryth's *vita* and cult, see Blanton, *Signs*. For more on texts standing in for saints' bodies, and St Æthelthryth's body in particular, see Robyn A. Bartlett, *Relics and Writing*. In particular, Bartlett shows the full transformation from the hagiographer's emphasis on the body to an emphasis on the text: the poet in *Vita S. Etheldredae Eliensis* (c. 1420) 'insists that Æthelthryth remained incorrupt in the tenth century, when some doubted the integrity of her body. He does so without giving the reader (or any character) a glimpse of the body itself. Instead, the poem relies on a punishment miracle included in the

Anglia, St Edmund (d. 869). In his *vita*, a group of Danish invaders send a messenger to St Edmund to demand his submission to Hinguar, their leader. St Edmund refuses this demand and, when the Danes arrive in response to this refusal, Edmund tosses his weapons aside in imitation of Christ. The saint is subsequently beaten, shot, and decapitated by the Danes. As they leave, the invaders hide the saint's head in the woods. This is not an obstacle for the loquacious martyr: his head calls out to the Christian search party, who then reunite and inter the saint's head with his body. Later, St Edmund is translated and, like St Æthelthryth, his body is found to be incorrupt.[7]

Despite the incorruption of their bodies, the *vitae* of both St Æthelthryth and St Edmund focus intensely on their healed wounds after their translations. For the former, the healed wound originates from a tumour that is excised before her death, whereas the latter's scar is the result of his decapitation.[8] I argue that in both *vitae*, these healed wounds are legible: they are written upon the body and can be read (or interpreted) by the people who view them. Here, I agree with Virginia Blanton and other scholars in viewing these healed wounds as part of the ways in which saints' bodies are read as texts. For example, Blanton identifies St Æthelthryth's body as a 'textual body' wherein the saint's scar, which appears in versions of the *vita* other than Ælfric's, can be read by others.[9] Thea Tomaini likewise argues that the body can be

Liber Eliensis, wherein a canon suffers for attempting to see whether Æthelthryth's body has in fact decayed. The *Etheldreda* poet thus understands what Æthelthryth's body is *from what is written about it*. And in turn, insofar as the *Vita*—not the body itself—enables us to interpret the relic, Æthelthryth's body exists as a discursive object: writing confirms its transcendent status' (p. 47, emphasis in the original).

7 For more on St Edmund's *vita* and the development of his cult, see the essays collected in Bale, ed., *St Edmund, King and Martyr*.

8 Ælfric, 'Natale Sancte Æðeldryðe Virginis', ll. 90–91a, 93–95; and 'Passio Sancti Eadmundi', ll. 178–183. St Æthelthryth is particularly noteworthy here, given the differences in the description of her healed wound between translators. In Ælfric, as we will discuss, the wound is mentioned but described as 'gehæled' (healed; l. 93, p. 201). Unless noted otherwise, all quotations of Ælfric's *vitae* are from Ælfric, 'Saint Æthelthryth' and Ælfric, 'Saint Edmund'; translations are by Mary Clayton and Juliet Mullins. However, Bede specifically mentions the presence of a postmortem scar: 'Sed et discooperto uultus indumento monstrauerunt mihi etiam uulnus incisurae, quod feceram, curatum, ita ut mirum in modum pro aperto et hiante uulnere, cum quo sepulta erat, tenuissima tunc cicatrices uestigia parerent' (They drew back the cloth which covered her face and showed me the wound I had made by my incision, now healed, so that instead of the open gaping wound which she had when she was buried, there now appeared, marvellous to relate, only the slightest traces of a scar); Bede, *Ecclesiastical History*, pp. 390 and 392; 391 and 393. For more on the scar—or lack thereof—for St Æthelthryth, see 'St Æthelthryth's Scar: Marking Crip Eschatology on the Saintly Body' in Parker, *Light of the Everlasting Life*.

9 Blanton, *Signs*, p. 31.

understood as a text, in addition to expanding her research to consider the gravesite itself as a text.[10] Similarly, Alicia Spencer-Hall argues for a connection between hagiographic bodies and media (specifically film) in her monograph *Medieval Saints and Modern Screens: Divine Visions as Cinematic Experience*.[11]

It is in this intersection of 'body as text' and 'wounded body' that we can see a potential for both mediality studies and disability studies to inform our understanding of the hagiographies. In mediality studies, bodies are viewed as intentional texts, 'installed' within the narrative to be read by other characters and by the audience.[12] Just as understanding a text is more than just reading the words on a page, so too is an understanding of the body's text influenced by outside factors. As Sarah Künzler states in *Flesh and Word: Reading Bodies in Old Norse-Icelandic and Early Irish Literature,* '[t]he messages that bodies provide can be *read* only within a social system and this system needs to be examined if one seeks to know how bodies can (and do) function as media.'[13] Here, mediality studies overlaps with disability studies, particularly the cultural model, which focuses on disability as a construction of bodily difference and social perception.[14] In order to understand how these bodies are installed as texts within their hagiographies, one must first understand the social perception of wounds and how the bearer's identity as a saint can impact that perception. The deceased body cannot (often) speak for itself, and some of the impairments visible on the postmortem body could be misread as divine or judicial punishment, particularly if viewed without the accompanying knowledge provided by the saint's hagiography.[15] If a saint is, as noted above, 'a person who [is] treated in a particular way', then this misinterpretation has the potential to negatively impact their postmortem treatment and their participation in society.[16] However, this is not the case for St Æthelthryth and St Edmund. While their recognition as saints is largely due to their continued productive postmortem participation in society, as recounted by their hagiographies, it is also

10 Tomaini, *Corpse as Text*. It is important to note here that Tomaini writes about the corpse as text in a later, non-medieval time period. However, similar arguments about the gravesite as text are also discussed in Williams, *Death and Memory*.

11 Spencer-Hall, *Medieval Saints*.

12 Künzler, *Flesh and Word*, p. 11.

13 Künzler, *Flesh and Word*, p. 23 (emphasis in original).

14 Eyler, 'Introduction', p. 8.

15 See Metzler, *Disability*, p. 47; and Appleton, 'Role of Æschere's Head', p. 432.

16 Bartlett, *Why Can the Dead*, p. 95.

supported by the narrative inscribed on their bodies.[17] Mediality theory is one lens through which we may examine how the saints' incomplete incorruption contributes to, rather than solely detracting from, their overarching hagiographic narrative.

For this essay, I use the language provided by Sarah Künzler in *Flesh and Word*. Künzler identifies three separate modes for bodily mediality. The first is expressive mediality, which 'denotes that bodies express the identity of a character and therefore enable social identification. Bodies thus function as a visible expression of identity and hence as a mediator between an individual character and the society (or societies) in a text'.[18] This type of mediality thus encompasses the whole body and focuses on the relationship between the body and identity. However, this type of mediality does not include deliberate alterations to the body. Instead, that is included in transmissive mediality, which includes bodies that 'mediate primarily through signs on their skin or in their flesh (such as scars or wounds), or more broadly, through alterations to the surface of the body'.[19] The final type of mediality identified by Künzler is mediality discourse of natural bodily matters, which addresses 'the natural processes of defecation, urination and menstruation'.[20] As I will show, the two most prominent forms of bodily mediality in Ælfric's *vitae* of St Æthelthryth and St Edmund are expressive mediality (evident in their incorruption) and transmissive mediality (evident in the postmortem interpretation of their healed wounds).

Writing Virginity and Sanctity: The Postmortem Healing of St Æthelthryth's Wound

Though her role in society shifts over the years, one aspect of St Æthelthryth remains the same: each new facet of her life is primarily defined in relation to her body, especially in terms of her bodily autonomy. As a wife, she is defined by her virginity. As a nun and an abbess, the focus shifts to her asceticism and the control of her body. As a saint, she is characterized by her bodily incorruption. Despite the prominent representation of St

17 See 'Reciprocity' in Bartlett, *Why Can the Dead*, pp. 106–12, and Rollason, *Saints and Relics*, pp. 3, 7.

18 Künzler, *Flesh and Word*, p. 24.

19 Künzler, *Flesh and Word*, p. 25.

20 Künzler, *Flesh and Word*, p. 26.

Æthelthryth's body throughout her *vita*, her physical embodiment of virtue is most evident in this lack of decay.[21]

In her *vita*, St Æthelthryth's body demonstrates both transmissive mediality in the form of her tumour and its postmortem healing, and expressive mediality in her incorruption revealed during translation. The mediality of the tumour is noteworthy because St Æthelthryth herself describes how it should be interpreted:

> She said: 'I know for certain that I well deserve that my neck should be afflicted with such sickness, because in my youth I adorned my neck with many necklaces. And it seems to me now that God's mercy may cleanse that guilt, when this tumor now shines in place of gold for me and this hot burning in place of precious gemstones.'[22]

According to Æthelthryth, then, the tumour is not just a present malady, but rather a physical echo of a former sin. Specifically, the location of the tumour serves as a reminder of her vanity, as is evident when St Æthelthryth states that the tumour 'shines in the place of gold for me and this hot burning in the place of precious gemstones'.[23] St Æthelthryth is afflicted by a disease that is located on the same part of the body which she associates with a past transgression, and it bears a physical resemblance to the sin in question. Consequently, the tumour assumes a positive role as a form of penance for the former sin.[24] The connection between the locational memory of the tumour and the opportunities it presents for penance are made clear by St Æthelthryth, who states that the tumour exists 'that God's mercy may cleanse that guilt'.[25] This connection between illness and penance is not unusual in hagiographical texts, particularly for female saints. For

21 The focus on incorruption and virginity is common to female saints in Old English hagiography. See Bartlett, *Why Can the Dead*, pp. 202–04, and Blanton, *Signs*, pp. 4–5.

22 Heo cwæð: 'Ic wat geare þæt ic wel wyrðe eom
þæt min swura beo geswenct mid swylcere untrumnysse
forðan þe ic on iugoðe frætwode minne swuran
mid mænigfealdum swur-beagum. And me is nu geþuht
þæt Godes arfæstnyss þone gylt aclænsige,
þonne me nu þis geswel scynð for golde
and þæs hata bryne for healicum gymstanum.'
Ælfric, 'Saint Æthelthryth', ll. 54–60.

23 '[Þ]is geswel scynð for golde / and þæs hata bryne for healicum gymstanum'; Ælfric, 'Saint Æthelthryth', ll. 59–60.

24 See Metzler, *Disability*, p. 47.

25 '[Þ]æt Godes arfæstnyss þone gylt aclænsige'; Ælfric, 'Saint Æthelthryth', l. 58.

example, this is often seen with leprosy. While it is possible for the medieval community to interpret leprosy as a physical indicator of a spiritual issue, it is also positioned by medieval hagiographers as a means of atoning for one's sins or for the sins of the community in an earthly, premortem form of purgatory.[26]

In establishing the connection between past vanity and present suffering, St Æthelthryth reads the tumour as a message about her former actions, as well as an opportunity for forgiveness. As a result, the tumour and the subsequent wound become what Blanton terms 'locational memory'—the injury has another layer of meaning in which past events are inscribed upon the skin in a way that can be read.[27] Here, though, the saint needs to read the injury for the elucidation of her fellow religious. This 'locational memory' is also a site of transmissive mediality. The tumour and its resulting wound alter St Æthelthryth's skin and inscribe her body with a narrative of her former sin that can be read by a Christian audience, though it needs glossing so that the community can understand the potential positive (rather than purely punitive) meaning of such a wound.

When St Æthelthryth is translated sixteen years after her death, one of the actions that the translators take is to examine the site where the tumour had been situated. The narrator describes St Æthelthryth's body thusly: 'There she lay in the coffin as if she were lying asleep, sound in all her limbs, and the doctor was there who had lanced the tumor, and he examined her intently. The wound had been healed then, which the doctor had made previously.'[28] For the witnesses and, by extension, the audience of the hagiographical text, the healed wound's meaning is much deeper than the locational memory: the site is a marker, not only of injury, but also the identity of the bearer.[29] This layering of meaning is particularly

26 For more on the connection between leprosy and penance, see Spencer-Hall, 'Christ's Suppurating Wounds'. On leprosy, see also chapters in this volume by Edwards (pp. 235–63) and Vargas-O'Bryan (pp. 115–46).

27 Blanton, *Signs*, p. 44. For more on scars as locational memory, see Frank, 'Macrina's Scar'.

28 Þa læg heo on ðære cyste, swilce heo læge on slæpe,
hal eallum limum and se læce wæs ðær
ðe þæt geswell geopenode and hi sceawode georne.
Þa wæs seo wund gehæled, þe se læce worhte ær.
Ælfric, 'Saint Æthelthryth', ll.90–93.

29 Spencer-Hall explores a similar (and more extensive) moment of hagiographic healing and scarification in the hagiography of the Franciscan beguine Douceline of Digne (c. 1215–1274). After Douceline heals Pellegrin (who was deaf, mute, and had 'putrefying cranial wounds'—the latter of which contributed to a mostly detached ear), the boy's mother recognizes him, in part due to the scarring of the reattached ear; Spencer-Hall, 'Chronic Pain and Illness', pp. 60, 62.

evident when we consider the physician's clear identification. The physician has not only seen the healed wound after the body was unearthed, but he was also the one who created the original wound in his attempt to heal St Æthelthryth's tumour. Consequently, out of everyone in the *vita*, the physician is in the best position to examine the site and ultimately to identify the body as belonging to St Æthelthryth.

One reason underpinning the requirement for formal identification of the saint's body is its apparent incorruptibility. The description of Æthelthryth as lying in her grave 'as if she lay in sleep' does not indicate mere peaceful repose. Rather, the miracle here lies in the inaction of the grave: the worms often associated with postmortem decomposition and decay did not visit the body. Instead, St Æthelthryth remains incorrupt and, indeed, her time in the grave has healed the earthly harms imposed on her body. St Æthelthryth's postmortem physical confirmation of virginity therefore answers an otherwise difficult question: how do you confirm virginity without endangering that choice? Sarah Salih observes that '[t]o read the body as virgin is difficult because one is looking for something which is not there, and if it is there, might be destroyed by looking'.[30] Incorruption confirms the presence of virginity without the concomitant threat of its destruction.

The use of St Æthelthryth's incorruption to identify her as one of the saintly virgins reveals her body's expressive mediality within the *vita*. The drastic difference between normal decaying corpses and the lack of decomposition evident in the incorrupt corpse signifies that the body in question belongs to a particular group: here, saints. This is reinforced within the *vita* by the narrator's comments regarding the confirmatory nature of St Æthelthryth's incorruption. The description of the body as miraculously incorrupt facilitates its identification as part of a group, particularly when its status as a member of the group could be called into question, as may be the case when one is twice married and yet claiming to be a virgin.

Within her *vita*, St Æthelthryth's body functions as a text in two separate ways. During her life, her neck tumour functioned as transmissive mediality, indicating St Æthelthryth's prior sins and allowing her to physically atone for them before her death. At this point, Æthelthryth is able to act as a primary reader for her own body as text, indicating the purpose of her illness to her fellow religious. This is not the case for her postmortem body—instead, it

This scarring is a locational marker of the act of healing, as well as a marker of identity for the boy. Moreover, as Spencer-Hall shows, Pellegrin's healing is conditional: the pain returns in adulthood when he does not follow the saint's instructions; ibid., pp. 62–63.

30 Salih, *Versions of Virginity*, p. 38.

needs to stand on its own as an easily interpretable text. This is primarily accomplished through the expressive mediality present in the incorrupt body. Æthelthryth's lack of decay confirms her virgin status and, through the miraculous nature of its appearance, identifies her as a saint. At the same time, the attention given to her healed wound—despite the incorruption evident in the rest of her body—serves as locational memory of her surgery, thereby recalling the illness—and its cause—that had plagued her at that site. The healed wound is ultimately a distant echo of a past sin forgiven, a reminder of the one who had read it before.

Dead Men Do Tell Tales: The Decapitation and Re-capitation of St Edmund

Just as St Æthelthryth's *vita* is marked by significant attention to her body, so too is St Edmund's body at the forefront of his *vita*. However, as a martyr, a great deal of attention is focused on the moment of his death and the postmortem body, rather than on the control of his body throughout his life.[31] This attention to the body is reflected in the scarring from St Edmund's decapitation and subsequent postmortem re-capitation, as well as his postmortem incorruption. The latter, as I will show, occurs twice in his *vita*: once when St Edmund's corpse is protected, rather than consumed, by a wolf, and the second time when he is translated.

St Edmund's postmortem scarring is an act of transmissive mediality in his *vita*. In many respects, the scar serves a similar function as St Æthelthryth's healed wound. For example, just as the healed wound from her tumour speaks to her identity and her former forgiven sins, so too can an audience find greater meaning in the scars on St Edmund's body. Most notably, St Edmund's translated body does not bear the marks from his premortem torture, but does have a scar where the incorruption extends to the point of reattaching his decapitated head to his body:

> And his neck, which had been cut through, was healed, and it was as if there was a red silken thread around his neck to reveal to people how he

31 Spencer-Hall explores this attention to the moment of death in martyrs' hagiographies and connects them to modern 'execution films'. In both cases, the importance is placed on the audience's ability to witness the death, and the ability to repeat that death: 'We need to see them die—and die and die and die—in order to grasp fully the moral imperative of their example'; *Medieval Saints*, p. 83.

> had been killed. Also, the wounds that the cruel heathens had inflicted on his body with repeated shots had been healed by heavenly God.[32]

By describing the mark around Edmund's neck as revealing 'how he had been killed', Ælfric makes apparent that the scar on St Edmund's neck is, like St Æthelthryth's scar, a mark of locational memory. The scar serves as a continual reminder to onlookers that St Edmund's head had, at one point, been separated from his body. Moreover, St Edmund's scar also acts as a statement about those who inflicted it upon him. For St Æthelthryth, her scar was a statement of forgiveness, a physical sign that she had been absolved of her former sin. This is not the case for St Edmund, whose scar is the result of an act of violence by an outside force, rather than penance for an earlier act. With this in mind, the scar's representation of the reunion of St Edmund's head and his body also serves as a statement against the Danes who caused his martyrdom. As Paul Cavill argues, 'The overall message is that physical and mental violence against saints, while infinitely varied, subtle and ingenious, does not ultimately work'.[33] In this case, the violence against St Edmund does not work because it does not last: the decapitation is reversed, with only a thin, red scar to show that it had happened, and the marks from the shots and the beatings are erased entirely. The postmortem healing obscures the violence and repairs the damage. Only the scar marking the decapitation—evidence of St Edmund's transition from king to martyr—remains. As such, St Edmund's scar can also be read as an everlasting testimony to the ineffectiveness of violence compared to the power found in the saint's faith.

St Edmund also experiences expressive mediality, the first moment of which occurs immediately after St Edmund's martyrdom. When St Edmund refused to submit to the Danish invader, Hinguar, and his forces, the saint was tortured and then decapitated. The Danes then threw the saint's head into the forest in order to prevent it from being found and buried with the rest of his body.[34] However, the saint's head is able to guide the Christian

32 [A]nd his swura wæs gehalod, þe ær forslagen wæs,
and wæs swylce an seolcen þræd embe his swuran ræd
mannum to sweotelunge hu he ofslagen wæs.
Eac swilce þa wunda þe þa wæl-hreowan hæþenan
mid gelomum scotungum on his lice macodon
wæron gehælede þurh þone heofonlican God[.]
Ælfric, 'Saint Edmund', ll. 166–71.

33 Cavill, 'Anglo-Saxon Saints' Lives', p. 83.

34 One reason why the Danes attempted to prevent the reunification of St Edmund's head and body could be the relationship between decapitation and the postmortem treatment of the criminal body; Marafioti, *King's Body*, p. 185.

search party to his location, calling out, 'Here, here, here'.[35] While the head's response is, in itself, miraculous, so too is its company: 'The gray wolf who guarded the head lay there, and he had clasped the head with his two feet, greedy and hungry, and for the sake of God dared not partake of the head, but guarded it against other wild animals'.[36] On the initial level of the text, the miraculous nature of this event is stated with relative clarity. The wolf, an animal already saddled with a negative connotation due to its predatory nature, is described as both 'greedy' (*grædig*) and 'hungry' (*hungrig*)—two states of being which ordinarily would not bode well for any prey that crossed its path, let alone a rather defenceless human head. Even so, the text states that the wolf 'had been sent at God's direction to guard the head'.[37] As a result of this miraculous intervention, the wolf acts contrary to its predatory nature and guards the saint's head, not only from itself, but from other animals as well.

The wolf being depicted as protecting, rather than consuming, the head is notable considering the wolf's inclusion in the larger 'beasts of battle' motif common in Old English literature. In this motif, animals like the raven, eagle, and wolf are included in descriptions of the battlefield and carry an ominous connotation. As Thomas Honegger states, 'The linking of the raven, the eagle, and the wolf with the battlefield originated in the factual appearance of these animals on the "wælstede" to feed on the corpses in the aftermath of a battle'.[38] By extension, the appearance of these beasts before the battle itself is a means of foreshadowing death: the beasts gather in anticipation of the feast to come. The decision to have the wolf *not* consume St Edmund is therefore a form of incorruption: just as the worm does not devour the interred body, the wolf likewise does not eat St Edmund's exposed head. This connection between non-consumption and incorruption is particularly evident when we consider other interpretations of the beast of battle motif. For instance, Victoria Thompson argues that the beasts of battle motif reinforces that death is 'part of everyday life', and serves as an acknowledgment of humanity's role in the food chain.[39] However, due to Edmund's body's incorruption, the saint is effectively removed from the food

35 'Her, her, her', Ælfric, 'Saint Edmund', l. 139.

36 'Þa læg se græge wulf þe bewiste þæt heafod / and mid his twam fotum hæfde þæt heafod beclypped, / grædig and hungrig, and for Gode ne dorste / þæs heafdes abyrian ac heold hit wið deor'; Ælfric, 'Saint Edmund', ll. 142–45.

37 '[W]earð asend / þurh Godes wissunge to bewerigenne þæt heafod'; Ælfric, 'Saint Edmund', ll. 133–34.

38 Honegger, 'Form and Function', p. 298.

39 Thompson, *Dying and Death*, p. 138.

chain. During translation this appears as the absence of decay, which would typically be described in terms of being consumed by worms.[40] The wolf, as well as other beasts of battle, plays a similar role in that it contributes to the destruction of the corpses left behind on the battlefield. Thus, the wolf's deviance from its usual role in the food chain allows St Edmund to remain 'incorrupt', insomuch as his head is protected from consumption by both the wolf and other passing predators, just as an incorrupt saint's body is protected from decay in the form of worms and other factors, like the passing of time.

St Edmund's incorruption is not solely limited to the non-consumption of his head. When the saint is translated some years later, the community discovers that his body was protected from the effects of time, just as it had been protected from the hunger of the wolf: 'Then it was a great miracle that he was as [incorrupt] as if he were alive'.[41] Ælfric connects this incorruption to St Edmund's virginity: 'His body, which lies undecayed, shows us that he lived without fornication here in the world, and with a chaste life departed to Christ'.[42] Here, the expressive mediality of the incorrupt body serves as evidence of the body's actions in life: St Edmund lived and died as a virgin and this otherwise difficult-to-prove status is made evident in his corpse's lack of decay.

While this incorruption functions similarly to that of St Æthelthryth (in that both incorrupt bodies are explicitly tied to their virginal status), it is important to note that its emphasis within the *vitae* differs, especially in the translation of their corpses. For instance, a great deal of build-up precedes the translation of St Æthelthryth's body, most notably the discovery of a marble tomb and the ceremony surrounding the body's translation and revelation of its incorruption.[43] In comparison, the decision to translate St Edmund appears rather perfunctory:

40 This is perhaps most evident in the Old English *Soul and Body* poems. These poems are present in both the Vercelli Book (*Soul and Body I*) and the Exeter Book (*Soul and Body II*). Both versions of the poem include a damned soul returning to speak to its deceased and decaying body, but *Soul and Body I* also includes an address from a blessed soul to its body. Notably, however, this blessed soul is not exempt from the decomposition process. See Moffat, *Old English Soul and Body*.

41 'Þa wæs micel wundor þæt he wæs eallswa gehal / swylce he cucu wære'; Ælfric, 'Saint Edmund', ll. 164–65. Mary Clayton and Juliet Mullins translate *gehal* as 'uncorrupt' here, but I have opted to use 'incorrupt' instead for consistency.

42 'His lic-hama us cyð, þe lið unformolsnod, / þæt he butan forligre her on worulde leofode, / and mid clænum life to Criste siþode'; Ælfric, 'Saint Edmund', ll. 174–76.

43 See in particular Ælfric, 'Saint Æthelthryth', ll. 78–89.

> Some time later, after many years, when the raiding had stopped and peace was restored to the oppressed people, then they joined together and built a church in magnificent fashion for the saint [...]. Then they intended to carry the saint's body with public honor and lay it to rest within the church.[44]

The narrator does not express a desire to find a specific tomb and does not describe the process of unearthing the body—there is not even a definitive span of time between St Edmund's original burial and his translation.[45] This difference is perhaps due to the clarity of St Edmund's status as saint through his martyrdom. St Æthelthryth needs the incorruption to prove her virginity, which forms the basis for her sanctity; conversely, though St Edmund's incorruption is also used as evidence for his virginity, the maintenance of virginity does not play as significant of a role in establishing his saintly status.[46] Instead of being the centre of St Edmund's hagiography, his identity as virgin amplifies the saintly qualities already present in the narrative.

Conclusion: Reading the Wounded, Incorrupt Saint's Body

St Æthelthryth's healed wound and St Edmund's scar identify their bearers as belonging to the category of 'saint'. As Irina Metzler notes, in early Christian theology martyrs were believed to be among the few who would be resurrected with scars as evidence of their wounds:

> In fact, re-reading in this light the eschatological statements that only saints and martyrs carry their impairments with them at the resurrection

44 'Eft þa on fyrste, æfter fela gearum, / þa seo hergung geswac and sibb wearð forgifen / þam geswenctan folce, þa fengon hi togædere / and worhton ane cyrcan wurðlice þam halgan, [...] Hi woldon þa ferian mid folclicum wurð-mynte / þone halgan lic-haman, and læcgan innan þære cyrcan'; Ælfric, 'Saint Edmund', ll. 156–59, 162–63.

45 Though the building of the church in honour of St Edmund could be considered equivalent to the discovery of St Æthelthryth's marble tomb, the two scenarios still differ in that the process of building the church is not described, whereas the process of locating the tomb is recorded in great detail. See Ælfric, 'Saint Æthelthryth', ll. 73–87, and Ælfric, 'Saint Edmund', ll. 167–72.

46 When male virginity is at the centre of a hagiographic text, it often takes the form of a trial to maintain or protect that virginity. John H. Arnold identifies four main narrative patterns in which male virginity is maintained through (1) bodily chastisement, (2) exercise of self-will, (3) revelation of the desired object's 'devilish' nature, or (4) divine intervention. See Arnold, 'Labour of Continence', pp. 104–07.

> shows just how special these cases are deemed to be: ordinary folk do not carry their impairments with them, whereas impairments sustained in martyrdom are special to the saints.[47]

In Ælfric, St Edmund's scar is quite clear—a thin, red line remains where his head has been reattached to his body. This is not the case for St Æthelthryth, whose tumour is healed without a mark. However, it does leave a mark in the text: despite being described as 'sound in all her limbs', the *vita* still stops for the doctor to examine the place where the wound had been.[48] The physical indication of the healed wound may no longer be visible, but the healed wound is still present in the text and St Æthelthryth still carries her impairment with her. In both *vitae*, St Æthelthryth's and St Edmund's healed wounds set them apart and provide a locational memory of the actions that caused its bearer's ascension to sainthood.

Through the abovementioned locational memories, one can see the intersection of disability studies and mediality studies. Both theories are concerned with the textual and physical marks inscribed upon St Æthelthryth's and St Edmund's bodies in their narratives, and how the readers' interpretation of these healed wounds are influenced by the cultural understanding of the body and its interactions with society. The incorporation of mediality studies, however, provides a deeper look into how the body is installed as a text within the *vitae* of the saints. Expressive mediality considers how the body as a whole can act as an expression of identity. For both St Æthelthryth and St Edmund, this is evident in their incorruption: they do not decay after death, and thus their body can be read as that of a saint. Their identity is further solidified through transmissive mediality, which considers alterations to the flesh. These alterations are evident in St Æthelthryth's and St Edmund's healed wounds, which indicate spaces where the flesh was marred by illness or by martyrdom and then stitched back together posthumously prior to the saints' translations. Through both forms of mediality, St Æthelthryth's and St Edmund's bodies are installed in their *vitae* as saints. These potential imperfections, though they may mar the text or their flesh, help to tell the stories of the saints' lives.

47 Metzler, *Disability*, p. 61. As Metzler notes, this belief is particularly clear in Augustine's *City of God*; see also Augustine, 'The City of God against the Pagans', pp. 157–61. For a thorough account of the medieval theologians' response to scarred martyrs, see Metzler, *Disability*, pp. 55–62.

48 '[H]al eallum limum'; Ælfric, 'Saint Æthelthryth', l. 91.

Bibliography

Primary Sources

Ælfric, 'Saint Æthelthryth', in *Old English Lives of Saints*, ed. and trans. by Mary Clayton and Juliet Mullins, Dumbarton Oaks Medieval Library, 3 vols (Cambridge, MA: Harvard University Press, 2019), II, pp. 193–203

Ælfric, 'Saint Edmund', in *Old English Lives of Saints*, ed. and trans. by Mary Clayton and Juliet Mullins, Dumbarton Oaks Medieval Library, 3 vols (Cambridge, MA: Harvard University Press, 2019), III, pp. 185–205

Augustine of Hippo, 'City of God Against the Pagans (413–26)', trans. by Leah Pope Parker, in *The Medieval Disability Sourcebook: Western Europe*, ed. by Cameron Hunt McNabb, (Earth, Milky Way: punctum books, 2020), pp. 157–61

Bede, *Bede's Ecclesiastical History of the English People*, ed. and trans. by Bertram Colgrave and R. A. B. Mynors (Oxford: Oxford University Press, 1969)

Moffat, Douglas, ed., *The Old English Soul and Body*, trans. by Douglas Moffat (Cambridge: D. S. Brewer, 1990)

Secondary Sources

Appleton, Helen, 'The Role of Æschere's Head', *The Review of English Studies*, 68 (2017), 428–47

Arnold, John H., 'The Labour of Continence: Masculinity and Clerical Virginity', in *Medieval Virginities*, ed. by Anke Bernau, Ruth Evans, and Sarah Salih, Religion and Culture in the Middle Ages (Toronto: University of Toronto Press, 2003), pp. 102–18

Bale, Anthony, ed., *St Edmund, King and Martyr: Changing Images of a Medieval Saint* (York: York Medieval Press, 2009)

Bartlett, Robert, *Why Can the Dead Do Such Great Things? Saints and Worshippers from the Martyrs to the Reformation* (Princeton, NJ: Princeton University Press, 2013)

Bartlett (Malo), Robyn A., *Relics and Writing in Late Medieval England* (Toronto: University of Toronto Press, 2013)

Blanton, Virginia, *Signs of Devotion: The Cult of St Æthelthryth in Medieval England, 695–1615* (University Park: Pennsylvania State University Press, 2007)

Cavill, Paul, 'Anglo-Saxon Saints' Lives—and Deaths', in *Visions and Revisions: The Word and the Text*, ed. by Roger Kojecký and Andrew Tate (Newcastle upon Tyne: Cambridge Scholars, 2013), pp. 79–93

Eyler, Joshua, 'Introduction: Breaking Boundaries, Building Bridges', in *Disability in the Middle Ages: Reconsiderations and Reverberations*, ed. by Joshua R. Eyler (Burlington, VT: Ashgate, 2010), pp. 1–8

Frank, Georgia, 'Macrina's Scar: Homeric Allusion and Heroic Identity in Gregory of Nyssa's *Life of Macrina*', *Journal of Early Christian Studies*, 8 (2000), 511–30

Honegger, Thomas, 'Form and Function: The Beasts of Battle Revisited', *English Studies*, 79 (July 1998), 289–98

Künzler, Sarah, *Flesh and Word: Reading Bodies in Old Norse-Icelandic and Early Irish Literature,* Trends in Medieval Philology (Berlin: De Gruyter, 2016)

Marafioti, Nicole, *The King's Body: Burial and Succession in Late Anglo-Saxon England* (Toronto: University of Toronto Press, 2014)

Metzler, Irina, *Disability in Medieval Europe: Thinking About Physical Impairment During the High Middle Ages, c. 1100–1400* (London: Routledge, 2006)

Parker, Leah Pope, *Light of the Everlasting Life: Disability and Crip Eschatology in Old English Literature* (Ann Arbor: University of Michigan Press, forthcoming 2025)

Rollason, David, *Saints and Relics in Anglo-Saxon England* (Oxford: Basil Blackwell, 1989)

Salih, Sarah, *Versions of Virginity in Late Medieval England* (Cambridge: D. S. Brewer, 2001)

Skinner, Patricia, *Living with Disfigurement in Early Medieval Europe,* New Middle Ages (New York: Palgrave MacMillan, 2017)

Spencer-Hall, Alicia, 'Christ's Suppurating Wounds: Leprosy in the *Vita* of Alice of Schaerbeek (†1250)', in *Wounds and Wound Repair in Medieval Culture,* ed. by Larissa Tracy and Kelly DeVries (Leiden: Brill, 2015), pp. 389–416

Spencer-Hall, Alicia, 'Chronic Pain and Illness: Reinstating Crip-Chronic Histories to Forge Affirmative Disability Futures', in *A Cultural History of Disability in the Middle Ages*, ed. by Jonathan Hsy, Tory V. Pearman, and Joshua R. Eyler (London: Bloomsbury, 2020), pp. 51–66

Spencer-Hall, Alicia, *Medieval Saints and Modern Screens: Divine Visions as Cinematic Experience,* Knowledge Communities (Amsterdam: Amsterdam University Press, 2018)

Thompson, Victoria, *Dying and Death in Anglo-Saxon England,* Anglo-Saxon Studies (Woodbridge, Suffolk: Boydell Press, 2004)

Tomaini, Thea, *The Corpse as Text: Disinterment and Antiquarian Enquiry, 1700–1900* (Woodbridge, Suffolk: Boydell Press, 2017)

Williams, Howard, *Death and Memory in Early Medieval Britain,* Cambridge Studies in Archaeology (Cambridge: Cambridge University Press, 2006)

About the Author

Aidan Holtan is an English professor and the Writing Center Coordinator at Grayson College. She completed her PhD at Purdue University in 2020, and her research interests focus on the body, mediality, and monstrosity in medieval literature. This is reflected in her dissertation, 'Reading the Body: Dismemberment of Saints and Monsters in Medieval Literature', which examines the use and interpretation of the dismembered postmortem body in Old English and Old Norse texts.

6. Sacred Spectacles? Eyeglasses, Iconography and the Holy Body

Rachael Gillibrand

Abstract: In the Middle Ages, sight loss—as signified by the wearing of spectacles—was used to indicate one of two things. On the one hand, the inclusion of spectacles in visual sources could signify that an individual had developed an ocular impairment as a result of their reading and writing of holy texts. On the other hand, spectacles could act as a visual indication that their wearer had damaged their sight by engaging in inappropriate behaviours. This chapter will investigate why, if sight loss could be considered to be a negative attribute within medieval Christianity, saints were so frequently depicted as having visual disabilities that required the use of spectacles.

Keywords: spectacles, imagery, sight loss, disability

In c. 1352, Tommaso da Modena produced a fresco for the chapter house of the Dominican monastery of San Nicolò in Treviso, Italy. In this image, Tommaso depicted forty renowned scholars, ecclesiastics, philosophers, and theologians of the Dominican order, including individuals such as Thomas Aquinas and Albertus Magnus. One of these men is the French cardinal Hugh de Saint-Cher (1200–1263) who is shown sitting at his desk writing, while surrounded by books (see Figure 6.1). He is dressed in cardinal's robes and is wearing a pair of rivet spectacles on his nose.[1] Initially, it does not seem unusual that Tommaso da Modena has depicted Hugh de Saint-Cher using spectacles. As a respected biblical commentator, Hugh would have spent long

1 Unlike the spectacles that we wear today, medieval rivet spectacles did not have 'arms' to go over the ears. Instead, they consisted of two framed lenses held together by a rivet. To use this kind of spectacles, the wearer had to either pinch them onto their nose or hold them up to their eyes by hand.

Grace-Petinos, Stephanie, Leah Pope Parker, and Alicia Spencer-Hall, eds. *Disability and Sanctity in the Middle Ages.* Taylor & Francis Group, 2025
DOI 10.5117/9789463724333_CH06

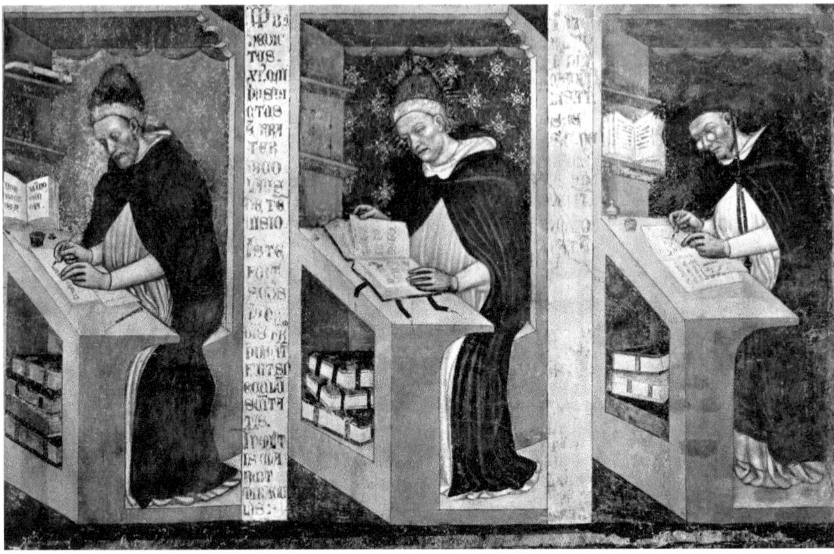

Figure 6.1: Hugh of St Cher (right), painted by Tommaso da Modena in a fresco, c. 1352. Image credit: Alamy.

hours reading, writing, and studying theology and, particularly in his later years, may very well have benefitted from the use of spectacles. However, Hugh de Saint-Cher died approximately twenty years before the invention of rivet spectacles. He would never have worn eyeglasses in his lifetime.[2] This raises an interesting question—if we can assume that Tommaso da Modena was interested in depictions of these figures as they were in life, why did he anachronistically represent Hugh de Saint-Cher as requiring spectacles?

For medieval image makers, spectacles provided an opportunity to make an individual's actions or character traits 'readable' upon their body. As David Hillman and Ulrika Maude explain, 'the body is notoriously difficult to theorize or pin down, because it is mutable, in perpetual flux, different from day to day and resistant to conceptual definition'.[3] This corporeal resistance to definition presented a challenge to medieval image makers

2 There are numerous examples of glass, water, and crystal being used as magnifying lenses prior to the medieval period—both within and beyond Europe. For example, as early as 65 CE, Seneca wrote that 'every object much exceeds its natural size when seen through water. Letters, however small and dim, are comparatively large and distinct when seen through a glass globe filled with water'—a theory that was built upon by Islamic scholars such as Hasan ibn al-Haytham in the eleventh century. See Seneca, *Naturales Quaestiones*, 1.6.5; Ibn al-Haytham, *Optics*. However, it was not until the 1280s that 'spectacles' as we might recognize them today—that is, two framed lenses designed to rest on the nose—appear in the historical record.

3 Hillman and Maude, 'Introduction', p. 1.

who were asked to represent elements of an individual's character, status, or life experiences through portraiture alone. To help viewers 'read' the bodies of the people depicted in their images, medieval artists relied on a network of visual 'signs' including objects, hairstyles, types of clothing, and certain colours to demonstrate the attributes of a particular individual. This concept of a visual 'sign' was coined by Ferdinand de Saussure (1857–1913) who suggested that a sign (defined as anything that communicates a meaning to the interpreter of the sign) is made up of two components: the signifier and the signified. The signifier consists of a sound, image, or word; whereas the signified is the concept associated with that sound, image, or word.[4] These two understandings come together to create a sign whose meaning is commonly understood within a particular time, place, and culture. Today, we engage with signs throughout the day without recognizing that we are doing so. We may, for example, encounter an image of skull and crossbones on a bottle of bleach (a signifier). Within popular consciousness, this image carries the meaning of 'danger to humans' (the signified). The signifier and signified then come together to create a sign, which indicates the contents of the bleach bottle may present a danger to people. St. Hugh's spectacles operate in much the same way.[5] It does not matter that Hugh could not have worn spectacles in his day-to-day life. Instead, they are included as a visual signifier that the monks who viewed the fresco would have been able to interpret and use to impose a stable interpretation on Hugh's otherwise mutable body. This chapter investigates why spectacles were used as visual signifiers in images of saints and holy figures, the meanings they carried as visual signs, and how they may have been 'read' by contemporary lay and monastic communities, with emphasis on images of the Four Evangelists. I argue that spectacles could visually signify both holiness and immorality in the iconography of late medieval Christianity, but the combination of spectacles with other signifiers, including scholarly activity and advanced age, assured viewers of instances in which they signified sanctity.

Scriptoria, Sight Loss, and Signs

In the years following the invention of spectacles in the 1280s, the main beneficiaries of this new technology were scholars and ecclesiastics whose

4 De Saussure, *Course in General Linguistics*, p. 68.

5 For a more expansive discussion of medieval iconography, see the essays in Liepe, ed., *The Locus of Meaning*.

professions required them to spend long hours bent over desks, reading and writing in dimly lit environments. The difficulty of this process is evidenced by scribes who complained about the long and uncomfortable nature of their work. For example, in a ninth-century copy of the Codex Theodosianus, one cleric included the following colophon:

> Oh, what weighty writing! It bends the back, makes the eyes foggy, and it breaks the stomach and ribs. And you Brother, who are reading this book, pray for Radulfo the cleric, God's servant, who wrote in the atrium of St Aignan.[6]

This short statement offers an insight into the pain and impairment experienced by the individuals who produced the texts that historians so heavily rely upon to access the Middle Ages.[7] Radulfo draws attention to the link between his work as a cleric and the physical suffering that the work causes him. He explains how writing for extended periods affected both his body and eyes, causing him such significant joint pain and eye strain that he requests all who read his work to pray for him specifically. If Radulfo only undertook this kind of work occasionally, his injuries would have been uncomfortable but brief. Having adequate time to rest between periods of writing would likely have helped to alleviate his symptoms. However, as a cleric, Radulfo was probably engaged in manuscript production on a regular basis—as Julia Barrow suggests, literacy was one of the defining features of the clergy.[8] By frequently putting his body under this kind of strain, Radulfo's acute impairments could have become chronic in nature.

6 'O quam grave pondus scriptura! Dorsum incurvat, oculos caliginem facit, ventrem et costas frangit. Et tu frater, qui legis istum librum, ora pro Radulfo clerico, famulo Dei, qui hoc scripsit in atrio Sancti Aniani'; Paris, Bibliothèque nationale de France, Latin 4415, fol. 111v. All manuscript translations and transcriptions, with scribal abbreviations silently expanded, are my own unless otherwise stated.

7 Such colophons and annotations are interesting examples of marginalized individuals speaking, quite literally, from the margins. The scribes and clerics who complained about their work-related pains and impairments at the edges of manuscripts both mirror and challenge the notion of disabled individuals operating on the edge of society. On the one hand, the voices of physically impaired individuals appearing 'on the edge' of a master text reflects their own marginal position within the dominant social structure. However, as Elaine Treharne expresses in relation to a colophon in the Lindisfarne Gospels, these scribal additions demonstrate a 'daring act that reflects the degree of ownership' that scribes and clerics felt over their work; Treharne, *Perceptions*, p. 92. The very fact that these scribes feel authorized to complain about their poor working conditions, and subsequent pains, provides a space for otherwise silent voices to be heard. In this sense, these colophons and annotations allow marginal figures to move into the more dominant discourse.

8 Barrow, *Clergy*, p. 170.

The development of early-onset vision impairments can also be caused by straining one's eyes in low light. Poor lighting conditions were a common problem in scriptoria—especially in the winter when the hours of natural light were limited. Florence Edler de Roover suggested that, 'Ordinarily, work by artificial light was not permitted [within a scriptorium] because of the greater possibility for errors or poor writing and the dangers of casualties to the costly books from grease and fire', and that subsequently scribes were only permitted to work during daylight hours.[9] That said, the number of scribal manuscript annotations that complain about writing at night or by low lamplight suggests that this rule was rarely followed. For example, in a ninth-century commentary on Cassiodorus's Psalms, a scribe included a marginal annotation in vernacular Irish, complaining that 'the light of the candle is not bright'.[10] Focusing on small, detailed work, for extended periods of time, in low or flickering lighting would likely have led to eyestrain, blurred vision, and ultimately hyperopia.[11] As Joy Hawkins suggests, 'the constant labour and poor light had a detrimental impact, and, as a result, many scribes would have suffered from poor sight'.[12] Based on the damaging effect of reading and writing in low light for extended periods of time, it makes sense that 'most of the accounts we have of [spectacle] use relate to churchmen and friars', as these would have been some of the most likely groups of people to develop hyperopia and to have subsequently purchased and used spectacles.[13] It is perhaps unsurprising, then, that many of the earliest visual representations of spectacles were commissioned and/or produced by the same group of people who initially benefitted from the technology. It was the Abbot who could approve the production of communal artworks in the monastery—such as Tommaso da Modena's Dominican fresco—while the monks and lay brothers were responsible for copying and illuminating manuscripts in the scriptoria, such as the Tilliot Hours and *Das Schachzabelbuch* (discussed below) in the scriptoriums. As such, these monastic image-makers played a significant role in the early development of spectacles as a visual sign.

9 Edler de Roover, 'Scriptorium', p. 605. One need only look to the Cotton Library Fire of 1731 or the Tre Kronor Palace Fire of 1697 to see the devastating impact of fire on medieval manuscripts.

10 'Nisorche suilse indítharni'; Laon, Bibliothèque municipale, MS 26, fol. 6v.

11 The development of long-sightedness as a result of detailed work in dim environments is still a problem today. In 2010, the American Optometric Association listed occupations that include 'near vision demands' as a common risk factor for hyperopia (long-sightedness). See American Optometric Association, *Optometric Clinical Practice Guideline*, p. 6.

12 Hawkins, 'The Blind in Later Medieval England', p. 116.

13 Kuulalia, *Childhood Disability*, p. 261.

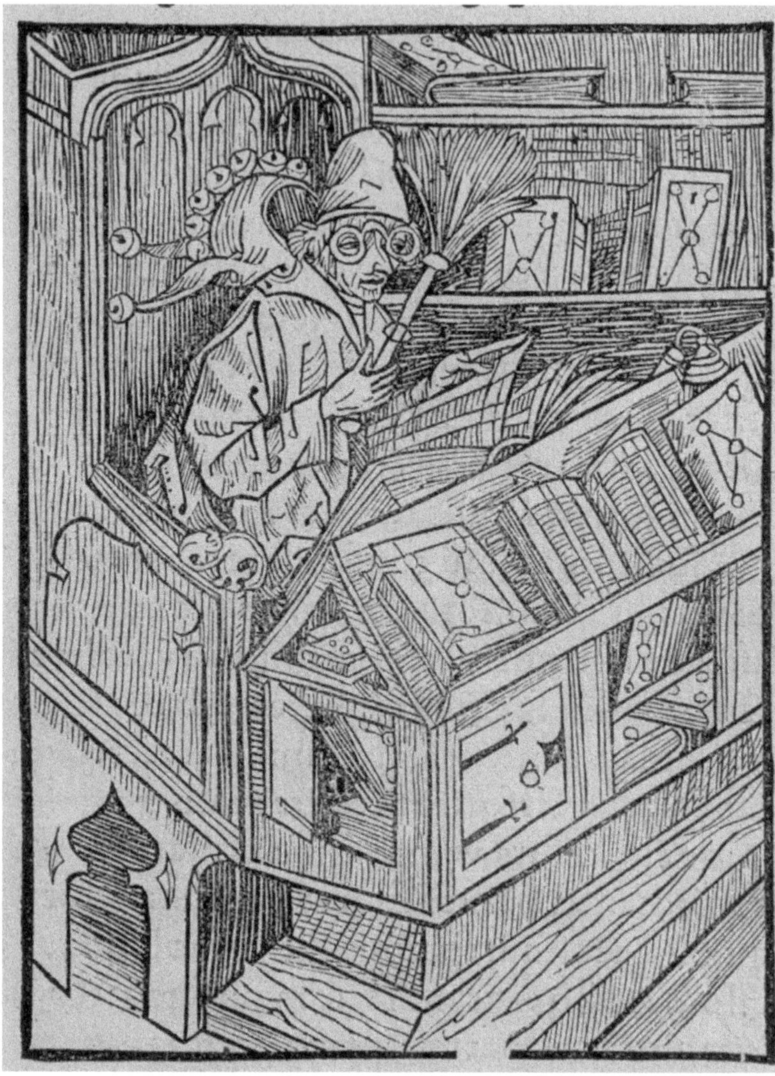

Figure 6.2: Haintz-Nar-Meister, illustration of *Das Narrenschiff* (Ship of Fools) by Sebastian Brant (Basel: Johann Bergmann, 1498). Special Collections, University of Houston Libraries.

Over the course of the Middle Ages, depictions of spectacles came to represent either of two things. On the one hand, in images of saints and respected religious figures, spectacles signified the 'venerable mark of wear of the eyes that read and reread the holy writings'.[14] On the other hand,

14 'Marque vénérable de usure des yeux qui ont lu et relu les écrits saints'; Margolin, 'Des lunettes et des hommes', p. 381.

when accompanying an image of someone exhibiting negative behaviours (such as getting drunk, gambling, or failing to pay attention in church) spectacles indicated that the wearer had spent too much time engaging in, or looking at, inappropriate things. An example of this is found in the second woodcut accompanying Sebastian Brant's *Das Narrenschiff* (Ship of Fools, see Figure 6.2).[15] In this image, a fool—indicated by his cap, decorated with bells and donkey-shaped 'ears'—sits at his desk surrounded by books. He peers into one of these books through a pair of rivet spectacles. The construction of this image is very similar to that of Hugh de Saint-Cher. Both images depict a man, surrounded by books, using spectacles to read or write at his desk. However, while we know that Hugh de Saint-Cher is engaged in 'appropriate' and pious activities, the fool is using his books to learn the Latin terms for 'inappropriate things'. In Brant's poem accompanying the woodcut, the fool says:

> Although my Latin isn't fine
> I know that 'vinum' stands for wine,
> 'Gucklus' a cuckold, 'stultus' fool,
> And I am 'doctor', that's my rule.[16]

Here, the fool admits that his knowledge of Latin is not very good. Despite that, he has prioritized learning the words for objects and activities that are connected to immoral behaviours; for example, 'wine' implying drunkenness, and 'cuckold' suggesting a man whose wife has been conducting an extra-marital affair. Unlike the image of Hugh de Saint-Cher, in which spectacles signify the wearer's engagement with holy teachings, the image of the fool demonstrates an interest in immoral or undesirable activities such as drinking or sexual affairs.

Following Saussure's definition of a sign, the spectacles in these images can be understood as the primary signifier, which, when combined with different secondary signifiers (i.e., the holy man and the fool) result in distinct interpretations. In the case of Hugh de Saint-Cher, spectacles (the primary signifier) signify reading, looking, and learning. However, as the person represented is a respected cardinal (the secondary signifier) the spectacles come to suggest that the wearer has been engaged in desirable Christian

15 Dürer, *Büchernarr* (woodcut), German, c. 1494; in Brant, *Das Narrenschiff*, Fool No. 1.

16 '[D]an ich gar wenig kan latin; / ich weiß, das vinum heißet win, / gucklus ein gouch, stultus ein dor / und das ich heiß domne doctor'. Brant, *Das Narrenschiff*, p. 64. Translation from Brant, *Ship of Fools*, trans. by Edwin H. Zeydel, p. 63.

behaviour. The overarching sign is that Hugh de Saint-Cher acquired his ocular impairment through the reading and production of holy materials. In the image of the fool, spectacles (the primary signifier) still signify reading, looking, and learning. However, the fact that the wearer of the spectacles is visually coded as a fool (the secondary signifier), the overarching sign is that the individual has acquired their ocular impairment through the pursuit of undesirable and potentially sinful activities.

In both the image of Hugh de Saint-Cher and the image of Brant's Fool, spectacles are applied as a visual signifier. However, the resulting sign conveyed to the viewer is dependent on their understanding of how an individual acquired an ocular impairment. The fool's eyesight is damaged through the pursuit of inappropriate knowledge—such as learning the Latin words for 'wine', 'cuckold', and 'fool'—whereas Hugh de Saint-Cher, as the biblical commentator responsible for directing the first revision of the Vulgate Bible, damaged his eyesight through the reading and rereading of holy texts. The fool's spectacles underscore his immorality, while Hugh's spectacles underscore his morality.

Bespectacled Saints

The visual tradition of depicting learned religious figures wearing spectacles developed quite quickly over the course of the fourteenth century, resulting in a wide range of saints being retrospectively depicted wearing spectacles, including St Peter, St Jerome, and St Ambrosius, to name but a few.[17] Unfortunately, there is neither the time nor space to discuss each individual or instance of spectacle use here. Instead, this chapter will consider the inclusion of spectacles in fourteenth- and early fifteenth-century representations of the Four Evangelists: SS Matthew, Mark, Luke, and John. As the men responsible for writing the Gospels included in the New Testament of the Bible, the representation of spectacles in images of

17 A clear example of St Peter wearing spectacles can be found at the bottom centre-left of the 'Twelve Apostles Altar' (produced 1466) at the church of St James, in Rothenberg. Similarly, an image of St Ambrosius wearing spectacles is currently held by the Belvedere Museum (Vienna, Belvedere, 4859), produced by the Master of Grossgmain, c. 1498. Images of St Jerome, on the other hand, are a little different. Although Jerome is very frequently shown with spectacles laid out on his desk—as depicted in Domenico Ghirlandaio's fresco painted for the Church of Ognissanti, Florence in 1480 or in the 1456 *Vie et miracles de Notre Dame* (Paris, Bibliothèque nationale de France, Français 9198, fol. 2r)—he is less frequently depicted as actively using his glasses.

the Evangelists demonstrates their prioritization of religious duties and scholarship over the needs of their physical bodies. Leaving aside St John for the moment, let us consider how St Matthew, St Mark, and St Luke are regularly represented wearing spectacles.

There are several privately commissioned religious manuscripts which contain one or more images of the Evangelists wearing spectacles. Eltjo Buringh defines these texts as 'books for personal devotion such as Book of Hours and prayer books' and explains how, despite beginning as a commodity exclusive to royal households, manuscripts 'eventually became virtually books for "everyone". That is, for everyone who was well off in the Middle Ages'.[18] A particularly good example of this kind of book is the Tilliot Hours, a French Book of Hours, illustrated by Jean Poyer, c. 1500.[19] This manuscript was produced after the advent of the printing press and consequently represents what Janet Backhouse refers to as one of the 'last decadent manifestations of a dying art'; it would have been an especially decadent commission given the availability of cheaper, printed alternatives.[20] Drawing on a sample of manuscripts housed in the Louvre, Carla Bozzolo and Ezio Ornato argue that the value of French manuscripts fell significantly in the fourteenth and fifteenth centuries on account of the financial difficulties posed by the Hundred Years War.[21] But that does not mean that manuscripts were 'cheap'. By the fifteenth century, an 'average' manuscript may cost around £2 5s (which would have the equivalent buying power of approximately US$2,319 as of May 2024).[22] Although the exact owner of the Tilliot Hours remains unknown, a manuscript such as this would have been commissioned by someone with access to significant personal wealth. The manuscript's calendar was also written for someone interested in the Franciscans and their feast days, which shows that the owner had some interest in or knowledge of the religious orders. Moreover, the primary language of the text is Latin, suggesting that the reader/s would have been familiar with the language.

In the Tilliot Hours, the Four Evangelists are depicted with their distinctive saintly attributes as they work on their gospels.[23] The images of the

18 Buringh, *Medieval Manuscript Production*, p. 128.

19 For an overview of the contents and image programme of Books of Hours, see the essay by Escobedo in the present volume, pp. 207–34.

20 Backhouse, 'Tilliot Hours', p. 211.

21 Bozzolo and Ornato, *Pour une histoire du livre manuscrit au Moyen Âge*, p. 25.

22 Buringh, *Medieval Manuscript Production*, p. 429.

23 London, British Library, Yates Thompson 5. For St Luke, see fol. 10; for St John, see fol. 9; for St Matthew, see fol. 11; for St Mark, see fol. 12. Throughout the Middle Ages (and still to this day) saints were commonly depicted with a defining 'attribute' so that individual saints could be

Evangelists are quite simple, showing only the saint, their gospel, and a single piece of scholarly apparatus. In the case of Matthew and Luke this scholarly equipment takes the form of a quill and in the case of Mark it is a pair of spectacles. While Matthew and Luke are presented as writing their gospels, neither are looking directly at their manuscripts. Instead, Matthew is cutting a quill and Luke is dipping his quill in an inkwell while looking up as though in thought. Mark is the only Evangelist actively involved in reading his gospel and is subsequently the only Evangelist depicted with spectacles. For this reason, the image of Mark could have been very easily 'read' within the broader context of medieval visual iconography. He wears spectacles to draw attention to his act of reading; his attribute identifies him as St Mark the Evangelist, allowing viewers to infer that his reading is an example of desirable Christian behaviour; and the two together allow the viewer/s to conclude that his visual impairment was acquired through moral means.

Some scholars have argued that, due to the magnifying function of spectacles, image-makers chose to include these devices in depictions of religious figures as a reference to the hymn known as the Magnificat, whose opening line states, 'My soul doth magnify the Lord'.[24] Stephen Hanley, for example, suggests that 'the tradition of depicting an apostle using spectacles to "magnify" text was a reference to the Virgin's supreme act of magnification as expressed in her canticle of joy'.[25] While a connection between spectacles and the Magnificat is possible, Hanley's interpretation presupposes a more thorough knowledge of liturgical hymns than some members of the laity might have had. For an individual to 'read' this visual metaphor they would need a very strong knowledge of both the scripture and canticles as well as a working knowledge of Latin. While it is likely that this connection would

quickly and easily recognized within visual material; much like spectacles, this attribute was a signifier that signposted the identity of a particular saint. Often, these attributes invoked elements of the saint's martyrdom, miracles, or broader hagiography. However, the devices which represent the Four Evangelists differ from these formats and instead represent the four-faced creatures from Ezekiel's Inaugural Vision. In this vision, Ezekiel describes witnessing four heavenly creatures residing in a flaming storm cloud. Each of these creatures had four faces: 'And as for the likeness of their faces: there was the face of a man, and the face of a lion on the right side of all the four: and the face of an ox, on the left side of all the four: and the face of an eagle over all the four.' (Ezekiel 1.10; Douay-Rheims Bible). Later, in his *Commentary on Matthew*, St Jerome attributes each of these 'faces' to the four gospels, suggesting that the face of a human man represented the Gospel of Matthew, that the lion represented the Gospel of Mark, that the ox (or calf) represented the Gospel of Luke, and the eagle represented the Gospel of John. See St Jerome, *Commentary on Matthew*, p. 55.

24 'Magnificat anima mea Dominum'; Luke 1.46–55 (Vulgate Bible; translation from the Douay-Rheims Bible).

25 Hanley, 'Optical Symbolism', p. 8.

have been clear to someone with a religious background and education in Latin (such as the owner of the Tilliot Hours), Hanley's suggestion does not account for the use of spectacles as a sign in images with a much broader lay audience.

One such image, for example, is the depiction of St Matthew on a fifteenth-century rood screen in St Agnes's Church, Cawston, England.[26] In this image, a balding and bearded St Matthew is depicted as reading from an open Bible in his hand, while holding a pair of rivet spectacles up to his face. St Matthew is part of a line-up of twenty influential saints depicted across the rood screen, facing into the nave, making him visible to members of the laity throughout church services. While it could be that the inclusion of spectacles in this image was intended to represent the Magnificat, it seems more likely that, given its location and audience, the portrait sought to demonstrate that St Matthew was so devout that he had damaged his vision through the noble pursuit of reading and writing of holy scripture, rather than through engagement in immoral or un-Christian activities. By rendering St Matthew's impairment legible through the inclusion of spectacles in the image, the portrait may have provided reassurance to individuals who were concerned about developing ocular impairments of their own.

The cause for this concern likely stemmed from contemporary understandings of ocular theory and the way in which this theory connected to religious practice and physical health. Throughout the Middle Ages it was accepted that the eyes emitted a substance known as 'visual spirit' that absorbed information about the objects it fell upon and returned this information back through the lens of the eye, to the brain. This theory built upon earlier Greek optics and was known as ocular 'emission' or 'extramission'.[27] As this visual spirit could carry external elements into the body and brain, any image seen could disturb the body's humoral equilibrium, for better or worse. Correspondingly, looking at beautiful or holy sights could have the opposite effect. By viewing religious imagery, a person could stimulate and strengthen both their physical body and their immortal soul.

Perhaps the most effective way to receive spiritual and physical healing through the act of looking was to witness the elevation of the Host during Mass.[28] As Edward Wheatley explains, 'the synodal statutes of Paris of

26 A 360-degree tour of St Agnes Church, which includes the painted rood screen, is available in Diocese of Norfolk, 'St Agnes, Cawston'.

27 For a more thorough overview of extramission theory and medieval optics, see Lindberg and Tachau, 'Science of Light and Color'.

28 Duffy, *Stripping of the Altars*, pp. 91, 101.

1205–8 mandated that the *elevatio* take place only after the bread was consecrated, so that the viewers would be looking not at bread but at the actual body of Christ'.[29] As the Host was believed to be the actual body of Christ, those who looked upon it would receive a form of humoral and spiritual cleansing and would have been protected by its blessing for the rest of the day. The benefits bestowed on those people who could witness the elevation of the Host were so important that several measures were implemented to make this possible. Some of these measures were legitimized by the Church; for instance, just before the event took place, a mass bell was rung to tell worshippers that they should look up from their prayers to see the moment of consecration. Similarly, it was not unusual for small holes called 'elevation squints' to be drilled into a church's rood screen at the height of a kneeling parishioner. These 'squints' allowed members of the congregation to look through the rood screen, bear witness to the elevation, and receive any associated physical or spiritual healing.[30]

Although the rood screen at the Church of St Agnes does not contain squints, its height is low, which allowed members of the laity to see over it while they were sitting or standing in the nave, but not when they were kneeling. As parishioners would have been encouraged to kneel for the elevation, they would only have been able to see the Host when the priest lifted it above his head and over the sightline imposed by the rood screen. Throughout the rest of the rite, kneeling parishioners would have found themselves face-to-face with the portraits of the saints depicted across the rood screen, including St Matthew wearing spectacles. The location of these portraits and their 'interactivity' in response to the physical movements associated with liturgical rites, would have provided viewers with an additional opportunity for spiritual reflection. The image of St Matthew wearing spectacles would have reminded members of the laity that visual disabilities need not be a barrier to faith at the very moment they were likely to have felt most concerned about this. Although sight loss or sight deterioration might prevent an individual from fully experiencing the elevation of the Host, these images demonstrated that, provided one's sight was weakened through their engagement in appropriate and pious activities, 'declining vision did not preclude them from having inner sight'.[31]

29 Wheatley, *Stumbling Blocks*, p. 15.

30 These elevation squints, also known as hagioscopes, still survive in many churches across Europe. For a more detailed discussion of hagioscopes, see Kemp, 'Out Past the Eye Mark'.

31 Hawkins, 'Seeing the Light', p. 156.

Another similarly reassuring image of an Evangelist depicted with spectacles is Maarten van Heemskerck's 'Saint Luke painting the Virgin and Child'. Completed in 1532, this image shows St Luke painting the Virgin Mary and the baby Jesus as, according to Christian tradition, Luke was believed to be the first painter of holy icons.[32] St Luke sits upon a carved block displaying his winged-ox attribute and wears a pair of rivet spectacles upon his nose. As stated in a note in the bottom left of the painting, Heemskerck produced this image for the Haarlem Painters' Guild Chapel in Saint Bravo, Haarlem, Netherlands, where it is referenced in the guild's archives as 'an altarpiece by Heemskerck'.[33] This is supported by the way in which Heemskerck has painted the image as though seen from a low viewpoint, suggesting that the image was hung above natural eye level over an altar.[34] Due to its location in the guild's chantry chapel, the primary audience for this image would have been members of the guild, comprising of a combination of painters, craftsmen, and members of associated trades (including paint-makers, engravers, and printers). Heemskerck's decision to paint St Luke with spectacles references the idea that Luke had developed long-sightedness because of extensive close work in the form of icon painting—a desirable Christian activity. This firmly positions the painting within the iconographic framework that spectacles, when worn by an individual engaged in desirable Christian behaviour, signifies an impairment that reflects morality, even holiness. As a result, this image would have been reassuring to the guild members who, as painters themselves, might also have experienced sight loss and have needed to wear spectacles. The image reminded painters that the production of Christian iconography was a noble pursuit and would have confirmed that any work-related impairments they developed as a result would be 'read' on their body in a positive way by their direct contemporaries.

However, not all the Evangelists were regularly depicted wearing spectacles. Although we frequently see Matthew, Mark, and Luke wearing spectacles, the same cannot be said for St John. Considering St John's reputation as the author of a gospel, Book of Revelation, and other books of the New Testament, coupled with the inclusion of spectacles in images of the other three Evangelists, it initially seems odd that the signifier of spectacles would not have also been applied to him. However, St John was already emmeshed in a complex web of visual signifiers that would have conflicted with the sign produced by spectacles. St John is regularly depicted in visual

32 See Bacci, *Il Pennello dell'Evangelista*.

33 'Een Autaarstuk door Heemskerk'; quoted in Taverne, 'Salomon de Bray', p. 62.

34 Images of the painting are available at Frans Hals Museum, 'Maarten van Heemskerck'.

source material as a youthful figure, who would not have been expected to use spectacles. As Sarah McNamer suggests, St John 'is always depicted without a beard; moreover, the artists call attention to his hair, portraying him with curly locks, often long and blond. These physical features have been interpreted in the scholarship as signs of John's youthfulness'.[35] The fact that St John is so frequently depicted with long curly hair, rosy cheeks, and without a beard, suggests that, in these images, he was not yet at the age of maturity, let alone of acquired long-sightedness.[36]

Medieval scientists, artists, and philosophers widely debated the ways in which the human lifecycle should be divided. However, as J. A. Burrow suggests, 'the physiological theory of the four ages of man [...] can claim to have provided the most powerful and the most influential of all attempts to explain scientifically the changes which human being go through in the course of their life'.[37] Allegedly, this division of the life course originated with Pythagoras, whom Diogenes Laetius claimed divided 'man's life into four quarters thus: "Twenty years a boy, twenty years a youth, twenty years a young man, twenty years an old man"'.[38] Building upon this sequence, Johannitus (whose *Isagoge* was translated into Latin at the end of the eleventh century) stated that:

> The ages are four, namely adolescence, maturity, old age, and decrepitude. Adolescence is of a hot and moist complexion, and in it the body grows and increases up to the twenty-fifth or thirtieth year. Maturity follows, which is hot and dry and preserves the body in perfection without any decrease in its powers; it ends in the thirty-fifth or fortieth year. After that follows old age, cold and dry, in which the body does indeed begin to lessen and diminish, but still without loss of power; it lasts until the fifty-fifth or sixtieth year. After that follows decrepitude, cold and moist through the gathering of the phlegmatic humour, during which a loss of power becomes evident; its years run to the end of life.[39]

35 McNamer, *Affective Meditation*, p. 143.

36 There are many examples of St John depicted according to these youthful tropes throughout the Middle Ages, from his image in the Lindisfarne Gospels in the eighth century (London, British Library, MS Cotton Nero D IV, fol. 209v) to representations in late medieval Books of Hours (see, for example, Paris, Bibliothèque Nationale de France, Latin 9474, fol. 16v; New York City, Morgan Library and Museum, MS M.1054, fol. 13r; The Hague, Koninklijke Bibliotheek, MS 74 G 28, fol. 13r).

37 Burrow, *Ages of Man*, p. 12.

38 Diogenes Laertius, *Lives of Eminent Philosophers*, 8.1, p. 329.

39 'Quattuor sunt etates, scilicet adolescentia, iuventus, senectus, et senium. Adolescentia complexionis videlicet calide et humide est, in qua crescit et augetur corpus usque ad 25

This work significantly influenced later Western scholarship pertaining to the lifecycle, coupled with Avicenna's *Canon*, which was translated into Latin at the end of the twelfth century, and divided the life course into Adolescence (birth to age thirty), the 'Age of Standing Still' (thirty to thirty-five or forty), the 'Age of Diminution' (thirty-five or forty to sixty), and the 'Age of Decrepitude' (over sixty).[40]

Following Johannitus and Avicenna, images of St John frequently depict him within the age of 'adolescence' and therefore below the age of thirty. Within Western medieval visual culture, the 'adolescent' period of life is usually marked by signifiers including blond hair and a clean-shaven face. 'Maturity' (or 'the Age of Standing Still') is marked by shorter hair and a beard. As spectacles were used as a visual signifier of a long career of pious reading and learning, St John cannot be known for both his youthfulness and the wearing of spectacles. Unlike the other Evangelists whose maturity aligns with the suggestion that they have spent many years reading or writing the holy scripture (to the point that their eyes had deteriorated), for St John the commonly understood reading of spectacles would contradict the signifier of youth.

In this way, age becomes another important visual signifier in the production of meaning. If a younger individual were to be presented with spectacles it may suggest that they had acquired their visual impairment through some means other than religious learning. This is depicted quite clearly in examples of 'fools' wearing spectacles. Although these later medieval fools—as seen in the woodcut accompanying Brant's 'First Fool' in the *Ship of Fools*—are not necessarily young, they are certainly more youthful than Matthew, Mark, and Luke, who are regularly depicted as white-haired, bearded, and aged. Unlike the elder Evangelists, whose ocular impairments demonstrate a lifelong commitment to the pursuit of religious learning, the inclusion of spectacles in images of fools who are visually coded as being in the 'adolescent' or 'mature' stages of life—rather than old age—suggests that they acquired their impairment through inappropriate means.

vel 30 perveniens annum. Hanc iuventus sequitur que calida est et sicca, perfectum sine diminutione virium corpus conservans, que 35 vel 40 anno nitur. Hinc succedit senectus, frigida et sicca, in qua quidem minui et decrescere corpus incipit, tamen virtus non decit, quinquagesimo quinto anno vel sexagesimo persistens. Huic succedit senium, collectione phlegmatis humoris frigidum et humidum, in quo virtutis apparet defectus, quod suos annos vite termino metitur'; *Isagoge Joannitii ad Tegni Galieni*, quoted and translated in Burrow, *Ages of Man*, p. 23.

40 Avicenna, *Canon*, bk I, fen i, doctr. 3, ch. 3.

Misbehaving Monks

Fools were not the only individuals for whom spectacles could be used as a visual signifier of inappropriate behaviour. Spectacles were also used in images to draw attention to religious individuals who are looking at, or participating in, things that are undesirable within the Christian worldview. In these instances, the individual's behaviour and associated ocular impairment demonstrates their distance from—rather than closeness to—God.

An example of this is depicted in a manuscript miniature located in a late fourteenth-century copy of Konrad von Ammenhausen's *Das Schachzabelbuch*.[41] This manuscript is a Middle High German verse translation of the *Liber de moribus hominum et officiis nobilum ac popularium super ludo scacchorum* (Book of the Customs of Men and the Duties of Nobles or the Book of Chess), a morality text written by Jacobus de Cessolis (c. 1250–c. 1322).[42] It was likely produced in the scriptorium of the monastery of Stein-am-Rhein, where Konrad von Ammenhausen lived and worked across the fourteenth century.[43] In this illustration, a tonsured and bespectacled monk is depicted playing dice with another man.[44] The monk's opponent represents a lower-status or unsavoury character: his hose are falling down, he has a hole in the toe of his left boot, and he is depicted with wild red hair and a red forked beard. These signifiers are anti-Semitic in nature and were frequently used in contemporary Western imagery to represent both Judas as an individual and Jewish people more broadly.[45] Engaging in gambling would have been against the monk's religious upbringing, as 'contemporary school texts and ecclesiastical rules t[old] young clerics to stay away from dice and malicious women'.[46] There is little doubt then that, by gambling with a roguish opponent, the monk depicted in *Das Schachzabelbuch* is focusing his attentions on the wrong kind of activity. As outlined towards the beginning of this chapter, monastic scribes and illuminators were integral to the early development of spectacles as a visual signifier. In this image, we see spectacles being combined with an individual engaged in undesirable behaviour. This changes the overall 'reading' of spectacles to

41 St Petersburg, National Library of Russia, NLR Germ. F.v. XIV.1.

42 Jacobus de Cessolis was an Italian Dominican friar who adopted chess as an allegory for the city, around which he composed this morality text. See Adams, *Power Play*; Luchitskaya, 'Chess as a Metaphor'.

43 National Library of Russia, 'Cultural Heritage of Europe'.

44 St Petersburg, National Library of Russia, NLR Germ. F.v. XIV.1., fol. 104v.

45 Boyarin, *The Christian Jew and the Unmarked Jewess*, pp. 87–88.

46 Warnar, 'Discovery', p. 70.

indicate the acquisition of an impairment through immoral means. As this manuscript is a morality text, originally written by a Dominican friar, it makes sense that the inclusion of spectacles was intended to render the monk's immorality as legible on his body—indicating that he should be applying himself to holy scripture, instead of a game of dice.

Another example of spectacles being used as a sign of immorality and bad Christian behaviour is depicted in a fourteenth-century French Psalter.[47] Much like the Tilliot Hours, this manuscript would have been commissioned by a wealthy member of the laity to facilitate their private worship. In this Psalter, an illuminated initial 'D' shows four tonsured monks reading from a prayer book in front of a cloth-covered altar. Whilst the three monks at the front of the group are looking at the text before them with scowls of concentration, the bespectacled monk at the back of the group is wistfully staring over his shoulder, away from the prayer book. The spectacles in this image thus critique their wearer's inappropriate behaviour. Unlike his pious brothers, who are actively engaged in reading the holy text in front of them, the bespectacled monk's mind and eyes have wandered away from his religious responsibilities. Spectacles are used in this image to demonstrate that the monk should be applying himself to the holy text, rather than idle daydreaming. It is also possible that this image served as a warning to the lay reader whose eyes had wandered away from the central text of the manuscript to focus, instead, upon the marginal illustrations. In this case, the monk's distraction actively mirrors the potential distraction of the reader, with his spectacles acting as a caution against misplaced attention.

Conclusion

Within medieval European image-making traditions, spectacles were a complex signifier whose meaning could shift and change depending on how they were combined with other signifiers. On the one hand, they could be combined with an individual engaging in desirable Christian behaviour to indicate the acquisition of impairment through moral means; on the other hand, they could be combined with signifiers of undesirable behaviour to condemn individuals who had spent too much time reading, looking at, or engaging with the wrong kinds of people and materials. As it was impossible for medieval people to determine how an individual had acquired a visual impairment, it was unclear whether the impairment resulted from moral and

47 Besançon, Bibliothèque municipale de Besançon, MS 0140, fol. 190r.

desirable Christian activities or from immoral and undesirable behaviours. Depictions of holy figures wearing spectacles helped clarify this ambiguity. These images made a more explicit connection between visual impairment and desirable Christian behaviour. By doing so, they stabilized the otherwise mutable and illegible bodies presented in medieval imagery.

Bibliography

Manuscripts

Besançon, Bibliothèque municipale de Besançon, MS 0140

The Hague, Koninklijke Bibliotheek, MS 74 G 28

Laon, Bibliothèque municipale, MS 26

London, British Library, MS Cotton Nero D IV

London, British Library, Yates Thompson 5

New York City, Morgan Library and Museum, MS M.1054

Paris, Bibliothèque nationale de France, Français 9198

Paris, Bibliothèque nationale de France, Latin 4415

Paris, Bibliothèque nationale de France, Latin 9474

Saint Petersburg, National Library of Russia, NLR Germ. F.v. XIV.1

Primary Sources

Avicenna, *Canon Medicinae* (Venice: Petrus Maufer de Maliferis et Socii, 1486)

Brant, Sebastian, *Das Narrenschiff* (Basel: Johann Bergmann von Olpe, 1494)

Brant, Sebastian, *The Ship of Fools*, trans. by Edwin H. Zeydel (New York: Dover, 1944)

Diocese of Norfolk, 'St Agnes, Cawston', Exploring Norfolk Churches <https://www.exploringnorfolkchurches.org/church/st-agnes-cawston/> [accessed 30 June 2024]

Diogenes Laertius, *Lives of Eminent Philosophers*, trans. by C. D. Yonge (London: Henry G. Bohn, 1853)

Frans Hals Museum, 'Maerten van Heemskerck', Frans Hals Museum <https://franshalsmuseum.nl/en/see-and-do/maarten-van-heemskerck> [accessed 12 August 2024]

Ghirlandaio, Domenico, 'Saint Jerome in his Study', 1480, Church of Ognissanti, Florence <https://www.wga.hu/html_m/g/ghirland/domenico/3fresco/1jerome.html> [accessed 17 August 2014]

Master of Grossgmain, 'Saint Ambrosius', 1498, Belvedere Museum (Vienna, Belvedere, 4859) <https://museums.eu/collection/object/239604/master-of-grogmain-st-ambrosius?pUnitId=358> [accessed 17 August 2024]

Herlin, Friedrich, 'Twelve Apostles Altar', 1466, Church of Saint James, Rothenberg, Bavaria <http://rothenburg-evangelisch.de/sites/www.rothenburgtauber-evangelisch.de/files/styles/max_1300x1300/public/media/img/bilder_manuskript_ballis_26.jpg?itok=m9wT9DSy> [accessed 17 August 2024]

Ibn al-Haytham, Hasan, *The Optics of Ibn Al-Haytham, Books I–III: On Direct Vision*, trans. by A. I. Sabra (London: Warburg Institute, University of London, 1989)

St Jerome, *Commentary on Matthew*, trans. by Thomas P. Scheck (Washington, DC: Catholic University of America Press, 2008)

Seneca, *Naturales Quaestiones*, trans. by John Clarke (Baltimore: Johns Hopkins University Press, 2004)

Secondary Sources

Adams, Jenny, *Power Play: The Literature and Politics of Chess in the Late Middle Ages* (Philadelphia: University of Pennsylvania Press, 2006)

American Optometric Association, *Optometric Clinical Practice Guideline: Care of the Patient with Presbyopia*, rev. by Nancy B. Carlson (St. Louis, MO: American Optometric Association, 2010)

Bacci, Michele, *Il Pennello dell'Evangelista: Storia delle immagini sacre attribuite a san Luca* (Pisa: GISEM-ETS, 1998)

Backhouse, Janet, 'The Tilliot Hours: Comparisons and Relationships', *British Library Journal*, 13 (1987), 211–31

Barrow, Julia, *The Clergy in the Medieval World: Secular Clerics, Their Families and Careers in North-Western Europe, c. 800–c. 1200* (Cambridge: Cambridge University Press, 2015)

Boyarin, Adrienne Williams, *The Christian Jew and the Unmarked Jewess: The Polemics of Sameness in Medieval English Anti-Judaism* (Philadelphia: University of Pennsylvania Press, 2021)

Bozzolo, Carla, and Ezio Ornato, *Pour une histoire du livre manuscrit au Moyen Âge: Trois essais de codicologie quantitative* (Paris: CNRS, 1980)

Buringh, Eltjo, *Medieval Manuscript Production in the Latin West: Explorations with a Global Database* (Leiden: Brill, 2010)

Burrow, J. A., *The Ages of Man: A Study in Medieval Writing and Thought* (Oxford: Clarendon Press, 1986)

Duffy, Eamon, *The Stripping of the Altars: Traditional Religion in England 1400–1580* (New Haven, CT: Yale University Press, 1992)

Edler de Roover, Florence, 'The Scriptorium', in *The Medieval Library*, ed. by James Westfall Thompson (Chicago: University of Chicago Press, 1939), pp. 594–612

Hanley, Stephen, 'Optical Symbolism as Optical Description: A Case Study of Canon van der Paele's Spectacles', *Journal of Historians of Netherlandish Art*, 1 (Winter 2009), 1–20

Hawkins, Joy, 'The Blind in Later Medieval England: Medical, Social and Religious Responses' (unpublished doctoral dissertation, University of East Anglia, 2011)

Hawkins, Joy, 'Seeing the Light', in *Saints and Sanctity*, ed. by Peter Clarke and Tony Claydon (Woodbridge, Suffolk: Boydell Press for the Ecclesiastical History Society, 2011), pp. 148–58

Hillman, David, and Ulrika Maude, 'Introduction', in *The Cambridge Companion to the Body in Literature*, ed. by David Hillman and Ulrika Maude (Cambridge: Cambridge University Press, 2015), pp. 1–9

Kemp, Emma, 'Out Past the Eye Mark', *X-tra: Contemporary Art Quarterly*, 2 (Spring/ Summer 2021), 116–29

Kuulalia, Jenni, *Childhood Disability and Social Integration in the Middle Ages: Constructions of Impairments in Thirteenth- and Fourteenth-Century Canonization Processes* (Turnhout: Brepols, 2016)

Liepe, Lena, ed., *The Locus of Meaning in Medieval Art: Iconography, Iconology, and Interpreting the Visual Imagery of the Middle Ages* (Kalamazoo, MI: Medieval Institute Publications, 2018)

Lindberg, David C., and Katherine H. Tachau, 'The Science of Light and Color, Seeing and Knowing', in *The Cambridge History of Science, Volume 2: Medieval Science*, ed. by David C. Lindberg and Michael H. Shank (Cambridge: Cambridge University Press, 2013), pp. 485–511

Luchitskaya, Svetlana, 'Chess as a Metaphor for Medieval Society', in *Saluting Aron Gurevich: Essays in History, Literature and Other Related Subjects*, ed. by Yelena Mazour-Matusevich and Alexandra Korros (Leiden: Brill, 2011), pp. 277–300

Margolin, Jean-Claude, 'Des lunettes et des hommes ou la satire des mal-voyants au XVIe siècle', *Annales: Économies, Sociétés, Civilisations*, 2 (1975), 375–93

McNamer, Sarah, *Affective Meditation and the Invention of Medieval Compassion* (Philadelphia: University of Pennsylvania Press, 2010)

National Library of Russia, 'Cultural Heritage of Europe in the Collections of the National Library of Russia: Switzerland', NLR Online Exhibitions <https://expositions.nlr.ru/eng/cult/switz.php> [accessed 30 April 2022]

Saussure, Ferdinand de, *Course in General Linguistics*, ed. by Charles Bally and Albert Sechehaye, trans. by Wade Baskin (New York: McGraw-Hill, 1966)

Taverne, E., 'Salomon de Bray and the Reorganization of the Haarlem Guild of Saint Luke in 1631', *Simiolus: Netherlands Quarterly for the History of Art*, 6 (1972–73), 50–69

Treharne, Elaine, *Perceptions of Medieval Manuscripts: The Phenomenal Book* (Oxford: Oxford University Press, 2021)

Warnar, Geert, 'The Discovery of the Dialogue in Dutch Medieval Literature: A Discourse for Meditation and Disputation', in *Meditatio—Refashioning the Self:*

Theory and Practice in Late Medieval and Ealy Modern Intellectual Culture, ed. by K. Enenkel and W. Melion (Leiden: Brill, 2011), 69–88

Wheatley, Edward, *Stumbling Blocks Before the Blind: Medieval Constructions of a Disability* (Ann Arbor: University of Michigan Press, 2010)

About the Author

Rachael Gillibrand is currently employed as a Lecturer in the Schools of English and History at the University of Leeds. Her research focusses on the ways that people have experienced, understood, and augmented their bodies throughout time, with a particular focus on the relationship between technology and the embodied experience.

Part II

Saints and the Disability Community

7. The Socio-Economic Value of Healing Miracles in the *Liber Miraculorum s. Fidis*

Elizabeth A. Wiedenheft

Abstract: This chapter discusses the relative socio-economic value of healings and punishment miracles as performed by St Foy at Conques. St Foy healed the dis-abled and impaired, and punished the able-bodied with physical disfigurements. After being healed, the formerly dis-abled were expected to direct their labour to outlets that contributed to the benefit of the saint, either through becoming a living relic, or donating directly to the community. Those who directed their work to their own economic benefit were punished. These miracles demonstrate the intersections between work and the power of the saint, and how this manifested the socio-economic value of the dis-abled and able-bodied in eleventh-century Aquitaine.

Keywords: St Foy, punishment, healing, labour, miracle, socio-economic

In the early eleventh century, a cleric in France recorded a story about a warrior named Raymond of Valières. Raymond had been wounded while putting down a rebellion on his lord's lands, and his wounds were said to be significant, causing his life to become a 'loathsome burden' (*plus tedio*) to his friends, who were forced to take care of him.[1] The cleric, Bernard of

An earlier version of this article was presented at the International Medieval Congress at Leeds in July 2015. I am grateful to the Hagiography Society for their helpful input during that session.

1 For the original text, see *Liber miraculorum sancte Fidis* (henceforth *Liber*), edited by Bouillet. Throughout, I use Pamela Sheingorn's English translation, *Book*. Sheingorn based her translation on Bouillet's edition, which was based on a manuscript now known as Bibliothèque Humaniste, MS lat. 22 (formerly Bibliothèque de la Ville MS lat. 95), fols 15r–104r, held at Sélestat in Alsace.

Grace-Petinos, Stephanie, Leah Pope Parker, and Alicia Spencer-Hall, eds. *Disability and Sanctity in the Middle Ages*. Taylor & Francis Group, 2025
DOI 10.5117/9789463724333_CH07

Angers, described the wounds in detail. Raymond's 'nose was cut in two about halfway down, his jaw was severed on one side and on the other almost cut off to the middle, and the root of his tongue was separated from his throat'.[2] Surprisingly, Raymond survived these wounds, and lived on for three more months, relying on others to take care of him. He communicated with them 'as best he could, in signs and by nodding his head' (*nutu quo posset, innueret*), and was fed by his companions who 'dripped thick liquids' (*distillarentur pinguia*) down his throat. Falling into a deep depression, he appealed to his local saint. St Foy appeared to him a dream and prayed over his body. When Raymond awoke, he was healed, and soon he travelled to see St Foy's relics for himself at their home in Conques, in order to give thanks.[3]

This healing was only one of many recorded by Bernard and the other compilers of the *Liber miraculorum s. Fidis*. The book chronicles the many miracles of St Foy, whose relics were housed at Conques in Aquitaine. The relics had been acquired (some said stolen) by the Conques community in 866, from a monastery at Agen, an event that was later recorded in a thrilling account.[4] By the time Bernard of Angers was invited to write a *miracula* (an account of the miracles performed by a saint) in 1013, St Foy had a large regional cult, and both he and the monks of her cult had a great desire to spread the news of the work the saint was undertaking. Bernard's contribution, written between 1013 and 1020, form the first two of the four books which comprise the completed *Liber*, while the final two books were compiled by a series of anonymous monks at Conques between 1020 and 1060.

This chapter examines the use of literary *topoi* in the *Liber miraculorum s. Fidis* to convey the socio-economic effects of long-term illness and disability in St Foy's healing and punishment miracles. Hagiographical records have been somewhat under-utilized in medieval disability studies, but they can offer some valuable insights.[5] Miracles have great utility because they form the fracture points in which liminal figures (e.g., the disabled) became

St Foy has also been the subject, either directly or indirectly, of numerous monographs and articles: see Ashley and Sheingorn, *Writing Faith*; Campbell, 'Sacrificial Spectacle'; Remensnyder, 'Legendary Treasure'; and Kao, 'Tomboyism'. For more information on the extant manuscripts, see *Book*, pp. 22–26. Quote from *Book*, p. 130; *Liber*, p. 112.

2 '[U]t nasus divisus per malarum medium, mandibularum quoque una in duo desecta, alteraque ad medium fere truncate, lingue etiam radical gutturi disjunctum, hiatum sub palpebris patefecissent in tautum immanem, ut divise faciei ossa horrerent pendula'. *Book*, p. 130; *Liber*, ii.7, p. 112.

3 *Book*, pp. 130–31; *Liber*, ii.7, p. 112.

4 See *Translatio metrica s. Fidis*.

5 For more on the use of hagiographical texts in disability studies, see Metzler, *Social History*, *Disability in Medieval Europe*, 'Disability in the Middle Ages'; Wheatley, *Stumbling Blocks*; Barasch, *Blindness*; and Porterfield, *Healing*.

able-bodied members of society (or, sometimes, vice-versa). In the same way that the disabled were liminal characters before being healed, so too was the set of relics that could not perform miracles. Not all relics healed supplicants, of course. But for those whose cult had installed them for the purpose of healing supplicants in exchange for donations, the saint who could not perform, or whose healings were ineffective, could be said to be disabled themselves. In the simplest terms, relics were valuable if they performed a large number of impressive miracles. Of course, a relic's value was influenced by other factors, including the number and relative commensurate value of 'competing' saints' cults nearby, the geographic position of the relics, and the ability of the cult to produce written or widespread oral accounts of miracles. These components combined to encourage pilgrimage to the saint's shrine and thereby increase donations.

The value of St Foy's relics was based on two things: their use-value (the ability to be used to perform miracles) and their exchange-value (the extrinsic structures that surrounded the relics). Use-value, being the amount of utility that the person consuming the commodity received from the object, and exchange-value (derived from the amount, usually in monetary terms, that can be exchanged in the market for the item) together make relics commodities. In this way, relics could be sold, bartered, traded, or gifted in the ecclesiastical and spiritual marketplace.[6] One of the best ways of establishing exchange-value was the production of written accounts such as the *Liber miraculorum s. Fidis*. Associated economic transactions, such as some of those mentioned in the *Liber*, including the donation of money or goods, allowed additional economic gains to be made by the community. The efforts of Bernard of Angers and his anonymous monk co-authors in building the exchange-value of the cult reinforced the use-value of the relics and the sanctity of St Foy.

This chapter examines healing miracles and their counterpart, punishment miracles, wherein St Foy would cause a disability or a long-term illness to appear in someone, and then heal them from their infirmities. Healings and punishment miracles, as presented in the *Liber*, had socio-economic consequences for those who were affected, manifesting attitudes towards long-term impairments or disabilities. Healings allowed those affected to return to work and reintegrate into society, and for the monastic community

6 See Marx, *Capital*; Hodges, 'Cosmology'; Pestell and Ulmschneider, *Markets*; and Geary, *Furta Sacra*. Some historians consider relics to be inalienable possessions; see Weiner, *Inalienable Possessions*; Theuws, 'Exchange'. Relics are in fact best defined as inalienable commodities: see Ferry, 'Inalienable Commodities'; Wiedenheft, 'Circulating Saints'.

at Conques to likewise define its place in society, either because the healed gave a gift in exchange, or because it allowed the monastery to acquire new lands and grow their patrimony. Punishment miracles also manifested exchanges that occurred between the disabled and the community at Conques, and like healing miracles, often ended with the cult of St Foy growing in esteem throughout the region. Examination of these miracles demonstrates that the monastic community at Conques consciously used the *topoi* of healing or creating disability and illness to create economic outcomes beneficial to their community, thereby increasing their wealth and improving their social power within the region.

Bernard of Angers and Healing the Disabled Social Body

Bernard of Angers was a highly educated cleric, having studied at Chartres under its abbot, Fulbert. By the time he visited Conques for the first time, he was the head of the cathedral school at Angers.[7] He was familiar with contemporary ideas about the ideal social structure for society, which, by the end of the eleventh century, was embodied as a tripartite. Adalbero of Laon's formulation, which Jacques Le Goff dated to the years 1025–1027, labelled the three components of this social body as the *oratores* (those who pray), *bellatores* (those who fight), and *laboratores* (those who work).[8] Bernard of Angers had a similar conception of the idealized social body, which I would term the *able* social body. The ideal society was one in which all three parts—*oratores, bellatores*, and *laboratores*—were performing their duties optimally. Those who did not perform in coordination with their role and the roles of others, whether this miscoordination was caused by a disability, a long-term illness, or an impairment, or by choosing a role that was outside the tripartite structure, remained liminal figures who were outside the able social body. They could be called the *disabled* social body.

The relative economic impact of a person's disability depended on their specific impairment and the degree to which it influenced their capacity to perform their presumptive social functions, understood here as their utility. To be distinct, disability was socially constructed in the medieval period. Disability (and long-term illnesses that resulted in disability) were differentiated from impairments, which did not necessarily prevent inclusion in the social body. There are therefore examples in St Foy's *miracula* wherein a disability

7 *Book*, p. 24.

8 Le Goff, *Time*, p. 54; see Adalbero of Laon, 'Carmen'.

for one is 'merely' an impairment for another. The consequences of the two could be quite different depending on the social role of the individual, and the ideal version of their work. The ideal performed utility of the *oratores*, for example, was expanded in Bernard's view from simply those who prayed to include roles such as that of the scholar, theologian, or those who laboured to support the monastic or clerical community.[9] Consequently, disability among the religious in the *Liber miraculorum s. Fidis* would include anything that impacted their ability to think or pray, including an illness that rendered them unconscious, 'dumb' (*mutus*), or mute. *Bellatores*, or those who fight, were meant to devote their work to protecting the innocent, including the *oratores* and *laboratores*; their ability to do so was impeded by disabilities including 'lameness' (*debilis*), a wound, or mental health issues including depression. Finally, the *laboratores* functioned as the roots that allowed the other parts of society to flourish, by providing sustenance and other goods necessary for life; most commonly in the *Liber miraculorum s. Fidis*, their utility was compromised by 'lameness', blindness, or by being struck mute or deaf.

In the first two books of the *Liber*, Bernard of Angers paints a vivid picture of the ways in which disabilities and long-term impairments impacted the economic and social standing of the individual. In his proto-ethnographer style, Bernard was careful to make a record of the ways in which those who received a miraculous healing had suffered from their impairments, and how it had impacted their lives and ability to perform their functions within society. The story of one young girl, whose information was given to Bernard after her miraculous healing while the relics of St Foy were on procession to Molompize, is a good example of the saint's healing powers. The girl had been born blind, deaf, mute, and lame, with her fingers 'perpetually closed into fists' (*cui etiam perpetui pugni, digitis in palma adhesis, inerant*).[10] She had previously been cured of the defects of her mouth, eyes, and ears, but was left with the 'birth defect of her fists' (*pugnis tantum in nativo vitio relictis*), which made her unable to open her hands.[11] Meeting the relics at Molompize, she prayed before the image of the saint. She cried out that her 'hands [were] still curled up and useless' and urged the saint: 'Bring it about that they may also perform their proper function from now on'.[12]

9 Ashley and Sheingorn, *Writing Faith*, pp. 22–45.

10 *Book*, pp. 123–24; *Liber*, ii.4, pp. 100–04.

11 Ibid.

12 'Sancte Fides, olim michi visum, auditum eloquiumque reddidisti, quod si vere fecisti, adde etiam, precor, ut et manus que hactenus inutiles contracteque fuerunt, amodo proprium expleant officium.' *Book*, pp. 123–24; *Liber*, p. 103.

Once healed, Bernard wrote that her hands 'that had been inflexible and not suited for work were unbound and reshaped by the highest Craftsman'.[13] The episode, with its emphasis on how the 'birth defect' (*nativo vitio*) made her 'useless' (*inutilis*) and unable to 'perform their proper function' (*amodo proprium expleant officium*) affected her, was significant for both the young girl, who was readmitted to society in her ability to perform her proper function, and for St Foy and her cult, because of the public and expressive nature of the miracle which would have allowed the news to spread throughout the region. The healed body is here a commodity itself, wherein the utility of the girl, devoted to St Foy now, is on display for a regional audience, and being exchanged for goodwill and donations to the community.

Molompize was a territory of the monastery at Conques, and the purpose of the relics' procession was, according to Bernard, 'to lay claim to the property for the use and sustenance of the abbey' (*ut ad usus supplementumque illud abbatie pervaderent*).[14] The use of such tours to claim lands was well established by this point. It is significant that at Molompize Bernard chose miracles that demonstrated the liminality of those with disabilities, and furthermore, miracles that demonstrated the utility of the person after their healing. The young girl, who complains of her useless hands, links the concept of utility to disability. Utility, or the lack of it, defined this miraculous healing; only once the healed were useful again could they rejoin the social body. In addition, once healed, the young woman is described again as 'reformed' (*reformationis*) and with her hands restored to their 'proper function' (*proprium expleant officium*). St Foy's utility is demonstrated by healing those who need her help, and in this way, these socially liminal figures are central to her ability to do her work.

Utility, however, had to be directed in the correct way—a person, once healed, had to use their healing to perform what was socially determined to be their proper function. If they did not, then their healings could easily be reversed. Thus it is that Bernard saves his strongest emotions (and denigrating comments) for those persons who failed in this regard, those who subverted their position as a healed person in order to 'take advantage' of others, and those who adopted roles outside the three orders. This is confirmed by Kathleen Ashley and Pamela Sheingorn, who write that 'in his social thinking, Bernard accepts the scheme of functional roles prevalent in his era [...] Bernard understands the roles of peasants, warriors and clergy

13 '[U]ltro illi pugni paulatim se erigentes, digitis per successionem singillatim micantibus, inflexibiles manus operique [in]habiles, summon fabricante opifice, resolute suat.' Ibid.

14 *Liber*, p. 100.

in society, but has no place for the entrepreneur or the money economy'.[15] Those who failed to conform to the three orders were punished by St Foy for their subversion. This starts with the first miracle that Bernard recorded in his *Liber*. It was St Foy's most famous miracle, the one that had established her cult and resulted in an abundance of donations: the healing of Guibert 'the Illuminated', an event that was said to have occurred in 983.[16] Guibert had been enucleated after submitting to a lustful relationship with his lord's wife. Thereafter, he began to work as a jongleur, at which he was apparently quite successful. In this sense, Guibert was impaired—but not professionally disabled—by his blindness; able to work as a jongleur, and a successful one at that, did not deny him a place in the social body.

It was, however, the enjoyment of monetary wealth that doomed Guibert. St Foy appeared to him in his sleep a year after he had been blinded, and instructed him to buy her two candles and to bring them to her shrine at Conques. When he asked Foy as to how he would afford the candles (a questionable assertion given his apparent success as a jongleur), Guibert was told to ask for alms outside the church. When Guibert went to Conques and begged for alms outside the church, as instructed, he received enough money to buy the requisite candles to facilitate his own successful healing. Yet this only provided him with another scheme to increase his own income. After St Foy had healed him, he returned to Conques, and stationed himself as a competitor to the monastic community outside the entrance, where he petitioned the crowds of pilgrims for donations.[17] The abbot at Conques, Arladus, granted Guibert leave to sell wax in addition to giving him a place to live, although it seems likely that Arladus imagined that Guibert would donate a good portion of his earnings to the church in exchange for his continuing good health. As a living witness to the power of St Foy, he could be understood as a living 'secondary' relic; like contact relics, he manifested the power of St Foy to others outside her shrine. It was likely understood by the community, therefore, that like other relics, he would bring his donations to them to use for the benefit of the community. According to Bernard, however, Guibert 'received much profit' (*unde cum multiplicem questum coegisset*) from this business venture and 'began [...] to grow arrogant' (*cepit* [...] *insolescere*). Profaning his miraculous healing with an 'unchaste woman' (*incestam mulierem*) he was punished by St Foy, and blinded in one eye; later, after slipping into sin again, he was blinded in the other eye. Only after he embraced his role as a living relic, and after

15 Ashley and Sheingorn, *Writing Faith*, p. 48.

16 *Book*, p. 10.

17 *Book*, pp. 49–50; *Liber*, i.1, pp. 6–15.

he became a monk, he was once again healed, but as an old man he lived in destitution, surviving 'on the common dole provided by the brothers' (*nunc fratrum publica alitur alimouia*).[18] Guibert's blindness, while nominally caused by his lust and unchaste behaviour, was deeply related to his lust for wealth and his greed. This explains why he required multiple healings, and why the saint punished him with blindness in the end. Only by performing his proper function (i.e., acting as a witness to his healing and living a good life impoverished and relying on charity as a member of the deserving poor) could he rejoin the able social body.

Greed is an overarching theme in the *Liber miraculorum s. Fidis*. The community at Conques felt threatened by their neighbours, who wanted to usurp their lands and who undermined the power of their saint and her cult. Written in the midst of the Peace of God movement, wherein clerics and monastics waged a spiritual fight against the castellans who were not fulfilling their idealized duties in protecting the other sections of society, it is unsurprising that Bernard and his compatriots believed that there was a crisis in society.[19] Bernard addressed this threat in his second miracle, presenting another man healed of blindness called Gerbert. Gerbert was a 'mounted warrior' (*milicie vitam redire*) who was prevented from returning to his former occupation after he was healed by the saint, who insisted he become a monk.[20] Both Guibert and Gerbert were punished for their attempts at using their healed bodies to make money, whether this was by presenting themselves for donations at the entrance to the monastery and thereby taking advantage of the pilgrim trade that travelled through the gates daily, or by attempting to return to their former life as a greedy castellan. Only by adopting lives of poverty or by joining the monastery could the two men fulfil their potential and keep their healed bodies. Only Raymond, the vassal of Peter, 'a cleric from Auvergne' (*ex Avernia clericum*), is healed from his massive facial trauma and retains his healing. It seems that by suppressing the rebellion on Peter's lands, Raymond reinforced his status as a 'good' castellan, protecting the lands and vassals of his lord and thereby the lands of the church.

Bernard includes more examples of those who were punished by St Foy, or who had their miraculous healings reversed, for adopting social roles that he believed subverted traditional norms. In one example, Bernard writes

18 Ibid.

19 For more on the Peace of God, see Nugent, 'Ritual Illness'; and Head and Landes, *Peace of God*.

20 This she does through advice given to Gerbert by Theotberg, the wife of Count Pons, 'that if he ever wished to become well, he should not abandon Sainte Foy nor refuse the yoke of her service'. *Book*, pp. 54–55; *Liber*, i.2, pp. 16–21.

about a 'poor girl who had been crippled in all her joints and had been carried to Sainte Foy's monastery' (*pauper puella, que emnium membrorum compage debilitate, in monasterium sancte Fidis fuerat allata*), where she was healed.[21] She subsequently began to work as a weaver in a nearby town. One day, the relics of St Foy were carried through the town in a procession, and 'according to the custom there all the people rushed out of their houses and fell prostrate before the image' (*cunctique de more, de propriis ediculis prosilientes, obviam ei procidererent*).[22] The girl refused to stop working, 'as if she were deeply devoted to her work' (*velut pro nimio operis studio*)—more likely, she was paid piecemeal for her work, and therefore would earn less if she stopped to watch the procession. St Foy punished her for her disobedience, making her muscles contract quickly—so quickly, in fact, that 'she didn't have the strength to let go of the tools of her loom—the very shuttle was held fast in her clenched fist'.[23] Only after following the saint's relics back to Conques and keeping vigil there for several nights was she healed again.[24] This was a common form of punishment in *miraculae*. Individuals would be punished for the failure to stop working in order to pay homage to the saint. The punishment that followed, of the symbolic fusing of the hand to the work tool, would be lifted once the supplicant recognized their transgression and prayed for forgiveness, after which the hand and the tool were separated and the supplicant would be healed. As a tradesperson, the girl in this miracle sought monetary rewards, and this devotion to money surpassed her devotion to the saint; she therefore deserved to be punished. Like Guibert and Gerbert, only by repenting of this monetary wealth by going to Conques on pilgrimage could she be healed.

Similarly, Bernard records the punishment of a merchant, 'an inhabitant of Auvergne' (*Arvernensis pagi incola*), who went on pilgrimage to Conques before noticing, like Guibert had before him, that 'there was a very brisk trade in wax' (*facillimum cere commertium*).[25] He sensed an opportunity for profit, and in Bernard's conception of his thoughts, sounds much like a modern businessman:

> 'What an easy profit! How stupid I am! If I had learned this before, I could have put my business on a sound footing and made myself rich! But now

21 *Book*, pp. 80–81; *Liber*, i.15, pp. 50–51.

22 Ibid.

23 '[N]ec tele utensilia abicere valens, cui ipse stricto pugno radiolus inherebat.' *Liber*, p. 51.

24 Ibid.

25 *Book*, pp. 91–92; *Liber*, i.24, p. 63.

> I'll make up for my ignorance! Frequent trips to and from Conques will make me a wealthy man in no time! It's time to act like a man and get this business underway.'[26]

He bought a 'great quantity of wax' (*plurima cere pondera diligentissime taxat*) for ten gold coins and believed his profit would be 'at least four times what he had paid for the wax' (*minimo sese vel quadruplum lucratarum*). St Foy punished him for his greed, however. He had put the wax into sacks, but one candle did not fit into the bags. This taper suddenly caught fire and began to burn his clothes, then his beard, and the hair on his head. On fire, the merchant ran to the shrine of St Foy, and as he dumped the wax before the saint's relics, the fire vanished. Unsurprisingly, 'he didn't complain about the loss of the money as long as he had escaped from torment' (*neque homo queritur de damno pecunie, dummodo a tormento potuit evadere*). Bernard summarizes the punishment with a moralizing tone: 'I don't think I would offend anyone by asserting that Sainte Foy's goodness is praiseworthy and marvellous also for this: that to prevent vile commerce from weakening her pilgrims, she punished greed and avarice'.[27]

In the first two books of the *Liber miraculorum s. Fidis*, Bernard of Angers places emphasis on the sins of greed, lust, and theft. Those who partake in mercantile activities, like the unnamed merchant trying to make a fortune on wax, and the young weaver girl, are subjected to punishment by St Foy for their actions. Similarly, those who take advantage of the pilgrims, like Guibert, or who use their positions for financial gain, like Guibert and Gerbert, are also penalized. They are also being punished for being liminal figures, outside the normal roles of the social body. Their choices of work, as tradespeople, merchants, jongleurs, and warriors, are outside the ideal structure. St Foy first punishes these characters, but then heals them, bringing them across the social boundary and back into the social fold. In this way, healing miracles are used as a tool by Bernard to promote the cult of St Foy throughout the region. The choice of merchants, tradespeople, and castellans—all groups of people who took money and kept it for themselves in the growing proto-capitalist economy—as the figures deserving of

26 'Quam facili questu, si hec stultus rescivissem, divitem me potuissem facere, ac meam rem constabilire! Sed quod hactenus ignorantia distulit, hoc ammodo pervigil recursus, frequensque repetiti itineris reditus brevi temporis spacio perficiet. Accingar ergo viriliter, reique exordium aggrediar.' Ibid.

27 'Hic ita gestis, nequaquam offendere putaverim, si bonitatem sancte Fidis laudabilem mirabilemque in hoc quoque predico, quod ne commercii vilitas deficeret peregrinis, improhibitatem avaricie castigavit.' Ibid.

punishment is significant. Only by joining the deserving poor and living off charity, or by directly devoting their work to the church, do these men and women deserve their healings. The healing miracle therefore functions as a promotional tool for the community, marking their saint, and their cult, as particularly powerful in the region through its ability to solicit more donations and gain further wealth (and land) for their community. Miracles were also a method of social control for those who adopted the wrong attitude or social role after being healed. This, for Bernard, emphasized the transactional nature of St Foy's miracles. For Bernard, healing miracles were an essential tool both in combatting sins, but also in surviving within the growing monetary economy.

Healing Miracles and Economic Gains at Conques after Bernard of Angers

The final two sections of the *Liber miraculorum s. Fidis* were written by a succession of monks from the Conques community who remain anonymous. The third book was likely written by a single author who had access to Bernard's notes, shortly after Bernard's death between 1020 and 1050, but more likely closer to 1020.[28] The fourth book, according to Pamela Sheingorn, was written closer to 1050 and was composed by several authors.[29] The monk-authors of the second half of the *Liber* were, like Bernard, concerned with those who 'steal goods from God's holy Church, or those who appropriate, as if it were legally their own, property that the saints have inherited, and unjustly claim the rents and services due its owners'.[30] The miraculous *topoi* of this section focus on the economic resources available to Conques and their efforts to increase these resources by increasing the exchange-value of their saint's relics. Healing miracles occur during processions to the monastery's extended land holdings and are therefore focused on the acquisition of new lands or the protection of the existing patrimony of the saint.

Economic gains could be substantial and did not always take the form of grants of land. One castellan was named Bernard, who lived at Valèilles. He defended his town against a pack of robbers and was injured in this effort with a lance that stabbed him in the centre of his eye. The wound

28 *Book*, p. 25; Frédéric de Gournay thought closer to 1020: see *Étude*, p. 398.

29 *Book*, p. 25.

30 '[I]llos vero qui sancta Dei ecclesie bona violenter diripiunt, vel sanctorum hereditates quasi jus suum reposcentes injuste ablatas possident perterrefaciat.' *Book*, pp. 70–73; *Liber*, i.11, p. 38.

became infected, and he promised St Foy a gold ring and a gold coin if she would heal him, which she did.[31] In Auvergne, she healed another 'brave warrior' (*eques* [...] *magnanimus*) named Bernard, who was from Gransoux. Returning from a pilgrimage to Rome, Bernard 'suffered a serious physical illness' that caused him to go bald (*gravi egritudinis molestia vexabatur*).[32] While he was ill, the other castellans began stealing his lands. After appealing to St Foy, he had three visions of the saint, and finally his mother helped him to travel to the monastery at Conques. While praying at St Foy's shrine, Bernard was healed, and he went back to his home at Valèilles to retrieve his lost lands. The granting of gold or wax in exchange for healings (which Bernard does not do) were solid economic gains for the Conques community, but healings could also function to increase their socio-economic power in softer ways. These healings functioned to extend the patrimony of the cult, creating landholders such as Bernard who were loyal to St Foy and thereby increasing the chances that the lands (or additional goods) would be donated to the community.

Alternatively, St Foy could punish those who tried to steal her goods, and it was often neighbouring castellans who felt the saint's wrath after encroaching on the monastery's lands. The anonymous monk-author of the third book records direct attacks against the encroachments of monastic lands, including their land at Molompize. There, a lord named Robert attacked the monk-guardian of the monastery's lands, but was 'repulsed by peasants and servants and he took flight with all his men' (*rusticorum atque servicatium obpugnatione victus, terga vertit cum suis omnibus*).[33] Incensed, Robert came back during the night, and while breaking into the house through the back door, was struck blind. After fleeing, his men found him, and 'his entire body had been stricken and his mouth was wrenched back toward one ear' (*quem toto corpore dampnatum oreque ad aurem retort factum obscenum*), forcing his men to carry him home on a litter. He was carried to the church at Molompize and spent a week praying there. Healed by St Foy through these efforts, he then travelled for three days on pilgrimage to Conques, and made peace with the monk-guardian of Molompize.[34]

The anonymous monk-author of part three of the *Liber* also featured the punishment of those castellans who made direct attempts to steal lands from

31 *Liber*, iii.3; *Book*, pp. 147–48.

32 *Book*, pp. 153–54; *Liber*, iii.7, p. 139.

33 *Book*, pp. 158–59; *Liber*, iii.10, p. 146.

34 Ibid.

the monastery. In Quercy, an unnamed noblewoman 'obsessively coveted the holy martyr's lands that adjoined her own fields' (*terram sancta martiris agris suis vicinam immoderate concupivit*).[35] She harassed the peasants working the fields, and after driving them off the land, 'arranged to have this field plowed with her own plowshare, and she dared to make it part of her own property'.[36] Upon doing so, 'her whole body shrivelled instantly and she croaked and hissed horribly' (*actutum toto corpore emarcuit, ac sic horrificus strideribus garriens*) before she died. Terrified, her peasants left the monastery's fields, so that 'after she was destroyed in this way, the holy martyr's land was henceforth safe from all who had designs on it and remained afterwards the property of the monks'.[37] The offence of the noblewoman, in taking the saint's lands, directly brought about her own death, and this 'miracle', with no mention of the opportunity for repentance or healing, would have served as a strict warning to those who desired to take property that belonged to the saint and her community.

Similarly, a man named Siger who lived at Conques 'stole everything he could from the holy martyr's property' and harassed 'her monks with vile insults, and he mutilated the men who worked on their lands' (*omnia quecumque poterat a ditione sancta martiris subripiebat, hominesque ejus membris diminuebat*).[38] In response, the monks brought out the saint's reliquary. The man was struck with an illness and subsequently died, as did his four sons. Likewise, two of the man's three daughters were also punished, one by paralysis, the second with 'a disease that caused swelling and sores' (*elephantine morbo ulcerosa pena dampnatur crudelissima*). Finally, his castle was struck down by a strong wind.[39] Siger's sins, in stealing from the monastery, harassing St Foy's peasants, and mutilating them, meant that his punishment had to be much harsher than that meted out to others: hence the destruction of his entire dynasty, his home, and his family.

The anonymous authors of the second half of the *Liber miraculorum s. Fidis* were highly concerned about the monastery's territories and patrimony. It seems that their aim in producing this part of the book was, in part, to identify their territories and remind readers (especially those in neighbouring monasteries or neighbouring castellans) that these lands

35 *Book*, pp. 165–66; *Liber*, iii.16, p. 156.

36 'Sequenti vero die proprio vomere en jugera sulcare fecit, sueque dicioni ea subjugare presumpsit.' *Liber*, p. 156.

37 'Qua tali modo extincta, terra sancta martiris tuta ab omnibus remansit, et in monachorum postea ditione jacuit.' Ibid.

38 *Book*, pp. 166–67; *Liber*, iii.17, p. 137.

39 *Book*, pp. 166–67; *Liber*, iii.17, p. 138.

were protected by St Foy. Thus the use of healing miracles, or the disabling, killing, or striking down of the offender with an illness that only the saint could cure, marked out St Foy's cult as a powerful and protective landowner. Many of the monastery's extended holdings are mentioned in the *Liber*; alongside lands at Molompize and in Quercy, they also held lands at Millau (approximately 100 km away from Conques), where the monks brought the relics of St Foy on procession.[40] Here, while conducting an outdoor service in a field, the monks were faced with a man named Lambert, who 'threw insulting abuse upon God's saint' (*suaque ec* [...] *avitia in sanctam Dei objectans*) and refused to display 'appropriate deference' (*dignaque obseqaia exhibentes*).[41] His son was struck down by St Foy, although when the baby's mother left him under the relics, the baby was healed.[42] Other miracles took place on somewhat distant territories of the monastery. In one village, 'above the torrent called Bromme in Rouergue' (*Rutenico in territorio, super torrentem Brogma*; likely Brommes in Mur-de-Barrez, which lies above the Bromme river in the Aveyron) there was a church dedicated to St Foy.[43] At the village, there was a seven-year-old girl, 'paralyzed from her waist to her feet' (*ab umbilico ad pedes usque premortuam*). She was carried by her father 'on a horse-drawn pallet' (*in equeo grabato*) to the shrine inside the small church (which presumably held secondary relics of St Foy) where she was healed in front of a large crowd.[44] In the *Liber*'s fourth book, St Foy healed a young man named William who was paralyzed with 'his left hand curved backward and permanently clinging to the side of his body. He could neither raise it to his mouth nor use it for any purpose'; he was healed at Calonge, where there was a church dedicated to St Foy (nearly 200 km away from Conques and close to Agen, where St Foy's relics were originally buried).[45] She also healed a man named Raymond of epilepsy, who was from Montpezat near Cahors (a distance of approximately 100 km, or a twenty-four-hour walk from Conques), although the healing took place at her shrine at Conques, and a young girl who was carried from Cayssac to Conques (an eight- or nine-hour walk in the best of conditions).[46] These healings at Conques emphasized that for those who

40 *Book*, pp. 169–71; *Liber*, iii.20.

41 *Book*, p. 169; *Liber*, iii.20, p. 161.

42 *Book*, pp. 169–71; *Liber*, iii.20.

43 *Book*, p. 173; *Liber*, iii.22, p. 165. Brommes is approximately twelve hours' walk from Conques.

44 Ibid.

45 '[P]aralisi percussus, sinistram manum a latere cui recurve inextricabiliter inherebat, neque ad os ducere, neque ad aliquod officium poterat convertere.' *Book*, p. 189; *Liber*, iv.6, p. 184.

46 *Liber*, iv.8; *Book*, p. 194; *Liber*, iv.12; *Book*, p. 200.

needed them, Conques (and consequently St Foy's tomb) was a worthy site for a miraculous intervention.

These miracles were performative and spectacular, designed to be witnessed by great crowds. This is emphasized by one of the authors of the fourth book, who wrote of the loud exclamations surrounding the healing of a young blind boy at Conques. The young boy received support from the monastery for the remainder of his lifetime, presumably receiving alms from the community in exchange for being a physical memorial and witness to his healing.[47] The great crowds were an integral part of the process of touring relics as it was practised by the monks of St Foy's cult. The display of St Foy's ability, manifested through the healed body of the young boy, made a spectacle of the disabled body. This spectacle was then replicated or discussed throughout the Auvergne and beyond. As the monks moved the relics of St Foy around the region, they were effectively sacralizing the trail and the land around them, differentiating it from the surrounding space. This was a territorializing process, one that created not only a common identity, but also a sense that the places where the relics had been and the trail that they had taken were essentially sacred and special; this allowed the people in the area to orient themselves and their communal identity around those places, even if temporarily. While the relics created a locus for devotion, they also increased the amount of power the relics had regionally. Thus, while we can point out specific places that were sanctified by the presence of the relics, these tours had the effect of bringing the entire region under the patrimony of St Foy.

Conclusion

Healing miracles as recorded in the *Liber miraculorum s. Fidis* not only underscored the value of being healed for the disabled or those suffering from a long-term illness, but also highlighted the value of healing relics for the monastic community. In portraying the disabled person as outside the able social body, the authors emphasized that utility was established by their ability to contribute to society. This utility was not formed by the straightforward labour/pay exchange, but instead through the display of the healed body as a sign of St Foy's holiness, bringing consequent fame and monetary gains for the community at Conques. Thus, healings had a real socio-economic value to those that were healed, in making them

47 *Liber*, iv.3; *Book*, pp. 183–84; *Liber*, pp. 178–79.

able-bodied and reintegrating them into the social fold. This utility, however, had to be directed towards their ideal role in society; those who chose work as merchants, tradespeople, or sought monetary gains after their healings, had their healings reversed by St Foy. These healing miracles in particular mark this as a choice between remaining a liminal figure, outside the idealized social structure, or reintegrating into the social fold by directing one's energies towards the Church. The authors who recorded these miracles, especially Bernard of Angers, thereby manipulated the *topoi* of disabilities, long-term illnesses, and their healing by St Foy, to promote their cult within the region. The healing miracles that St Foy performed established the utility of her own relics and promoted them throughout the region, leading to commensurate economic gains for the monastic community. Bernard and his co-authors made every effort to produce a valuable product for consumption by the pilgrims who visited the shrine, or who saw it while it was on tour to their area. In so doing, they used healing miracles as a means to establish their relics as a high-value commodity within the region, and as a consequence reaped concrete socio-economic gains including lands, monetary wealth, and luxury goods.

Abbreviations

AASS	*Acta Sanctorum*
BHL	Bibliotheca Hagiographica Latina

Bibliography

Manuscripts

Liber miraculorum sancte Fidis, Sélestat, Bibliothèque Humaniste, MS lat. 22 (formerly Bibliothèque de la Ville, MS lat. 95), fols 15r–104r

Primary Sources

Adalbero of Laon, 'Carmen ad Rotbertum regem', poem II, in *Poème au roi Robert*, ed. by Claude Carozzi (Paris: Les Belle Lettres, 1979), pp. 295–96

The Book of Sainte Foy, trans. by Pamela Sheingorn (Philadelphia: University of Pennsylvania Press, 1995)

Liber miraculorum sancte Fidis, publié d'après le manuscrit de la Bibliothèque de Schlestadt avec une introduction et des notes par M. l'abbé A. Bouillet, ed. by

Auguste Bouillet (Paris: Alphonse Picard et Fils, 1897; repr. Paris: Hachette Livre BnF, 2012)

Translatio metrica s. Fidis virg. et mart. ad monasterium conchacense [BHL 2941], AASS, October III, pp. 289–94

Secondary Sources

Ashley, Kathleen, and Pamela Sheingorn, *Writing Faith: Text, Sign and History in the Miracles of Sainte Foy* (Chicago: University of Chicago Press, 1999)

Barasch, Moshe, *Blindness: The History of a Mental Image in Western Thought* (New York: Routledge, 2001)

Campbell, Emma, 'Sacrificial Spectacle and Interpassive Vision in the Anglo-Norman Life of Saint Faith', in *Troubled Vision: Gender, Sexuality and Sight in Medieval Text and Image*, ed. by Emma Campbell and Robert Mills (London: Palgrave Macmillan, 2004), pp. 97–115

Ferry, Elizabeth, 'Inalienable Commodities: The Production and Circulation of Silver and Patrimony in a Mexican Mining Cooperative', *Cultural Anthropology*, 17.3 (2002), 331–58

Geary, Patrick, *Furta Sacra: Thefts of Relics in the Central Middle Ages* (Princeton, NJ: Princeton University Press, 1978)

Gournay, Frédéric, *Étude du Cartulaire de l'abbaye de Conques (actes postérieurs à 1030)*, 2 vols (unpublished master's thesis, Université de Toulouse–Le Mirail, 1988)

Head, Thomas, and Richard Landes, eds, *The Peace of God: Social Violence and Religious Response in France around the Year 1000* (Ithaca, NY: Cornell University Press, 1992)

Hodges, Richard, 'The Cosmology of the Early Medieval Emporia?', *Archaeological Dialogues*, 10.2 (2004), 138–44

Kao, Wan-Chuan, 'The Tomboyism of Faith: Spiritual Tomboyism in the Cult of Sainte Foy', *Journal of Lesbian Studies*, 15.4 (2011), 412–49

Le Goff, Jacques, *Time, Work and Culture in the Middle Ages*, trans. by Arthur Goldhammer (Chicago: University of Chicago Press, 1980)

Marx, Karl, *Capital*, vol. 1 (London: Penguin, 2004)

Metzler, Irina, *Disability in Medieval Europe: Thinking about Physical Impairment during the High Middle Ages, c. 1100–1400* (New York: Routledge, 2006)

Metzler, Irina, 'Disability in the Middle Ages: Impairment at the Intersection of Historical Inquiry and Disability Studies', *History Compass*, 9.1 (2001), 45–60

Metzler, Irina, *A Social History of Disability in the Middle Ages: Cultural Considerations of Physical Impairment* (London: Routledge, 2013)

Nugent, Patrick, 'Ritual Illness and Ritual Healing: Miracle Stories and the Peace of God in Eleventh-Century Europe' (unpublished doctoral dissertation, University of Chicago, 1999)

Pestell, Tim, and Katharina Ulmschneider, *Markets in Early Medieval Europe: Trading and Productive Sites, 650–850* (Macclesfield: Windgather Press, 2003)
Porterfield, Amanda, *Healing in the History of Christianity* (Oxford: Oxford University Press, 2005)
Remensnyder, Amy, 'Legendary Treasure at Conques: Reliquaries and Imaginative Memory', *Speculum*, 71.4 (1996), 884–906
Theuws, Frans, 'Exchange, Religion, Identity and Central Places in the Early Middle Ages', *Archaeological Dialogues*, 10.2 (2004), 121–38
Weiner, Annette, *Inalienable Possessions: The Paradox of Keeping-While-Giving* (Berkeley: University of California Press, 1992)
Wheatley, Edward, *Stumbling Blocks before the Blind: Medieval Constructions of a Disability* (Ann Arbor: University of Michigan Press, 2010)
Wiedenheft, Elizabeth, 'Circulating Saints: A Study of the Movement of Corporeal Relics in Three Regions of Western Europe, c. 800–1200' (unpublished doctoral dissertation, University of Nottingham, 2017)

About the Author

Elizabeth A. Wiedenheft received her BA in History and the Study of Religion from the University of Northern Iowa in 2011, her MA in History from the University of Connecticut in 2013, and her PhD in Medieval History at the University of Nottingham in 2017. Her thesis, 'Circulating Saints: A Study of the Movement of Corporeal Relics in Three Regions of Western Europe, c. 800–1200', examined the socio-economic benefits of moving saints' relics in France, England, and Flanders in the High Middle Ages. She is interested in the medieval economy and its impact on religious behaviour, including popular devotional practices, the economics of saints' cults, and the intersections between trade networks and ecclesiastical communities. Dr Wiedenheft is now an independent researcher.

8. Disability and Healing Touch in Representations of the Midwife with the Withered Hands in Late Medieval Books of Hours

Libby Karlinger Escobedo

Abstract: The addition of the doubting midwife Salome to scenes of the nativity in late medieval French Books of Hours provides an opportunity to examine the perception of disability, piety, and faith among the owners of these books. Salome doubted Mary's ability to maintain her virginity after giving birth and insisted upon examining her. As a result of her lack of faith, Salome's hands withered when she touched Mary, only to be miraculously healed when she touched the Christ Child. Through a study of the iconography of the doubting midwife and its role in personal prayer books, this chapter explores ideas about disability, divine punishment and miraculous healing, and the changing professional, social, and medical contexts that might prompt the appearance of Salome in this particular place and time.

Keywords: leprosy, midwife, nativity, Salome, withered

In the Middle Ages, non-normative bodies were often linked to sin, a concept that can be traced to Old Testament stories in which God meted out physical punishment.[1] At the same time, miraculous healing, often

1 Old Testament physical punishments sent by God include disability, deformity, and disease. For example, God sends a pestilence to the Israelites in 2 Samuel 24; he sends bears to maul disrespectful children in 2 Kings 2; and the men of Sodom are blinded in Genesis 19. See also Exodus 4, 1 Kings 13, Psalm 38, and Zechariah 11. Leviticus 26 also references physical punishments handed down by God, as well as barring people with non-normative embodiments like blemishes, blindness, lameness, or scurvy from entering God's temples (Leviticus 21). Apocryphal

Grace-Petinos, Stephanie, Leah Pope Parker, and Alicia Spencer-Hall, eds. *Disability and Sanctity in the Middle Ages.* Taylor & Francis Group, 2025
DOI 10.5117/9789463724333_CH08

through the medium of touch, features prominently in the New Testament and medieval saints' lives.[2] The physical body, therefore, carried particular spiritual and philosophical meaning in the Middle Ages.[3] Moreover, Ephraim Shoham-Steiner comments that the biblical book of Leviticus is explicit in its requirement that priests be unblemished, which reflects the 'fundamental view that wholeness is a prerequisite for holiness'.[4] While this requirement was not enforced for Christian clergy in the Middle Ages, there was a distinction made between able-bodied individuals capable of work and individuals without capacity and thus unable to work.[5] The interrelationships between divine punishment, disability, touch, and miracles are represented in some late medieval images of the Nativity. In addition to the usual cast of characters and animals, these images sometimes include one or more midwives, one of whom doubted the possibility of a virgin birth. The midwife insisted upon examining Mary, but when she did so, her hands withered.[6] This acquired disability was represented as a direct result of her lack of faith. Upon touching the Christ Child with her withered hands, the midwife's hands are restored to their previous state, thus embodying the concept of the miraculous cure through touch. The appearance of the midwife in the text and images of late medieval Books of Hours suggests a shift in attitudes about physical embodiments of the

texts contain more such stories. Particularly interesting for the purposes of this essay is the story of Jephonias. At the deathbed of the Virgin, Jephonias doubts that Mary is the mother of God. When he touches her bier, his hands are cut off with a sword of flame wielded by an angel. Recognizing his error, he begs forgiveness and proclaims his faith. His hands are then restored to his body. See St John the Theologian, 'Book of John', p. 591. Biblical references throughout this chapter are taken from the Douay-Rheims 1899 American Edition.

2 For example, Jesus cures lepers by touch in Matthew 8.3 and heals a bleeding woman and revives a child through touch in Mark 5. St Francis, who lived vainly until the Lord corrected him with sickness, cured a man's lame leg with his touch. See Jacobus de Voragine, *Golden Legend*, pp. 606–16.

3 Pearman, *Women and Disability*, p. 1. See also Spencer-Hall, 'Chronic Pain and Illness'; and Skinner, *Living with Disfigurement*.

4 Shoham-Steiner, *On the Margins*, p. 142.

5 Stiker, *History of Disability*, p. 85. See also Dubourg, *Disabled Clerics*.

6 For the sake of consistency, the term 'withered' will be used throughout, since that is the description given in the textual sources; see, for example, Jacobus de Voragine, *Golden Legend*, p. 38. The term 'withered' was also adopted as the descriptor for this iconography by subsequent scholars and later the Index of Medieval Art, though 'withered' hands can appear variously in visual sources as missing, shrunken, or misshapen. The midwife story appears in several versions, from apocrypha to popular sermons, with varying details. For example, sometimes it is one hand that is damaged, rather than two, or the healing results specifically from touching the garments of the Christ Child, rather than his body. For a summary of various iterations, see Swann, '"By Expresse Experiment"', pp. 2–5.

sacred that corresponds to larger social and cultural changes; this essay argues that such a shift reflects the increasing professionalization and masculinization of medical practice, a rise in literacy and access to books, particularly Books of Hours, and greater emphasis on the suffering of the body in popular piety.

The story of the midwife with the withered hands—usually identified by the name Salome, sometimes written Zelomi—sometimes seems to have been conflated with that of St Anastasia, a handless girl Joseph brought to the stable to tend to Mary and her newborn, whereupon her missing hands were miraculously restored by touching the Christ Child. While the midwife story seems to conflate several different women and girls found in saints' lives and pseudo-Gospels—not just Anastasia's *vita*—the core elements of disability removed through faith and physical touch remain consistent and highlight the ways medieval audiences viewed links between sin, faith, disability, and healing. Just as sin could be punished with physical ailments, miraculous healing was seen as a sign of faith, worthiness, and God's mercy.

While images of the Nativity are a standard feature of Books of Hours from the early fourteenth century onwards, the addition of the midwives to that visual narrative (and with them the story of the withered hands) does not appear until a century later. The iconography is not entirely new, however, and has a long history in other media and locales.[7] The addition of these elements to the visual tradition of the Nativity in late medieval Books of Hours produced in northern France and its environs corresponds to the expanded availability of prayer books to a wider and more diverse audience, the same audience that engaged with mystery plays, sermons, and other events we might think of as popular culture. These Books of Hours illustrate shifts in the perception of sanctity, disfigurement, and divine punishment in a post-plague, war-torn Europe experiencing the nascent professionalization of medicine. This chapter will begin with a description of late medieval Books of Hours and patterns of book ownership (since Books of Hours are both highly personalized and illustrative of late medieval piety), before examining the iconography of the midwife with the withered hands and placing it in a broader historical and social context. Finally, this

7 A manuscript of the *Evangelica historia* in the Ambrosiana Library, MS L. 58 Sup., has a sequence of images on fols 2v–4r showing Salome's story. She is shown arriving after the birth; with her hand withered and hanging limply; touching the Christ Child with the hand returned to normal; and preaching to a group of women. British Library, Additional MS 47682 (the Holkham Bible Picture Book) has a nativity scene that shows a midwife holding the Christ Child, with a disembodied hand dangling by her side, on fol. 12v. For textual sources, see *Canonical Histories*, pp. 2–4, and Jacobus de Voragine, *Golden Legend*, p. 38.

chapter will link the iconography of the midwife to shifts in popular piety that placed greater emphasis on physical experience and the trend towards professionalization, and masculinization, of medical practice occurring at this particular time and place.

An Introduction to Books of Hours

The Nativity was a standard subject in the sequence of images associated with the Hours of the Virgin in late medieval Books of Hours throughout Western Europe. The contents and overall iconography remained virtually unchanged and the Book of Hours remained the standard book of popular devotion right to the end of the Middle Ages, even after the advent of printing.[8] The standard text featured the Office of the Virgin Mary, a set of psalms, scriptural readings, and hymns to be said at each of the eight canonical hours—Matins, Lauds, Prime, Terce, Sext, None, Vespers, and Compline—throughout the day. In many examples, each of the eight hours was marked by a miniature with a predictable sequence of images from the infancy of Christ, including the Nativity for the hour of Prime, or somewhat less frequently, a sequence of images from the Passion.[9] In addition to the Office of the Virgin Mary, a Book of Hours typically contained a calendar that recorded feasts and saints' days, which could be personalized to a user's individual devotions and were usually illustrated with the occupations of the months and/or the signs of the Western zodiac. Books of Hours might also contain the Hours of the Holy Spirit and the Cross; the seven Penitential Psalms; the Office of the Dead; various prayers, such as the *Obsecro te* and *O intemerata*; and suffrages to saints. Decoration in the form of miniatures, borders, and initials could be found throughout. The

8 Backhouse, *Books of Hours*, p. 3. The Office of the Virgin, originally said by the clergy, became increasingly popular among the laity in the late twelfth and early thirteenth centuries. Early on, the text was bound with a Psalter. By the mid-thirteenth century, Books of Hours were appearing as independent manuscripts, and their popularity continued to grow throughout the Middle Ages. Guillaume Fichet, a member of the Collège de Sorbonne of the University of Paris, co-founded the first printing press in France in 1470 for the purpose of printing the works of the Italian humanists, particularly Petrarch. Printing presses had been established in Lyon by 1473, and in around twenty other French cities by 1500; see Bridge, *History of France*, pp. 238–40.

9 Matins is typically illustrated with the Annunciation; Lauds with the Visitation; Prime with the Nativity; Terce with the Annuciation to the Shepherds; Sext with the Adoration of the Magi; None with the Presentation in the Temple; Vespers with the Flight into Egypt; and Compline with the Coronation of the Virgin. See Harthan, *Book of Hours* for an excellent account of this category of prayer books.

extent of the decoration was largely determined by the wealth and status of the book's owner; generally speaking, the more heavily decorated and personalized a book was, the more it would cost.

Books of Hours are unique among late medieval manuscripts in that they were owned by people from all but the poorest sectors of society. As John Harthan writes, 'Books of Hours were the vehicle of both intellectual Christianity at its loftiest and of popular devotion on the most primitive level'.[10] While a Book of Hours might be just one of the dozens of books owned by a bishop or nobleman, a merchant or craftsman frequently owned just one book, and that book was nearly always a Book of Hours, as Albert Labarre's study of book ownership in early sixteenth-century Amiens has demonstrated.[11] His findings and conclusions are likely an accurate reflection of book ownership trends in the late Middle Ages within the larger context of northern France, including places like Rouen and Paris. Many of the book owners in Labarre's study were members of the middle class: merchants, shopkeepers, craftsmen, and artisans, many of whom owned just one or two books, nearly always a Book of Hours.[12] The Books of Hours created for this middle-class, lower end of the market differ markedly from those produced for the elite. While elite manuscripts were often highly personalized commissions from artists working with the newest artistic ideas coming from Renaissance Italy, middle-class books tend to be more conservative and formulaic, closely following established iconographic expectations. These Hours are also much more numerous, and their sheer number constitutes a substantial segment of the artistic output of French illuminators in the fifteenth and early sixteenth centuries. And because they were produced in large numbers for ordinary people, they reflect late medieval popular piety and social norms.

Books of Hours, particularly these mid-range examples, are the most numerous of manuscripts to survive from late medieval France. A manuscript from the Pierpont Morgan Library in New York (MS M.220) is typical of these 'near mass-produced' Books of Hours.[13] The predominantly Latin text of

10 Harthan, *Books of Hours*, p. 31.

11 Refer to Labarre, *Le Livre*.

12 Labarre, *Le Livre*, p. 105. About nine hundred of the more than four thousand inventories examined by Labarre mentioned books. Books of Hours were the most widely owned books, representing approximately thirty per cent of the identifiable books; of the 764 Books of Hours listed in the inventories, 282 were the only book a particular individual owned (for summaries of Labarre's findings, see lists in *Le Livre*, pp. 139–42). See also Chartier, *Cultural Uses of Print*, pp. 147–50.

13 Harthan, *Books of Hours*, p. 22.

the 111-folio manuscript includes the Hours of the Virgin, intercalated with the Hours of the Cross and the Hours of the Holy Spirit; a calendar; gospel sequences; the seven Penitential Psalms and litany; and the Office of the Dead. The manuscript also includes the Fifteen Joys of the Virgin, in French rather than in Latin like the rest of the text. The book was intended for a woman; she is depicted in a donor portrait on fol. 104v, where she kneels before the Virgin Mary and Christ Child at the start of the text of the Fifteen Joys. This is one of fifteen large miniatures, attributed to a follower of the Master of the Rouen Échevinage, a leading illuminator in Rouen in the mid-fifteenth century. His work made a profound impression on manuscript illumination in Rouen throughout the second half of the fifteenth century and well into the sixteenth.[14] The first miniature, on fol. 13r, marks the start of the gospel sequences and depicts the four evangelists. The next ten miniatures accompany the Hours of the Virgin, Cross, and Holy Spirit. Following the Hours of the Virgin are the seven Penitential Psalms, with a miniature of King David praying before God on fol. 66r. The iconography and compositions of these miniatures are consistent with most other examples of this type of manuscript. Produced for what has been characterized as the 'middle range' of the market, Morgan MS M.220, and the many other manuscript Books of Hours like it, are notable for several reasons. First, the number in which they survive attests to their popularity and marketability, even after printing became commonplace in France in the late fifteenth century. Second, these manuscripts show remarkable consistency in their iconography. In fact, it can be difficult to precisely date these manuscripts because there is such consistency over the period from about 1425 to 1525. Therefore, as visual documents of a particular time and place, these middle-range Books of Hours clearly reflect the popular culture of late medieval northern France.

Standard Iconography in Books of Hours

The iconography of the middle-range Rouen Books of Hours is consistent in part because Books of Hours contained a standard group of scenes, mostly from the life of Christ and the Virgin Mary. With such standardized requirements, the illuminators quite naturally repeated the same compositions over and over. Such a practice had several advantages: it saved time, since

14 For a discussion of the Master of the Rouen Échevinage, see Rabel, 'Artiste et clientele', pp. 48–60.

there was no need to imagine and execute a new composition; and illuminators of lesser skill or experience could execute adequate copies of a fixed composition, so that the master of a workshop was free to work on other, possibly *de luxe* or custom projects, that were therefore more lucrative. The repetitive compositions indicate that the standard miniatures of a Book of Hours were copied using an available manuscript as a model, or from pattern books or other exempla available in the workshops. In fact, there seems to have been an entire community of artists working from the same patterns or models.[15] No other practice fully accounts for the homogeneity of the miniatures over such an extended period of time and it is known that pattern books were used by illuminators.[16] While the pattern books certainly must have contained entire scenes, they probably also included examples of kneeling figures, drapery, and other illustrative motifs that could be incorporated into a variety of different scenes.

A comparison of representations of the Annunciation to the Virgin Mary illustrates this consistency. Many surviving examples are based on the style and compositions of the Master of the Rouen Échevinage; the original models for these illustrations date to the first half of the fifteenth century, such as the Annunciation by the Master of Sir John Fastolf in the so-called Porter Hours (New York, Morgan Library, MS M.105, fol. 19r), dated 1420–1425. The Virgin Mary, kneeling at a draped prie-dieu, with her arms crossed on her breast, turns to face the archangel Gabriel, kneeling before her; their dialogue appears on scrolls. The scene takes place in a room reminiscent of a church, with its dome and turret visible beside God in the arch at the top of the miniature. Many of these same features appear at mid-century in a miniature by the Talbot Master (New York, Morgan Library, MS M.202, fol. 38r); here Mary and Gabriel again kneel in an ornate room, though they face each other directly and Mary's hands are raised. Gabriel's announcement to her is recorded on a scroll held in his right hand. By the last third of the century, certain of these iconographic features, most

15 Watson, *Playfair Hours*, p. 54.

16 Harthan, *Books of Hours*, p. 23. A famous example of a pattern book is the Göttingen Model Book (Kunsthistorisches Museum, Vienna Kunstkammer, KK 5003, KK 5004), dated to the fifteenth century, which contains written instructions as well as painted examples. The model book consists of fourteen small wooden panels that fold up accordion-style to fit into a leather case; each panel is divided into quadrants, each containing a sample head depicting a person or animal. As the catalogue accompanying the Metropolitan Museum's exhibition 'Prague, the Crown of Bohemia' notes, '[d]espite the artist's virtuosity, evident in the artful variation of hairstyles and beards, and skillful observation of nature, particularly in the portraits, the types left relatively little room for individuality'; Boehm and Fajt, *Prague*, p. 275.

notably the scroll indicating Gabriel's speech, Mary's position with a book at a prie-dieu, and the architectural setting, have been adopted by the producers of the middle-range Books of Hours, where they are reproduced again and again with remarkable consistency.[17] Overall, these miniatures show a startling similarity, and this faithfulness to the model continues in subsequent decades.

This consistency of composition appears in other miniatures in Rouen manuscripts, for example in representations of the Nativity.[18] Mary and Joseph kneel flanking the Christ Child, with their hands joined in prayer. Mary is on the left, Joseph on the right. The Christ Child is nude, laying on the ground and emanating rays. Just to the background are one to three angels, kneeling with their hands joined, witnessing the scene, which takes place in or before a shed, frequently with a single hole in the roof.[19] Rowan Watson, in his work on the Playfair Hours, remarks on a similar consistency in the calendar illustrations.[20]

For middle-range Books of Hours it would seem that innovative style or iconography was simply not necessary; rather, the preference seems to have been for a product that was competent, consistent, and familiar. While the archbishop and other dignitaries might commission a Book of Hours from a famous individual artist, the majority of the population, judging by the number of surviving middle-range Hours, seems to have acquired their books from commercial workshops that specialized in a standardized product. By the fifteenth century, most manuscript production had long been carried out by commercial workshops, rather than the monastic scriptoria that characterized book production in the early Middle Ages. The various tasks necessary to produce a manuscript were carried out by specialists—scribes

17 For example, three manuscripts from the Pierpont Morgan Library illustrate this consistency: M.167, fol. 29r, dated 1465–1475; M.1093, fol. 24r, dated c. 1470; and M.137, fol. 27r, dated c. 1470–1480. In each miniature, Mary kneels on the left-hand side with her hands joined in prayer before an open book; in two cases the book is on a prie-dieu, and in the third on a sort of lectern. In both M.167 and M.137, Mary is beneath a canopy, with the curtain tied back. In each miniature Gabriel, wearing a brocade cope, kneels on one knee before Mary, his words recorded on a scroll that curls in the air between them. Above, filling the arch of the miniature, is an architectural structure. In M.167 and M.1093, this canopy is elaborately carved with pinnacles, and in M.1093, two statues of prophets. M.137 has a similar, though simpler, architectural canopy above the main scene.

18 See, for example, Morgan Library MSS M.220, fol. 45r and M.151, fol. 34r.

19 Refer to Morgan Library MSS M.137, fol. 51r; M.151, fol. 34r; M. 220, fol. 45r; M.129, fol. 35r; Princeton University Library, MS Garrett 56, fol. 29r; and Victoria and Albert Museum, MS L.475–1918, fol. 59v.

20 Watson, *Playfair Hours*, pp. 47–53.

to copy the text, illuminators to decorate it, and so forth.[21] Production could thus proceed in a sort of assembly line.[22] All of these production techniques served to speed up and standardize production. Furthermore, the consistency of the product meant that they could be produced for a speculative market, rather than the individual commission that characterized high-end manuscript production. With their general content and likely much lower production cost, the middle-range Books of Hours found a wide market in the growing middle class of professionals, merchants, and craftspeople. They reflect popular tastes. And significantly, these books were made to serve this specific audience, a point to which I will return later.

The Iconography and Sources of the Midwife with Withered Hands

While the Nativity is a standard scene, the addition of the midwife is an innovation that appears around the middle of the fifteenth century, and it warrants greater scrutiny because it represents a deviation from the norm. Changes to the iconography of these ubiquitous Book of Hours suggest changes in popular culture.[23] Stylistically, the Nativity scenes featuring the midwife with the withered hands, and indeed the manuscripts of which they are a part, are like those made in large quantities for the middle range of the market in places like Paris and Rouen in the fifteenth century. Getty MS 57 (94.ML.26), dated to c. 1420, is an early example of this variation (Fig. 8.1).

The artist depicts Mary and Joseph kneeling before the Christ Child, who is surrounded by cherubs. Behind Mary kneels the midwife, Salome, her hands withered and visibly smaller than those of the other figures. An angel appears from the left holding a pair of hands which will be restored to the midwife. God is above in heaven and shepherds stand in a shed on the left. New York, Morgan Library MS M.7, which originated in Paris c. 1490, is another example of this variation (Fig. 8.2).

21 Millard Meiss has done a great deal of work separating out the individuals responsible for the various parts of miniatures. See Meiss, *French Painting*.

22 Production could be further expedited by inserting miniatures painted on single folios into the quires of book. The trade in individual miniatures was in fact so widespread that it required ordinances in places like Bruges, where the importation of single folio miniatures was seen as a threat to the livelihood of local illuminators: see Hindman and Farquhar, *Pen to Press*, pp. 28–29.

23 A modern analogy would be television shows or movies. Viewer interest in a particular genre (for example, crime procedurals or superhero action films) will result in more of such shows or films being produced, while less popular genres will be abandoned.

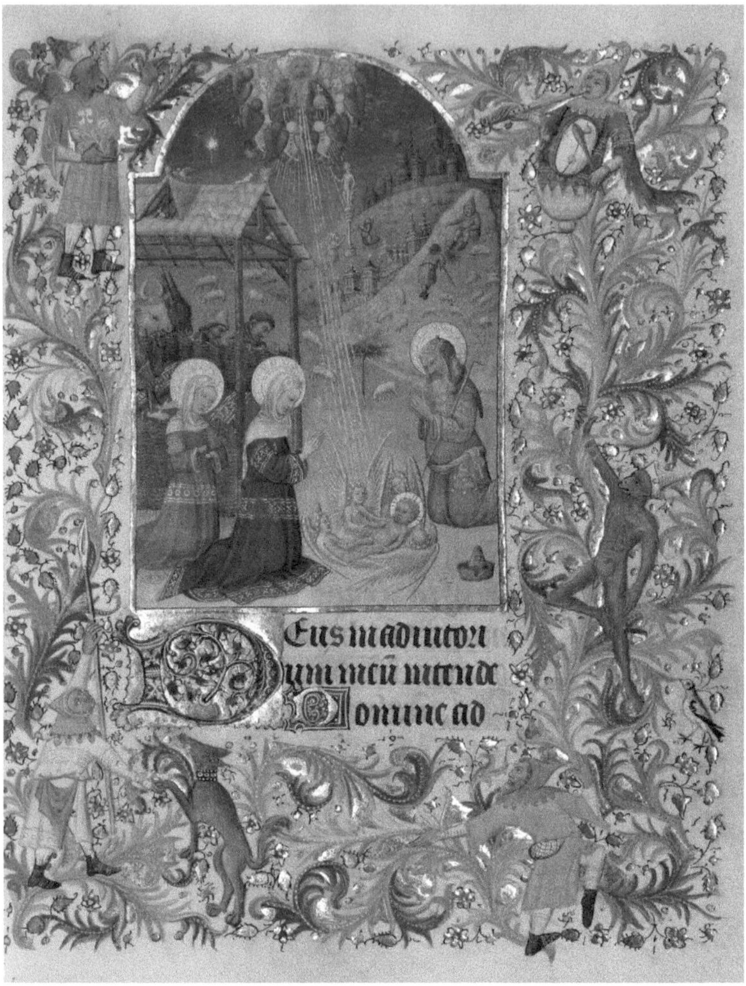

Figure 8.1: Spitz Master (French, active c. 1415–1425), *The Nativity*, c. 1420. Tempera colours, gold, and ink; leaf: 20.2 × 14.9 cm (7 15/16 × 5 7/8 in.). MS 57 (94.ML.26), fol. 84. The J. Paul Getty Museum, Los Angeles, MS 57, fol. 84.

In the miniature on folio 14r, Mary kneels with the Christ Child lying on her mantle on the floor of the stable. Joseph stands behind her. To Mary's right is the midwife, kneeling on one knee and holding out her arms, which end in stumps. An angel flies in from above holding a pair of hands to restore those the midwife has lost.

This variation on the depiction of the nativity has textual roots. The story of the midwife and the withering of her hands is found in the Proto-Gospel of James, dating from the late second century, and its Latin reworking, the Gospel of Pseudo-Matthew. Though widely read in the East, the Proto-Gospel

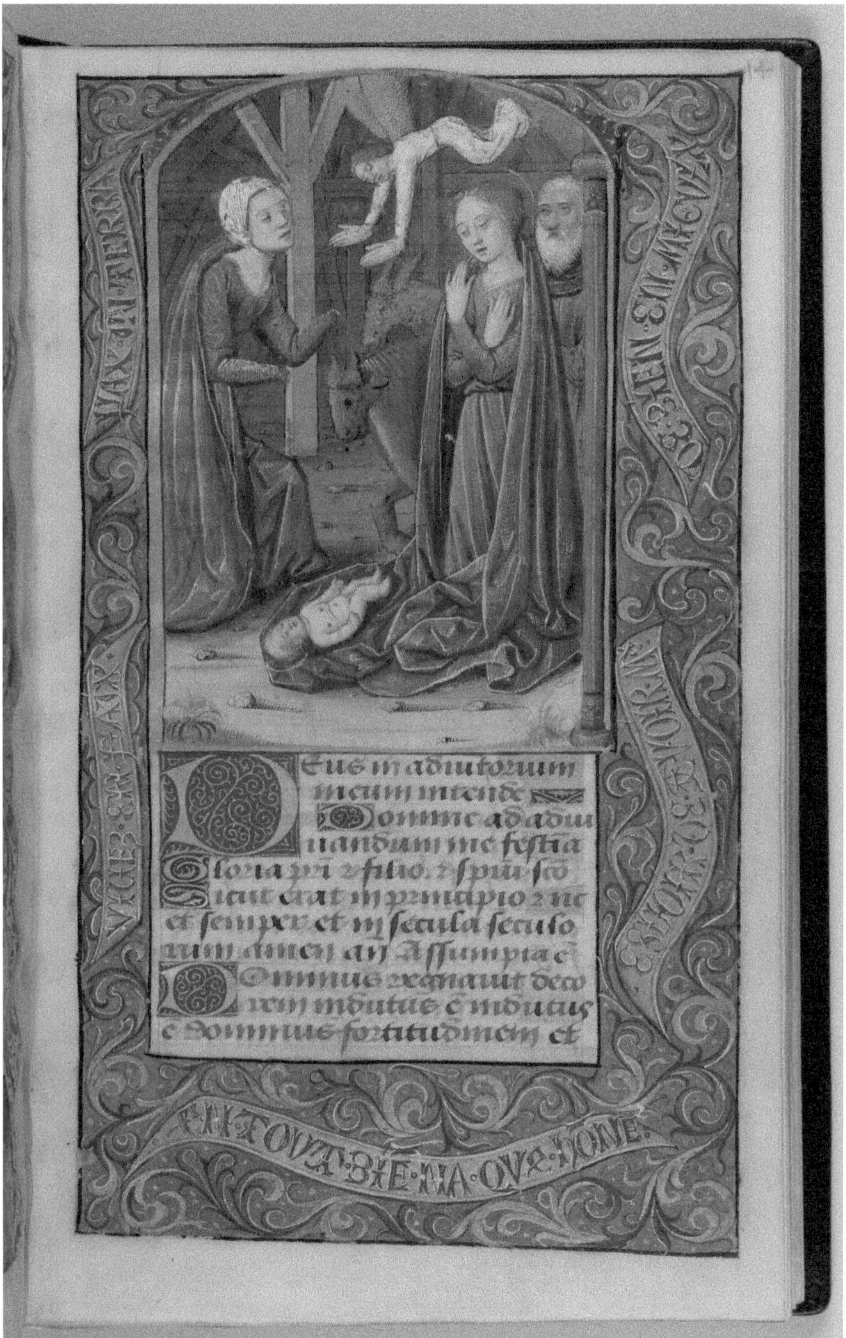

Figure 8.2: *The Nativity*, 1490–1500. Tempera colours and ink. The Pierpont Morgan Library, New York, MS M. 7, fol. 14r.

of James was not disseminated in the West because St Jerome and others condemned its mention of Jesus's brothers, Joseph's sons from a previous marriage. The Proto-Gospel was formally condemned by Pope Innocent I in 405 CE.[24] The Gospel of Pseudo-Matthew is probably based on now-lost Latin versions of the Proto-Gospel of James. During the Middle Ages, the Gospel of Pseudo-Matthew was one of the main sources for stories about the infancy of Christ, such as the miracles that occurred during the Flight into Egypt.[25] These Gospels, referred to collectively as the Infancy Gospels, contain much more detail about the events of Christ's birth than is related in the canonical Gospel of Luke. They tell the story of Mary going into labour on the road near Bethlehem. After finding shelter in a cave, Joseph goes in search of a midwife. Ultimately two midwives attend Mary; the first, Zahel, immediately recognizes the miraculous nature of the birth, but the second, Salome, doubts. When Salome examines Mary to prove her virginity, her hand withers. As Salome laments and repents her lack of faith, a figure appears to her and tells her to touch the Child to be healed. Once healed, Salome goes forth to preach about her miraculous experience and the coming of Christ.[26]

The story of Salome found new audiences in the later Middle Ages, when it appeared in sermon collections, devotional texts, and nativity plays, such as the N-Town plays. Jacobus de Voragine included Salome in his account of the birth of Jesus in the *Golden Legend*, a hagiographic collection compiled in the thirteenth century.[27] By the mid-fourteenth century, the midwife was referenced in an anonymous religious poem, the *Stanziac Life of Christ*.[28] The story also appears in a collection of homilies by John Mirk in 1380—the *Festial*—and in John Lydgate's *Life of Our Lady*, composed in 1420, as well as in the nativity scenes of some fifteenth-century cycle plays.[29] Alaya Swann attributes this renewed interest to a culture engaged 'in examining and evaluating sensory evidence in both medical and religious contexts'.[30] The appearance of the midwife, in text followed by image, in the later Middle Ages suggests a shift in attitudes about physical embodiments of the sacred

24 *Other Gospels*, pp. 18–19.

25 *Other Gospels*, pp. 37–38.

26 See *Other Gospels*, pp. 33–34 (Proto-Gospel of James); 51–52 (Gospel of Pseudo-Matthew); and 65–67 (Latin Infancy Gospels—J composition).

27 Jacobus de Voragine, *Golden Legend*, p. 38.

28 *Stanziac Life of Christ*, p. 27.

29 Powell, *John Mirk's* Festial, p. xlii; and Lauritis, *Critical Edition of John Lydgate*, pp. 107–08. See also Swann, "'By Expresse Experiment'", p. 5.

30 Swann, "'By Expresse Experiment'", p. 2.

that corresponds to larger social and cultural changes, for example in popular piety and medical practice.

Understanding the Meaning of the Midwife's Withered Hands

The midwife's withered hands and miraculous healing elucidate medieval attitudes towards faith, punishment, and disability. The story of the midwife Salome's doubt is reminiscent of that of the Apostle Thomas. Thomas doubted his fellow Apostles when they told him that Jesus had risen from the dead, saying that he would need to touch the wounds himself to believe. When Jesus appears before him, he believes and is forgiven for his lack of faith.[31] However, the divine response to the midwife's doubt is markedly different. After insisting on physically examining Mary to ascertain her virginity, Salome is immediately punished with the withering of her hands, which not only disfigures but also disables her. It is a physical manifestation of her lack of faith. Salome's loss of her hands renders her both disfigured and incapable of continuing to work as a midwife, and that loss occurs as a direct result of her physical engagement with the divine.

Physical punishment had the potential to cause permanent impairment and also played an important role in medieval society, in both secular and religious contexts. Both physical and sensory punishments were meted out to convicted criminals. Legal texts of the later Middle Ages make clear distinctions and justifications for mutilation as punishment, demonstrating first (as Irina Metzler has noted) a willingness to apply physical punishment, and second, a continuity with earlier judicial traditions.[32] In this context, the mutilation of the limbs of the midwife as a punishment fits firmly within the secular tradition of physical punishment for transgressions. However, the midwife's transgression was spiritual, not criminal in nature, suggesting additional religious nuance and meaning to this particular punishment. These associations bear further exploration.

31 John 20.24–29.

32 Metzler, 'Reflections on Disability', p. 20. See also Dean, *Crime in Medieval Europe*; Graves, 'From an Archaeology of Iconoclasm', p. 40; and Skinner, 'Marking the Face', p. 185. Dean writes that, beginning in the fourteenth century in France, a second offence of blasphemy was punished with a session in the pillory and the slitting of the upper lip. A third offence resulted in the slitting of the lower lip, the fourth in the amputation of the lower lip, and the fifth in the amputation of the tongue. The most serious crimes were punished with the most serious mutilations. See Dean, *Crime in Medieval Europe*, p. 56.

Salome's withered hands recall leprosy, the medical condition strongly associated with loss of sensation or even limbs in the Middle Ages.[33] Leprosy was greatly feared in the Middle Ages as a disease that not only disfigured and disabled sufferers, but also resulted in their removal from their communities.[34] Medieval lepers were routinely ostracized out of fear of contagion, as well as because leprosy had associations with sin and punishment going all the way back to biblical times. In her seminal essay on illness as metaphor, Susan Sontag notes that, 'In the Middle Ages, the leper was a social text in which corruption was made visible; an exemplum, an emblem of decay. Nothing is more punitive than to give a disease a meaning—that meaning being invariably a moralistic one'.[35] Medieval Jewish rabbinical texts identify leprosy as one of the signs that God gave to Moses. God afflicted Moses' hand with *tzara'at*, often translated as leprosy, and then cured him as a sign that Moses had sinned in asking God what would happen if the children of Israel didn't believe him.[36] Yet the perception of lepers was not exclusively negative in the Middle Ages. In the story of Alice the Leper (Alice of Schaerbeek), her affliction is characterized as a reward from God for her goodness. Her suffering is not seen as punishment for her own sins, but as a means of expiating the sins of others.[37]

Loss of limbs was associated with lepers simply as a result of the way the disease, today known as Hansen's disease, progresses. In actuality, the limbs or digits are not lost, but shortened, as sensation and blood supply are compromised and the body reabsorbs cartilage, causing withering or shrinking of the extremities.[38] Thus, the withering of Salome's hands is not unlike the withering of limbs associated with leprosy, a process described in the *Life of Alice the Leper*: 'Her hands, so needed for even her restricted uses, were long since all shrunken from the illness. Their skin was fissured with multiple wounds, like the bark of a tree'.[39] Rather than a slow progression, of course, the withering of Salome's hands happens all at once. Nevertheless, the similarity between the effect of her punishment

33 On leprosy, see also the chapters by Edwards and Vargas-O'Bryan in the present volume, pp. 235–63 and pp. 115–46 respectively. Edwards discusses Alice of Schaerbeek at pp. 252–55.

34 See Brenner, 'Between Palliative Care and Curing the Soul'; Orlemanksi, 'How to Kiss a Leper'; and Richards, *Sex, Dissidence, and Damnation*, pp. 150–63.

35 Sontag, *Illness as Metaphor*, p. 39.

36 Shoham-Steiner, *On the Margins*, p. 29.

37 See *Life of Alice the Leper*; and Spencer-Hall, *Medieval Saints*, p. 102. On this, see also Edwards's chapter in the present volume: pp. 252–57.

38 Bennett, Parker, and Robson, 'Leprosy', p. 201.

39 *Life of Alice the Leper*, 2.31.31.

and the physical effects of leprosy, a disease long associated with divine intervention, is compelling.

Leprosy and disfigurement also related to medieval ideas of the monstrous. The word monstrous was attributed by Isidore of Seville to come from the Latin 'to show forth' and monstrosity was often seen as symbolic.[40] As David Williams has noted, in the Middle Ages, the non-normative body functioned as 'a complementary, sometimes alternative, vehicle for philosophical and spiritual inquiry during this intellectually speculative period of Western civilization'.[41] At least as far back as Isidore in the seventh century, medieval thought had defined the monstrous in terms of the human body. His taxonomy of monstrosity lists twelve categories, all of which define a type of monstrousness in terms of human bodies.[42] Similarly, physically impaired children were sometimes connected with the idea of monsters and monstrosity. In one case, a mother said the child was immobile like a monster; in another, a father is recorded as having drawn back from the child as if from a monster.[43] The healthy, well-formed body, created in the image of God, represented order, while the monstrous represented disorder. Any transgression of the healthy, well-formed body was likewise associated with disorder and therefore sin. Salome's monstrous withered hands are symbolic, a physical sign of her spiritual transgression.

If the whole and intact body was the perfect vessel with which to worship, then physical impairment or disfigurement was often interpreted as an expression of sin, a tradition rooted in the Old Testament, where God often imposes physical punishment.[44] These ideas found their way into late medieval popular literature. As David King notes in his study of the *chansons de geste*, loss of limb was a suffering reserved for the villains of such tales, in which dismemberment highlights the moral corruption of these characters.[45] Like the midwife Salome, who is punished for her

40 Isidore of Seville, *Etymologies*, XI.iii.

41 Williams, *Deformed Discourse*, p. 3. Relatedly, Alice the Leper's biographer likens her to a 'horrible monster' (*Life of Alice the Leper*, 2.31.31).

42 See Williams, *Deformed Discourse*, pp. 107–08. Isidore's categories of monstrosity are atrophy of the body; hypertrophy of the body; excrescence of bodily parts; superfluity of bodily parts; deprivation of parts; mixture of human and animal parts; animal births by human women; mislocated organs of the body; disturbed growth; composite beings; hermaphrodites; and monstrous races.

43 Kuuliala, *Childhood Disability*, p. 82.

44 Shoham-Steiner, *On the Margins*, pp. 141–47.

45 See King, 'Meaning of Amputation', pp. 35–51. See also Mitchell and Snyder, *Narrative Prosthesis*. In an interesting inversion of this pattern, the story *Manekine* has the heroine cutting off her own hand to avoid an incestuous marriage to her father. Her hand is miraculously restored

spiritual transgressions with the loss of her hands, so too are the often non-Christian villains of these medieval epics the victims of limb loss. The literary use of disability serves to help define a character, but it can also serve as a metaphor for social ills, in part because disabled bodies are outside the norm.[46]

Salome's miraculous healing following her physical punishment is the more significant part of the story, however. It is that healing that ultimately results in her conversion and her desire to go out to preach the coming of the Messiah. Her miraculous story mirrors biblical stories such as John 5.14, in which Christ heals a man and tells him, 'Go and sin no more'. Physical impairment and miraculous healing also feature in the stories of saints. Jacobus de Voragine's popular *Legenda aurea* (*Golden Legend*), a collection of saints' lives written around 1260, is full of stories of miraculous healing.[47] Proof that a would-be saint had performed cures was in fact central to the canonization process.[48] Additionally, as Edward Wheatley argues in his work on blindness and disability, physical impairment provided an opportunity for a saint or holy figure to prove his or her holiness. Like in the story of Alice the Leper, physical suffering was seen to assist a saint on the path to holiness. These concepts made their way into popular culture in the later Middle Ages, when miraculous healings were re-enacted as stage performances and images of miraculous cures permeated art in virtually all media.[49] The story of Salome needs to be viewed amid this cultural backdrop.

While Salome is not a saint, the arc of her story is a familiar one of sin/doubt, physical redemption/restoration, and reinvigorated faith. The key moment comes not with the imposing of her disability through the withering of her hands, but with their healing. The restoration is the ultimate miracle, and it is that miracle that is featured in visual representations of the midwife with the withered hands. In the late medieval Books of Hours where she appears, Salome is shown in the moment after her realization, when she repents and receives mercy. The physical impairment creates the opportunity for her to ask and receive forgiveness, acts visualized by the arrival of an angel with replacement hands in these scenes of the Nativity.

years later after it is found in a fountain, perfectly preserved from having been kept in a vessel put into the belly of a sturgeon by the Virgin Mary. In the course of her story, some characters express concerns that the protagonist might be a criminal due to her mutilation. See Phillippe de Remi, *Roman de la Mankine*.

46 Pearman, *Women and Disability*, p. 21.

47 See Jacobus de Voragine, *Golden Legend*.

48 Kuuliala, *Childhood Disability*, pp. 3–4.

49 Wheatley, *Stumbling Blocks*, p. 11.

Disability and Faith in the Late Middle Ages

The seemingly sudden appearance of Salome in the Nativity scenes of late medieval Books of Hours reflects a cultural shift in the perception of piety, disability, and sanctity. It also coincides with the growing professionalization, and masculinization, of medicine, including the practice of midwifery. Women were an increasingly powerful force in Christian piety, in spite of the persistent misogyny of medieval culture. As Caroline Walker Bynum notes, late medieval views about women became more complex due to more positive female figures and feminine metaphors: for example, the increase in devotion to the Virgin Mary and to female saints and the use of childbirth and marriage as metaphors for spiritual advancement, trends which began in the twelfth and thirteenth centuries.[50] Women's piety in the late Middle Ages tended to be very much oriented towards the body and included bodily miracles such as stigmata, incorruptibility of the body after death, subsistence on the Eucharist alone, mystical lactation, and visions of bleeding hosts. Suffering and illness were often interpreted as religious experience.[51] Margery Kempe's well-known fifteenth-century narrative of her suffering from various ailments supports this perception of the intertwining of physical suffering and religious experience.[52] Female saints and mystics endured and were empowered by physical suffering, in imitation of Christ, and medieval people tortured their own bodies to achieve their religious goals.[53] Holy people spit or blew into the mouths of others to effect cures or convey grace, and, following St Francis of Assisi, kissed lepers and ate lice from the poor or sick, while sick people drank or bathed in the dirty bathwater of would-be saints.[54]

Illness and suffering were not necessarily something to be cured; their endurance was thought to increase holiness and closeness to Christ. According to Bynum, this physicality was especially the purview of women's piety; in turn, women's piety was a product of increased clerical control that pushed women's spirituality in the direction of mysticism, and Church reforms that emphasized the separation between priests and laypersons and augmented

50 Bynum, *Fragmentation*, pp. 151–52.

51 Ibid., p. 154.

52 See Kempe, *Book of Margery Kempe*.

53 Marshall, 'Politics of Self-Mutilation', pp. 12–13. See also Juárez-Almendros, *Disabled Bodies*.

54 Bynum, *Fragmentation*, p. 184. For example, St Catherine of Siena, after being repulsed by a patient's stinking ulcer, immediately pressed her mouth and nose over the sore. See Raymond of Capua, *Life of St. Catherine*, p. 149. On Catherine, see also the chapter by Edwards in the present volume, pp. 251–52.

clerical dignity. As a result, Bynum concludes, the only outlet for women, who lacked clerical office to authorize their speech, was to stress the experience of Christ and his suffering and to emulate it themselves.[55] There is some evidence to suggest that the somatic experiences of female mystics might be a clerical projection onto these women, since their own writing emphasizes the spiritual, much more so than the corporeal, as Amy Hollywood's research has demonstrated.[56] At the same time, the rise in vernacular literature and its greater availability to women created a language of feeling and emotion that crossed over into religious life. Literary characterizations of women were not always positive. For example, female characters were used to personify many of the Seven Deadly Sins in Guillaume de Deguiville's *Pelerinage de vie humaine*.[57] Tory V. Pearman notes: 'Medieval texts frequently construct socially unruly female characters as the deviance that prompts narrative, often by basing that unruliness on the defectiveness of the female body. Thus, the narrative busies itself with attempts to control that deviance'.[58] The physical nature of Salome's suffering is therefore a significant part of her spiritual journey from unbeliever to convert. Her redemption comes about through her physical suffering.

At the same time as these shifts in medieval piety were occurring, midwifery, long the purview of elder women in the community, was coming to be increasingly professionalized and the purview of men, as was the rest of medical practice. Hospitals were monastic institutions from their earliest beginnings, and medical practice developed within them in the Middle Ages. By the late medieval period, medicine had expanded from the monasteries and had become a standard part of the medieval university curriculum. It is not uncommon to find reference to clerics requesting medical books or dispensing medical advice.[59] However, women were neither permitted to attend the universities nor able to be clerics. Nevertheless, women clearly did practice medicine, particularly in the specialized area of obstetrics, and nuns often provided care at institutions like charity hospitals.[60] A 1421 petition put before the English Parliament included measures to protect (male) physicians, ensuring their hegemony and making

55 Bynum, *Fragmentation*, pp. 195–96.

56 Hollywood, *Soul as Virgin Wife*, pp. 26–56.

57 See Morgan Library MS M. 1038; for the text, Guillaume de Deguileville, *Pilgrimage of Human Life*.

58 Pearman, *Women and Disability*, p. 14.

59 Amundsen, 'Medieval Catholic Tradition', p. 82. See also Bowers, *Medieval Hospital and Medical Practice*.

60 Fissell, 'Introduction', p. 16.

sure that no women practised medicine.[61] The existence of this petition suggests two things: first, that there were female medical practitioners, probably trained through practical experiences and therefore not actual physicians; and second, that these female practitioners were common enough that male physicians sought to limit their ability to practise, seeing them as direct competitors.

Most female practitioners were probably midwives, though it can be difficult to trace them in historical records. As Monica Green points out, midwives had no institutional identity, unlike those in male-dominated medical fields. There were no formal guilds and no formal system of licensing before the fifteenth century. Additionally, the terminology used to refer to women functioning as birth attendants varies. For example, medical authors refer to *vetulae* (old women), but frequently as stereotypes in caricatured fashion; women acting in the role of birth attendants are mentioned frequently, but rarely by name.[62] Nevertheless, childbirth in the Middle Ages seems to have been almost completely attended by women, whether or not they were trained midwives. There is no evidence to suggest that midwives attempted to regulate themselves through a guild system or other institution before the fifteenth century.[63] The first known licensing imposed on midwives by municipal or ecclesiastical authorities in medieval Europe was in Regensburg in 1452. As Green points out, the timing of midwife regulations coincides with the first instances of witch persecutions, though she cautions against trying to connect the two.[64] Midwives were sometimes accused of being witches or of causing stillbirths or newborn deaths, but in general, society valued the role female birth attendants played in childbirth, as well as their specialized skills.[65] Pseudo-Albertus Magnus's *De secretis mulierum*, for example, praises midwives for their ability to turn a baby with a bad presentation or treat a woman who suffers tearing during the birth.[66] The regulation of midwifery, which often addresses the moral character of midwives as opposed to their medical skill, also corresponds to the secondary position that physicians tried to enforce on female medical practitioners. Women were increasingly restricted to the role of assistants and subordinates by male practitioners who wanted to expand their practice into the lucrative and very routinely required field of obstetrics. Male physicians still required female assistants

61 Green, *Women's Healthcare*, essay I, p. 54.
62 Ibid., essay II, pp. 336–40.
63 Ibid.
64 Ibid., essay I, pp. 54–56.
65 Ibid.
66 Pseudo-Albertus Magnus, *Women's Secrets*, pp. 57–107.

to act as the interface between doctor and patient, since notions of propriety restricted their physical contact with female patients.[67]

Regulation in the late Middle Ages also helped to professionalize midwifery as an independent profession for women, as did greater educational opportunities brought about by higher literacy rates.[68] However, better education and greater literacy for women does not seem to have translated into the creation of medical texts for women. The *Trotula*, a group of three texts written in the twelfth century, is often cited as a work of women's medicine, but there is no indication that the texts were necessarily written by or for women. Green suggests that the vernacular translations of the *Trotula*, which gradually begin to appear in the thirteenth century and then at a faster rate in the fourteenth and fifteenth centuries, might have been addressed to women in response to the increasing male intrusion into women's medical care in the later Middle Ages.[69]

Unfortunately, there is not much evidence of women owning medical books, even as women's literacy and the quantity of medical literature in both Latin and the vernaculars were increasing. Wills from Tournai document ninety-five female, middle-class book owners between 1266 and 1500; only one woman was in possession of a medical book and that was on loan to her.[70] The wills show the same general pattern of book ownership as Labarre's study of wills from Amiens. Women who owned books at all tended most commonly to own Books of Hours, Psalters, saints' lives, and other books of religious instruction.

Secular society expected nursing and nurturing to be done by women, even with the increasing professionalization and accompanying male dominance of medical care in the late Middle Ages. As Bynum writes, 'Women retained the right and the obligation to nurse the aged, the young, and the ill, and especially to provide what little obstetrical and gynecological care there was'.[71] Women transferred their nurturing roles into their religious experiences, so that the same somatic experiences that defined their everyday lives became part of their bodily experience of religion.[72] Late medieval women's piety incorporated views of sickness and suffering as a path to penitence and redemption, and embraced physical manifestations of holiness. Society and the Church had long associated women with fleshiness and sin, and

67 Green, *Women's Healthcare*, essay I, pp. 77–78.
68 Piper, 'Professionalization of Midwifery'.
69 Green, *Women's Healthcare*, essay I, pp. 65–67.
70 Ibid., essay VII, pp. 4–10.
71 Bynum, *Fragmentation*, p. 197.
72 Ibid., pp. 197–98.

sin with physical punishment, and so the body became intertwined with holiness and religious revelation. Salome receives a physical punishment; she suffers for the sin of lacking faith. When her faith is restored, her physical affliction and suffering likewise comes to an end. The appeal of her story to late medieval people, who saw a powerful religious experience to be had through physical suffering and miraculous cure, is readily apparent. They, too, endured suffering and doubt and prayed for forgiveness and deliverance, just like Salome, whose repentance was rewarded by God. At the same time, as medicine became increasingly professionalized in the later Middle Ages and as civic and ecclesiastical institutions sought greater control, midwifery practice became both more regulated and more visible as a profession. For these reasons, the appearance of Salome and her story in Books of Hours, particularly Books of Hours intended for the very middle-class people most affected by such societal shifts, marks a logical progression of ideas and iconography.

Salome or Anastasia?

The midwife in literary and visual sources is consistently identified as Salome. There is, however, a related story of the nativity that includes a handless girl, Anastasia. According to the story, found in texts of *Life of the Virgin and of our Lord*, Joseph went out to find someone to attend Mary in her labour and met a girl with no hands. She nevertheless went with Joseph and attempted to tend to the newborn Christ Child. As soon as she touched Him, she received hands. When she returned home with her miraculous hands, her father, a priest in the temple, was angry and threatened to cut them off. Instead, he was instantly blinded and Anastasia went out to preach about the miracle she had experienced.[73] If the woman with withered hands is not in fact Salome, but is instead the handless girl Anastasia, the possible meaning of the iconography shifts. While the story of Salome resonates as one of lack of faith resulting in a physical punishment that is in turn miraculously healed by renewed faith, the story of Anastasia is instead about the simple and absolute faith of a child rewarded with miraculous healing. As M. R. James pointed out more than a century ago, the stories of Anastasia and Salome were likely conflated in the Middle Ages, in part because the feast

73 *Life of the Virgin and of our Lord* (Cambridge, Fitzwilliam Museum No. 20). This text is unedited in any modern edition, but is summarized in M. R. James, 'Legends of SS. Anne and Anastasia'.

of St Anastasia of Sirmium falls on December 25 and because both stories are about attending at the birth of Christ. James saw the story of Anastasia as an exaggeration of the miracle enacted upon the midwife Salome.[74] Salome's story continues with her taking up preaching the coming of Christ to the Jews, for which she was likely killed. Cambridge, Fitzwilliam Museum No. 48 illustrates her fate. This manuscript, the Carew-Poyntz Hours, dated to c. 1360, illustrates both Salome with her withered hands, and a scene of a woman about to be beheaded: Salome's subsequent martyrdom.

While M. R. James makes a convincing argument for the conflation of the stories of Anastasia and Salome, it is worth taking a moment to consider the implications to a discussion of disability and sanctity if the midwife is identified as the child Anastasia instead of the adult Salome. Children in the Middle Ages were some of the most common recipients of miraculous healing, phenomena well represented in canonization records. Jenni Kuuliala's study of canonization documents highlights several important themes. First, the illnesses and impairments of children are much less likely to be characterized as punishment for deviance or sin. Additionally, healing miracles were fundamental to the idea of sainthood for the uneducated laity and form a large portion of the testimony given in canonization proceedings. While theologians tended to emphasize the virtuous lives of the saints, lay people considered miracles the most visible and essential aspect of sainthood.[75] Finally, veneration of the saints was a part of everyday life and physical impairment was intimately connected with sainthood and the miraculous.[76] The miraculous healing of an innocent child, as in the story of Anastasia, would have been less didactic than the story of Salome. Salome's initial punishment and physical suffering, followed by her miraculous restoration, was likely the more powerful story to a medieval audience primed to expect physical punishment for transgressions and attuned to Christian attitudes towards impairment, punishment, and restoration. The entire sequence of Salome's story provides the more powerful lesson about the costs of sin and the rewards of repentance and suffering.

The story of the midwife with the withered hands makes its way into Books of Hours in the late Middle Ages because the story had particular relevance to the owners of these books. The addition of her narrative to

74 James, 'Legends of SS. Anne and Anastasia', pp. 201–02. There are several saints named Anastasia, all of them martyred in early Christian times. The story of the Anastasia in question does not appear to be the same individual as any of these earlier Anastasias.

75 Kuuliala, *Childhood Disability*, pp. 2–4.

76 Ibid., pp. 4–9. See also Metzler, 'Disabled Children', pp. 161–80.

the standard scene of the Nativity is multifaceted and reflects the complex cultural shifts at work in late medieval France and elsewhere in Europe. As Jean Delumeau has written of the fourteenth to sixteenth centuries, 'Since most people's minds were now preoccupied with the fear of Deadly Sin, artists contrived all sorts of representations for it'.[77] Physical impairment was perceived as both a punishment for sin, as well as a physical expression of it. Physical impairment also provided an opportunity for redemption and holiness. According to Shoham-Steiner, 'The learned elite and the authors of ethical manuals sought to see physical deformity as an opportunity for soul searching, a call to inventory one's deeds in an attempt to identify a correspondence between a person's deformity and the actions for which he or she were presumably punished'.[78] The midwife with the withered hands embodies late medieval conceptions of the spiritual value of suffering and miraculous healing. The healing occurs with direct physical contact with the Christ Child, who will grow up to suffer and die for humanity's sins, a continuation of this cycle of impairment and empowerment.[79] The iconography illustrates the increased emphasis on the intersection of the spiritual and physical in the late Middle Ages. The presence of this iconography specifically within the context of Books of Hours made for the bourgeoisie of merchants, craftspeople, shopkeepers and others of the increasingly educated middle class—some of which were perhaps even made for female medical practitioners—suggests that the story resonated with conceptions of popular piety and the particular power of healing miracles as evidence of holiness.

Bibliography

Manuscripts

Baltimore, Walters Art Museum, W. 719 (Book of Hours)
Cambridge, Fitzwilliam Museum, MS 20 (*Life of Our Virgin and of Our Lord*)
Cambridge, Fitzwilliam Museum, MS 48 (Carew-Poyntz Hours)
London, British Library, MS Add. 47682 (Holkham Bible Picture Book)
London, Victoria and Albert Museum, MS L. 475–1918 (Playfair Hours)

77 Delumeau, *Sin and Fear*, p. 240.
78 Shoham-Steiner, *On the Margins*, p. 149.
79 A Flemish Book of Hours in the Walters Art Museum (W.719), dated to c. 1450, highlights this healing touch, showing the first midwife with her hands joined in prayer while Salome reaches out to touch the Christ Child (fol. 41v).

Los Angeles, Getty Museum, MS 57 (94.ML.26) (Spitz Hours)
Milan, Ambrosiana, MS L. 58 Sup. (*Evangelica historia*)
New York, Pierpont Morgan Library, MS M.7 (Book of Hours)
New York, Pierpont Morgan Library, MS M.105 (Porter Hours)
New York, Pierpont Morgan Library, MS M.129 (Book of Hours)
New York, Pierpont Morgan Library, MS M.137 (Book of Hours)
New York, Pierpont Morgan Library, MS M.151 (Book of Hours)
New York, Pierpont Morgan Library, MS M.167 (Book of Hours)
New York, Pierpont Morgan Library, MS M.202 (Book of Hours)
New York, Pierpont Morgan Library, MS M.220 (Book of Hours)
New York, Pierpont Morgan Library, MS M.1038 (*Pèlerinage de vie humaine*)
New York, Pierpont Morgan Library, MS M.1093 (Book of Hours)
Princeton, Princeton University Library, MS Garret 56 (Book of Hours)
Vienna, Kunsthistorisches Museum, Vienna Kunstkammer, KK 5003, KK 5004 (Göttingen Model Book)

Primary Sources

Canonical Histories and Apocryphal Legends Relating to the New Testament, ed. by A. M. Ceriani and Angelo della Croce (Milan: J. B. Pogliani, 1873)

Guillaume de Deguileville, *The Pilgrimage of Human Life*, ed. by Eugene Clasby (New York: Garland, 1992)

Isidore of Seville, *Etymologies*, trans. by Stephen Barney, W. J. Lewis, J. A. Beach, and Oliver Berghof (Cambridge: Cambridge University Press, 2006)

Jacobus de Voragine, *The Golden Legend*, trans. by William Granger Ryan (Princeton, NJ: Princeton University Press, 2012)

St John the Theologian, 'The Book of John Concerning the Falling Asleep of Mary', in *The Ante-Nicene Fathers: Translations of the Writings of the Fathers down to A.D. 325, Vol. VIII*, ed. by Alexander Roberts and James Donaldson (Edinburgh: T & T Clark, 1885; repr. Grand Rapids: Wm. B. Eerdmans, 1995), pp. 587–91

Kempe, Margery, *The Book of Margery Kempe*, trans. by Anthony Bale (Oxford: Oxford University Press, 2015)

Lauritis, Joseph, *A Critical Edition of John Lydgate's 'Life of Our Lady'* (Pittsburgh: Duquesne University Press, 1961)

The Life of Alice the Leper, trans. by Martinus Cawley (Lafayette, OR: Guadalupe Translations, 1994)

The Other Gospels: Accounts of Jesus from Outside the New Testament, ed. and trans. by Bart Ehrman and Zlatko Pleše (Oxford: Oxford University Press, 2014)

Powell, Susan, *A Critical Edition of John Mirk's 'Festial'* (Oxford: Oxford University Press, 2010)

Pseudo-Albertus Magnus, *Women's Secrets: A Translation of Pseudo-Albertus Magnus' 'De Secretis Mulierum' with Commentaries*, trans. by Helen Rodnite Lemay (Albany: State University of New York Press, 1992)

Raymond of Capua, *Life of St Catherine* (Gastonia: Tan Books, 2009)

Philippe de Remi, *Le Roman de la Manekine*, trans. by Barbara Sargent-Baur (Leiden: Brill, 1999)

A Stanziac Life of Christ, Compiled from Higden's 'Polichronicon' and the 'Legenda Aurea', edited from MS. Harley 3909, ed. by Frances Foster (London: Early English Text Society, 1926; repr. 1971)

Secondary Sources

Amundsen, Derrel, 'The Medieval Catholic Tradition', in *Caring and Curing: Health and Medicine in the Western Religious Traditions*, ed. by Ronald Numbers and Derrel Amundsen (Baltimore: Johns Hopkins University Press, 1986), pp. 65–107

Backhouse, Janet, *Books of Hours* (London: British Library, 1985)

Bennett, B., D. Parker, and M. Robson, 'Leprosy: Steps Along the Journey of Eradication', *Public Health Reports*, 123.2 (2008), 198–205 <https://doi.org/10.1177/003335490812300210>

Boehm, Barbara Drake, and Jirí Fajt, *Prague, the Crown of Bohemia, 1347–1437* (New York: Metropolitan Museum of Art, 2005)

Bowers, Barbara, ed., *The Medieval Hospital and Medical Practice* (London: Routledge, 2007)

Brenner, Elma, 'Between Palliative Care and Curing the Soul: Medical and Religious Responses to Leprosy in France and England, c. 1100–c. 1500', in *Medicine, Religion and Gender in Medieval Culture*, ed. by Naoē Kukita Yoshikawa (Cambridge: D. S. Brewer, 2015), pp. 221–35

Bridge, J., *A History of France from the Death of Louis XI to 1515*, 5 vols (Oxford: Oxford University Press, 1921–1936), v

Bynum, Caroline Walker, *Fragmentation and Redemption: Essays on Gender and the Human Body in Medieval Religion* (New York: Zone Books, 1991)

Chartier, Roger, *The Cultural Uses of Print in Early Modern France*, trans. by Lydia Cochrane (Princeton, NJ: Princeton University Press, 1987)

Dean, T., *Crime in Medieval Europe, 1200–1500* (Harlow and London: Longman and Pearson Education, 2001)

Delumeau, Jean, *Sin and Fear: The Emergence of Guilt Culture, 13th–18th Centuries*, trans. by Eric Nicholson (New York: St Martin's Press, 1990)

Dubourg, Ninon, *Disabled Clerics in the Late Middle Ages: Un/suitable for Divine Office?*, Premodern Health, Disease, and Disability (Amsterdam: Amsterdam University Press, 2023)

Fissell, Mary, 'Introduction: Women, Health, and Healing in Early Modern Europe', *Bulletin of the History of Medicine*, 82, Special Issue: Women, Health, and Healing in Early Modern Europe (2008), 1–17

Graves, Patricia, 'From an Archaeology of Iconoclasm to an Anthropology of the Body: Images, Punishment, and Personhood in England, 1500–1600', *Current Anthropology*, 49 (2008), 35–60

Green, Monica H., *Women's Healthcare in the Medieval West*, Variorum Collected Studies Series (Aldershot: Ashgate, 2000)

Harthan, John, *Books of Hours and their Owners* (London: Thames and Hudson, 1977)

Hindman, Sandra, and James Douglas Farquhar, *Pen to Press: Illustrated Manuscripts and Printed Books in the First Century of Printing* (Baltimore: Johns Hopkins and University of Maryland Press, 1977)

Hollywood, Amy, *The Soul as Virgin Wife: Mechthild of Magdeburg, Marguerite Porete, and Meister Eckhart* (South Bend, IN: University of Notre Dame Press, 2000)

James, M. R., 'Legends of SS. Anne and Anastasia', *Proceedings of the Cambridge Antiquarian Society, with Communications Made to the Society*, 9, new series 3.38 (1895–96), 173–204

Juárez-Almendros, Encarnación, *Disabled Bodies in Early Modern Spanish Literature: Prostitutes, Aging Women, and Saints* (Liverpool: Liverpool University Press, 2017)

King, David S., 'The Meaning of Amputation in the *Chansons de Geste*', *Symposium*, 62 (Spring 2008), 35–51

Kuuliala, Jenni, *Childhood Disability and Social Integration in the Middle Ages: Constructions of Impairments in Thirteenth- and Fourteenth-century Canonization Processes* (Turnhout: Brepols, 2016)

Labarre, Albert, *Le Livre dans la vie amiénoise du seizième siècle: L'enseignement des inventaires après décès 1503–1576* (Paris: Nauwelaerts, 1971)

Marshall, Claire, 'The Politics of Self-Mutilation: Forms of Female Devotion in the Late Middle Ages', in *The Body in Late Medieval and Early Modern Culture*, ed. by Darryll Grantley and Nina Taunton (Aldershot: Ashgate, 2000), pp. 11–22

Meiss, Millard, *French Painting in the Time of Jean de Berry: The Late Fourteenth Century and the Patronage of the Duke* (London: Phaidon, 1967)

Metzler, Irina, 'Disabled Children: Birth Defects, Causality, and Guilt', in *Medicine, Religion and Gender in Medieval Culture*, ed. by Naoē Kukita Yoshikawa (Cambridge: D. S. Brewer, 2015), pp. 161–80

Metzler, Irina, 'Reflections on Disability in Medieval Legal Texts: Exclusion—Protection—Compensation', in *Disability and Medieval Law: History, Literature, Society*, ed. by Cory James Rushton (Newcastle upon Tyne: Cambridge Scholars, 2013), pp. 19–53

Mitchell, David, and Sharon Snyder, *Narrative Prosthesis: Disability and the Dependencies of Discourse* (Ann Arbor: University of Michigan Press, 2000)

Orlemanski, Julie, 'How to Kiss a Leper', *postmedieval: a journal of medieval and cultural studies*, 3 (2012), 142–57.

Pearman, Tory Vandeventer, *Women and Disability in Medieval Literature*, New Middle Ages (New York: Palgrave Macmillan, 2010)

Piper, Leanne, 'The Professionalization of Midwifery in the Late Middle Ages', *Canadian Journal of Midwifery Research and Practice*, 9.1 (2010), 21–34

Rabel, Claudia, 'Artiste et clientele à la fin du Moyen Age: Les manuscrits profanes du Maître du Maître de l'échevinage de Rouen', *Revue de l'Art*, 84 (1989), 48–60

Richards, Jeffrey, *Sex, Dissidence and Damnation: Minority Groups in the Middle Ages* (London: Routledge, 1994)

Shoham-Steiner, Ephraim, *On the Margins of a Minority: Leprosy, Madness and Disability among the Jews of Medieval Europe* (Detroit: Wayne State University Press, 2014)

Skinner, Patricia, *Living with Disfigurement in Early Medieval Europe*, New Middle Ages (New York: Palgrave Macmillan, 2017)

Skinner, Patricia, 'Marking the Face, Curing the Soul? Reading the Disfigurement of Women in the Later Middle Ages', in *Medicine, Religion and Gender in Medieval Culture*, Gender in the Middle Ages, ed. by Naoē Kukita Yoshikawa (Cambridge: D. S. Brewer, 2015), pp. 181–200

Sontag, Susan, *Illness as Metaphor* (New York: Random House, 1979)

Spencer-Hall, Alicia, 'Chronic Pain and Illness: Reinstating Crip-Chronic Histories to Forge Affirmative Disability Futures', in *A Cultural History of Disability in the Middle Ages*, ed. by Jonathan Hsy, Tory V. Pearman, and Joshua R. Eyler (London: Bloomsbury, 2020), pp. 51–66

Spencer-Hall, Alicia, *Medieval Saints and Modern Screens: Divine Visions as Cinematic Experience*, Knowledge Communities (Amsterdam: Amsterdam University Press, 2018)

Stiker, Henri-Jacques, *A History of Disability*, trans. by William Sayers (Ann Arbor: University of Michigan Press, 1999)

Swann, Alaya, '"By Expresse Experiment": The Doubting Midwife Salome in Late Medieval England', *Bulletin of the History of Medicine*, 89 (2015), 1–24

Watson, Rowan, *The Playfair Hours: A Late Fifteenth Century Illuminated Manuscript from Rouen* (London: Victoria and Albert Publications, 1984)

Wheatley, Edward, *Stumbling Blocks before the Blind: Medieval Constructions of a Disability* (Ann Arbor: University of Michigan Press, 2013)

Williams, David, *Deformed Discourse: The Function of the Monster in Mediaeval Thought and Literature* (Montreal and Kingston, Ontario: McGill-Queen's University Press, 1996)

About the Author

Libby Karlinger Escobedo is Associate Professor of Art History at Aurora University, where she has taught since 2007. After receiving her bachelor's degree in Art History at UCLA, she received her master's and PhD in the history of art from Bryn Mawr College. Many of her research interests engage with visual culture and books from late medieval western Europe, interests nurtured by four years as a reader/cataloguer for the Index of Medieval Art at Princeton University. Her recent publications include essays on late medieval macabre imagery, and on the relationships between books and their owners. She is currently researching representations of nature in late medieval manuscripts as they relate to textual sources and to the ideas of monstrosity and sin.

9. Holy Women and Leprosy: Communities of Care

Jennifer C. Edwards

Abstract: Medieval saints' texts frequently describe encounters with 'lepers' but, oddly for miracle tales, rarely depict holy people curing leprosy. Instead, saints, especially holy women, offered care to the leprous by bathing, soothing, feeding, or clothing, or kissing—not curing—them. Leprosy deeply interested the saints, but not because of their holy power to cure. Instead, by treating leprosy saints demonstrated their faith, humility, and care for the Christian community. This chapter examines stories of female religious figures as they engaged with leprosy as a ritual practice demonstrating humility and faith. Holy women engaged intimately in caring for leprous bodies to prove their devotion and spiritual authority, and to bring incurably ill people into their communities.

Keywords: saints, leprosy, holy women, spiritual communities, Radegund, Kōmyō

Leprosy intensely interested saints and their cults during the Middle Ages, especially during the eleventh through thirteenth centuries, when much of Western Europe was concerned about this disease.[1] Saints offered charitable

This chapter began as conference papers presented at the American Association for the History of Medicine and the International Congress on Medieval Studies, on a project greatly encouraged by Monica Green and Rachel Scott at the National Endowment for the Humanities Summer Seminar on 'Health and Disease in the Middle Ages' at the Wellcome Institute in 2012. The work was supported by a Manhattan College sabbatical and Fordham University Center for Medieval Studies visiting fellowship. The author is grateful to this volume's editors for generous, insightful, and expert comments and suggestions that vastly improved the work. As ever, all errors and imperfections remain the author's own.

1 Several significant studies of leprosy have appeared recently, including Rawcliffe, *Leprosy in Medieval England*; Brenner, *Leprosy and Charity*; Touati, *Maladie et société au Moyen Âge*;

Grace-Petinos, Stephanie, Leah Pope Parker, and Alicia Spencer-Hall, eds. *Disability and Sanctity in the Middle Ages.* Taylor & Francis Group, 2025
DOI 10.5117/9789463724333_CH09

care and holy healing both during their lives and posthumously at their shrines, which were tended by cult devotees who received pilgrims and penitents seeking cures and other miracles. Hagiographical texts associated with saints, such as holy biographies and miracle tales, record numerous encounters between saints and leprous people. Some of these encounters included miraculous healings of the disease, but many did not, and simply narrated charitable work performed by the saints in bathing, feeding, clothing, treating, and comforting people with leprosy. The collector of the miracles of St Milburga of Much Wenlock (d. 715) defensively reported the complaint of a woman he called a 'Jezebel'. According to his report, she said: 'I have seen the saints perform many miracles, but it is very rarely that they heal leprosy'.[2] While Milburga did go on to cure the disease, such cures are surprisingly rare within hagiographical texts discussing leprosy. While the holy power of the saints to work intercessory miracles was otherwise nearly unlimited—the same saints' holy power cured blindness and deafness, restored mangled limbs, and even brought the dead back to life—they rarely cured leprosy, and medieval people noticed. When Symeon Stylites the Younger (d. 592) cured a man suffering from leprosy near Antioch, he told the man to go show himself to the priests 'who do not believe that it is possible for lepers to be cured'.[3] Eutychios (d. 582) anointed the hands and eyes of a man with leprosy, and advised him not to drink wine, but the supposed miracle is lacklustre: the disease had not advanced a year later, perhaps entering a remission—not exactly a cure.[4] Hugh of Lincoln (d. 1200) dropped by a leprosarium to kiss male patients, but claimed that these kisses were to heal his own spirit.[5]

Leprosy interested the saints and their cults, but not always as a way to demonstrate their holy power to work miracles, which may seem peculiar in texts such as *vitae* and miracle tales devoted to relating the wonders of saintly interventions. Instead, saints engaged with this disease to demonstrate their faith, humility, and care for the Christian community. This treatment of leprosy remained remarkably consistent across time and region, as the

Demaitre, *Leprosy in Premodern Medicine*; Brenner and Touati, *Leprosy and Identity*; and Krolikoski, 'Neither Sinner Nor Outcast'. In the present volume, see chapters by Escobedo (pp. 207–34, esp. 220–23), and Vargas-O'Bryan, (pp. 115–46).

2 Edwards, 'An Early Twelfth Century Account', p. 150.

3 'Life of Symeon Stylites the Younger'.

4 Eustratius, *Life of Eutychios*. For partial cures, see Spencer-Hall, 'Chronic Pain and Illness', especially pp. 62–63; with thanks to the author for this reference.

5 Rawcliffe, *Leprosy in Medieval England*, p. 175; Garton, *The Metrical Life of Saint Hugh of Lincoln*.

examples above suggest, particularly since hagiographical texts rely so often on existing narratives. Many of the saints who performed this labour of treating, but not curing, leprosy were female, indicating that care-work was gendered even among the cult of the saints.[6] This essay examines the treatment of leprosy by religious women, as they engaged with what was perceived as one of the riskiest, most incurable of diseases in order to provide the ultimate proof of their devotion and spiritual authority. Even if their ritual care of leprous people did not result in cures, their work displayed their humility and self-sacrifice, revealing not miraculous power but pious humility. Women's devotion and caring labour remained consistent tropes in descriptions of holy women's encounters with leprosy over time and over space, even beyond Christian Europe.

Leprosy is a disabling chronic illness, incurable before the development of modern drug therapies. It is not that easy to transmit leprosy—it involves very close contact over a long time, and while transmission is probably by droplets, the necessary period of contact appears to be much longer and requires closer proximity than that for COVID-19, for example.[7] It presents with a wide variety of symptoms, including muscle and bone weakening, discoloured skin, lesions, nerve damage, hoarse voice, destruction of cartilage, sterility, and general disability. Patients who stay clean, dry, warm, and well-nourished can slow the progress of the disease, even indefinitely. These were precisely the treatments offered in medieval leprosaria, whose patients stood a better chance of slowing the disease's progress than those who did not receive these benefits. When saints cared for leprous people by feeding, cleaning, and clothing them, they offered the most effective treatment available.

I examine leprosy, a chronic illness, as a disability here for a variety of reasons, despite the separation between illness and impairment in historical studies. First, to admit a personal bias, I am diabetic, and the experience of a chronic illness that disables, both physically and socially, has been profound. The constant threat of impairment, such as loss of sight, teeth, or feet, the failure of various organs, and loss of mobility, looms and is compounded by the risk of severe COVID-19 infection that continues to

6 The data for this observation comes from my work in progress *Holy Healing: Medieval Saints and Leprosy.*

7 *Mycobacterium leprae* (*M. leprae*) and *Mycobacterium lepromatosis* (*M. lepromatosis*) bacilii are most likely transmitted by infectious aerosols and direct contact with droplets, as well as by anthroponotic and zoonotic transmission: see Ploemacher, et al., 'Reservoirs and Transmission Routes of Leprosy'; and Kendall et al., 'A Social Network Approach for the Study of Leprosy Transmission'.

isolate and endanger diabetics as we watch others return to pre-COVID life. The inclusion of diabetes, and other chronic illnesses, as a disability covered by the Americans with Disabilities Act has offered crucial workplace protections, especially since 2020. Similarly, leprosy is a chronic illness that disabled physically and socially during the Middle Ages. Its many symptoms caused impairments such as bone loss, compromised mobility and finger dexterity, a hoarse voice that complicated speech and communication, and facial changes that made the illness obvious, unlike many chronic illnesses that might remain invisible. The leprous are most visible in medieval miracle tales when their disease was also most apparent, and most disabling. Further, as Julie Orlemanski has argued, the leprous have 'come to be the grotesque embodiment of historical alterity itself. [...] To think about lepers in the context of disability studies is to think about the "temporal incongruity" of bodies'.[8]

While many today believe that medieval Europeans feared those with leprosy, in truth, Christian communities in the Central Middle Ages, from about 1000 to 1300, reacted to the disease with pity, charity, and support.[9] While texts reveal saints' confessors' and companions' anxiety about saints engaging with leprous people and possibly becoming infected as well, actual transmission of the disease is rarely described. The narratives focused instead on risk and bravery to emphasize the saints' charity and humility. The leprous were not depicted as segregated, systematically isolated, or feared, but as people with a serious infectious illness that could be transmitted through close contact offered by saints. Fears about leprosy and contagion were not notably present in Europe until the thirteenth century, and not widespread until the fourteenth century, at which point the majority of the energy for charitable care in a sort of leprosy crisis had passed; even leprosy hospitals became repurposed for general care.[10] As Elma Brenner notes:

> [T]he widespread charitable patronage for leper houses in the twelfth and thirteenth centuries [...] may reflect not a wish to exclude lepers, but rather a concern to support them in the pursuit of their religious vocation. Indeed, the attachment of leper communities to prominent monasteries such as Fontevraud and Le Grand-Beaulieu at Chartres reflected a concerted drive to integrate lepers into the religious life.[11]

8 Orlemanski, 'How to Kiss a Leper', p. 144.
9 Brenner, 'The Leprous Body'. See also Touati, 'Saint-Lazare', pp. 225, 236.
10 Brenner, *Leprosy and Charity*, p. 2.
11 Brenner, 'The Leprous Body', p. 241.

Rather than flee the disease or isolate all leprous people, as modern communities did in the nineteenth and twentieth centuries, medieval communities saw leprous people as opportunities for Christian charity, even considering the possibility that they might, in truth, be Christ in disguise.[12]

Leprosy's visibility and obvious presence concerned medieval communities, especially from the eleventh through fourteenth centuries. During this time in Western Europe, patrons founded leprosaria in large numbers, ecclesiastical and secular leaders established rules to shape interactions between their communities and leprosy sufferers, and saints lavished attention on leprous men and women. While saints' texts include encounters with leprosy throughout the medieval period, these centuries saw a marked increase in saintly interest in the disease. This chapter focuses on the various ways that saintly attention manifested and how leprosy proved to be both a challenge and an opportunity to the medieval cult of the saints.

For several holy women, leprosy became an opportunity to display their faith and devotion through narratives of selfless care for the ill, and a chance to push the boundaries of their spiritual communities to include leprous members.[13] Hagiographical texts, whether depicting cure or care, used leprosy as narrative prosthesis, 'a crutch upon which literary narratives lean for their representation power, disruptive potency, and analytic insight'.[14] The purpose of a leprous person's appearance in a saint's *vita* or miracle tale was to demonstrate the holy person's sanctity. For some saints, this meant a healing miracle, for others it meant charitable treatment, but in either case the experience of disease and disability by the leprous person was inconsequential to most saints' narratives. Both care and cure were transactions in which the leprous person possibly received some relief, and the saint received boosts to their holy reputation. For the women discussed below, the desire to serve led them to shocking acts that earned them the censure of their immediate community, but eternal celebration in the pages of their *vitae* or miracle tales. The leprous recipients of these saints' attention appear for a moment only as objects of attention, the 'crutches' to holy women's glory. Nevertheless, partial glimpses of the leprous experience of holy encounters are visible in the documents, as discussed below.

The persistence of disease and disability in these non-miraculous holy encounters offers more opportunities to consider the leprous person as

12 Rawcliffe, *Leprosy in Medieval England*; Moran, *Colonizing Leprosy*.

13 On leprosy and gender, see also the chapter by Vargas-O'Bryan in the present volume, especially pp. 130–37.

14 Mitchell and Snyder, *Narrative Prosthesis*, p. 224.

historical subject than the successful healing miracle. In many leprosy miracles, leprous people turn out to be Christ, to be a test, and/or to vanish altogether as a result of the miracle. In more traditional cures the leprous person, health restored, disappears from the narrative once the disease and impairments are removed. In the encounters focused on non-miraculous ministrations the illness and impairments remained, potentially providing more space for the leprous person's subjectivity through continued narration.

The resistance of leprosy to cure in miracle tales and the choice of many saints to offer care rather than cure demonstrates the limitation of the medical model of disability for understanding medieval saintly encounters with leprosy. These holy women did not offer cures that failed; instead they saw cure as irrelevant to their treatment of leprosy. Encounters with leprous people focused instead on comfort, community, and care, transactions improving holy reputations. These texts suggest that a cure for leprosy was not simply too difficult to achieve, but instead an outcome that was not even desirable, for either side of the experience. The persistence of leprosy made this especially true, as the opportunity for care remained, offering saints ongoing, lifelong opportunities to build their holy dossiers, much more so than a singular instance of miraculous cure might do. While the hagiographical texts offer limited evidence from the perspective of the leprous, their participation in non-curative saintly care appears to have treated saintly care on a spectrum with secular medical care, which likewise offered little promise of cure of leprosy. Care and community offered a great deal to both the saints and leprous people they treated, making room for leprosy to remain present, visible and, quite literally, be embraced.

Palliative Care

The treatment saints offered demonstrated holy charity: they provided material assistance that did not cure leprosy, but certainly improved the health and comfort of those with the disease. Saints' lives and miracles reflect the significance of leprosy in the medieval period. While some saints continued to channel God's miraculous power over leprosy, the disease became an opportunity for all Christians to practise Christ-like charity and suffering, a chance to sacrifice themselves for the good of the larger Christian community.

An early example of this palliative care is the sixth-century Thuringian princess Radegund (d. 587), who was kidnapped by the Franks and eventually married King Clothar. The marriage was an uneasy one, with Radegund spending more time acting as a nun than a wife. She used her charity to moderate her husband's commands, such as by pleading for Clothar to reverse a death sentence, and freeing prisoners who sought her help.[15] After Clothar executed Radegund's brother, however, she fled Clothar's court in order to found a monastery in Poitiers, a house later known as the Abbey of Sainte-Croix. Radegund demonstrated her holiness in a number of ways, according to her contemporary biographer, the Italian poet Venantius Fortunatus. Radegund was an ascetic who denied herself food, wore a hairshirt, and even practised self-mortification in secret throughout her life. She devoted herself to prayer and care of the altar, as well as to works of service for prisoners and performing servile tasks for her fellow nuns. At one point she decided to enclose herself inside a small chapel, and it is through the chapel's window that she worked her most notable miracles, including healings, exorcisms, and resurrections.[16] Radegund was a miracle worker capable of healing injury and illness, which she demonstrated many times over.

Venantius Fortunatus's *vita* for the saint, completed at the end of the sixth century, also describes Radegund offering palliative care to a group of leprous people:

> When lepers arrived [...] she prepared a table [...] and she followed behind, sending supplies in furtively so that no one would see her. Then she seized some of the women spotted with leprosy in an embrace and kissed their faces, with a loving spirit. Then, sitting at table, bearing warm water she washed their faces and hands, she applied oil to their ulcers, and fed each one. When they were leaving she offered gold or clothing, with hardly anyone witness to this munificence. Her assistant nevertheless presumed to admonish her, accusing her thus: 'Most holy lady, who would kiss you when you embrace the leprous?' Radegund responded kindly, 'Really if you won't kiss me, that is not any concern of mine.'[17]

15 Fortunatus, 'Vita Radegundis', ch. 10–11.

16 Edwards, *Superior Women*, pp. 109–33.

17 Fortunatus, 'Vita Radegundis', ch. 19, 370–71: 'Cum leprosi venientes, signo facto, se proderent, iubebat adminiculae, ut, unde vel quanti essent, pia cura requireret. Qua sibi renuntiante, parata mensa, missorium, cocleares, cultellos, cannas, potum et calices scola subsequente, intromittebatur furtim, quo se nemo perciperet. Ipsa tamen mulieres variis leprae maculis conprehendens in amplexus, osculabatur et vultum, toto diligens animo. Deinde, posita mensa, ferens aquam calidam, facies lavabat, manus, ungues et ulcera et rursus administrabat, ipsa pascens per singular. Recedentibus praebebat auri vel vestimenti, vix una teste, munuscula. Ministra tamen praesumebat et blandimentis sic appellare: "Sanctissima domina, quis te

In Radegund's *vita*, this moment falls in the transition between her acts of charity and her miracles. In the next paragraph she miraculously cures wounds, fevers, and diseases; six paragraphs later comes a list of Radegund's miracles, in which she cures several illnesses, restores sight to a blind woman, and brings the dead back to life. Radegund was an intercessory miracle worker but she did not provide cures for the leprous women she kissed.[18]

The story invites the audience to shudder in awe of the saint, as Fortunatus remarks: 'Doesn't this thing that she accomplished sweetly make one shudder?'[19] Fortunatus secures his audience's attention by signalling that his next story will entertain and shock, ensuring that he will also have their ears when he instructs them on Radegund's worthiness for sainthood.[20] He establishes that Radegund's actions were outside the norm, as her attendant chided her for kissing leprous people, but also deeds to admire. Her humility is spotlighted in the contrast of both her able-bodiedness and her social status as princess, queen, and monastic founder acting as servant for low-status leprous recipients of charity. Radegund's kiss marked her leprous guests as members of her circle of Christian fellowship, regardless of their illness. Fortunatus indicates that these visitors had some expectation of receiving charity when he says that 'when lepers arrived, [they made] a sign, and approached'.[21] We do not receive further indication of their experience, beyond this description of leprous people travelling together, alerting a community to their presence and then approaching to receive charity, a process they likely repeated daily. Radegund's assistant did not object to Radegund engaging with the leprous visitors, only with her intimate physical contact. Yet the attendant's remarks led Radegund to note that she could do without the assistant's membership in that community, given her discomfort with whom Radegund chose to embrace. Radegund's lack of concern about her own safety as she put the care of others ahead of the health of her own body was another demonstration of her holiness and of Christian charity. Radegund's mark of inclusion for the leprous people was also a demonstration of courage and faith.

osculetur, quae sic leprosus amplecteris?" Illa respondit benivole: "Vere, si me non osculeris, hinc mihi cura ne ulla est"'.

18 Catherine Peyroux also noted Radegund's ability to perform other miracles, but not in this case; Peyroux, 'The Leper's Kiss', p. 181.

19 Fortunatus, 'Vita Radegundis', ch. 19, p. 370: 'Hanc quoque rem intremescendam qua peragebat dulcedine'.

20 For the dual purpose of hagiography to educate and entertain, see Spencer-Hall, *Medieval Saints*, especially pp. 43–44, 49.

21 Fortunatus, 'Vita Radegundis', ch. 19, p. 370: 'Cum leprosi venientes, signo facto, se proderent'.

Radegund's charity is an *imitatio Christi*, replicating Christ's attention to people with leprosy. We see this in Matthew 8.1–4:

> [W]hen he was come down from the mountain, great multitudes followed him: And behold a leper came and adored him, saying: 'Lord, if thou wilt, thou canst make me clean'. And Jesus stretching forth his hand, touched him, saying: 'I will, be thou made clean.' And forthwith his leprosy was cleansed. And Jesus saith to him: 'See thou tell no man: but go, shew thyself to the priest, and offer the gift which Moses commanded for a testimony unto them.'[22]

And later, in Matthew 10.5–8: 'These twelve Jesus sent, commanding them, [...] "Heal the sick, raise the dead, cleanse the lepers, cast out devils: freely have you received, freely give"'.[23] The biblical example sets expectations for saints to also cleanse people of leprosy, but Radegund's encounter requires an alternate description. Since she does not cure the disease, Fortunatus instead emphasizes holy charity.[24]

The offer of a kiss to leprous people was a hagiographical topos, as has been studied extensively.[25] For Radegund and Fortunatus, St Martin was the obvious exemplum for her sainthood, a local saint whose work in Tours shaped many of Radegund's actions. Martin kissed and miraculously cured a leprous man, imitating Christ by physically touching the man to cure him, but enhancing the touch with an embrace. The kiss itself was a significant gesture, an intimate contact laden with meaning, here indicating community, acceptance, and charity. Leprosy's effect on the face made the kiss especially significant as a point of contact between the saint and the

22 Douay-Rheims Bible; Vulgate: 'cum autem descendisset de monte secutae sunt eum turbae multae, et ecce leprosus veniens adorabat eum dicens Domine si vis potes me mundare, et extendens manum tetigit eum Iesus dicens volo mundare et confestim mundata est lepra eius, et ait illi Iesus vide nemini dixeris sed vade ostende te sacerdoti et offer munus quod praecepit Moses in testimonium illis'. The same incident is described much the same way in Mark 1.40–45 and Luke 5.12–14, with the addition that the healed man spreads the news. Consider also Luke 17.11–19, when Christ sends a group of ten leprous people to be healed by the priests.

23 Matthew 10.5–8: 'hos duodecim misit Iesus praecipiens eis [...] infirmos curate mortuos suscitate leprosos mundate daemones eicite gratis accepistis gratis date'.

24 Although not prevalent in the narratives examined here, Christ also charged the leprous man he healed with a task essential to healing miracles: once cured, the miracle's recipient is charged with reporting the story, often with evidence of their previous illness and current health. Miracle tale collections especially stress the importance of this crucial task, for the ill or disabled person, once healed, to thank the saint in person at the shrine and advertise the saint's intercession by reporting it.

25 Orlemanski, 'How to Kiss a Leper'; Peyroux, 'The Leper's Kiss'.

leprous person. Lesions with ulceration or necrosis can develop on the face, flattening or destruction of the nose, and loss of eyebrows and eyelashes can result in *leonine facies*, a change to the face that makes it appear like that of a lion. These facial changes were key to diagnosing leprosy, and became the disease's key identifying features culturally.[26] The kisses Radegund gave the leprous were not only intimate gestures of community and care, they also signified her saintly courage and charity by placing her lips on the body part most associated with the disease.[27]

This approach to leprosy on the part of saints, in which the disease served as a narrative prosthesis, remained consistent for centuries. St Elizabeth of Hungary, who died in 1231 at the age of twenty-four, was canonized in 1235. Born a princess, Elizabeth married and had children, but was widowed young and became a Franciscan tertiary, allowing relatives to raise her children. Elizabeth devoted herself to the sick and poor, working in a hospital and living under the spiritual authority and control of her confessor Conrad of Marburg (d. 1233). Conrad reported her interest in treating leprosy:

> She [Elizabeth] took on, without my knowledge, the care of a leprous girl and hid her in her own quarters, taking upon herself every duty dictated by humanity. She humbled herself by feeding her, laying her down, washing her, and even removing her shoes, imploring the other members of her household not to be offended by such things. When I discovered this, I punished her severely—may the Lord forgive me—because I feared she would be infected by contact with the girl. After I had sent away the leper and then left to preach in far-off places, she took in a poor little boy who was so mangy that he did not have a single hair on his head. Her intent was to cure him. And indeed by bathing and treating him she succeeded in curing him, and this boy was seated at her bedside when she died.[28]

26 Orlemanski, 'How to Kiss a Leper', pp. 148–49.

27 Though beyond the scope of this essay, it is also significant that kisses were extended only to leprous people of the same sex as the saint: for Fortunatus this is a way for Radegund to avoid any hint of sin, particularly as a married woman whose virginity could not be used to establish her saintly credentials. This larger project (see n. 6 above) will consider queer readings of the leper's kiss.

28 Conrad von Marburg to Gregory IX, pp. 33–34: 'Quo mortuo virginem sibi leprosam me nesciente assumpsit procurandam et in domo sua abscondit, omne humanitatis officium sibi impendens, ita quod non solum ad cibandam et ei sternendum, lavandam, sed etiam ad discalciandam se humiliavit, specialiter sue supplicans familie, ne super hiis offenderetur. Quo percepto, parcat michi dominus! Quia verebar eam infici inde, gravissime castigavi. Tandem leprosa per me rejecta et me ad laborem predicationis ad remotas partes recedente puerum pauperculum omnino scabiosum, ita quod ne unum pilum in capite habuit, a scabie curandum

We may wonder at the perspectives of this girl and boy, at being brought into the home of a princess for personal services. While Conrad depicts Elizabeth acting as their nurse and servant, what agency did her patients have in receiving this care or, for the leprous girl, being hidden away? Were they willing participants in this transaction of saintly care? What happened to the girl after Conrad evicted her? Elizabeth moved on, but would the girl have been able to find alternate care?

Conrad's contrast between the girl and the boy marks the differences in the ways that saints approached leprosy from their approaches to other illnesses they treated. While Elizabeth was confident of curing mange with bathing and treatment, Conrad did not identify this as a goal or even a hope she had for the leprous girl. Elizabeth's curing was not miraculous for either patient—she intended to nurse the boy to health with good hygiene and medical care—but there was also no delusion that such care would do the same for the girl. Elizabeth's charity to her leprosy patient was an exercise in humility, particularly for someone of Elizabeth's high social status, one that might offend her staff, and one requiring punishment because of the risk it posed to Elizabeth's health. All the same, she urged her household to accept her care for the girl among them. Like Radegund, Elizabeth humbled herself by caring for the leprous body, as well as by humbling herself to perform servile tasks despite her elevated status. Building a reputation for sanctity from such a position of privilege was facilitated for Elizabeth by the narrative position of the leprous girl.

The saint's disregard for her own health is similar to Radegund's, demonstrating her Christian charity and humility. Each holy woman offered the leprous people they tended excellent treatment, bathing them, offering them peace and comfort. And each faced the revulsion and censure of observers for their contact with leprous people. Conrad makes explicit what Radegund's assistant hinted at: 'I feared she would be infected by contact with the girl'. That fear of contracting the disease kept others from demonstrating the courage that made Radegund and Elizabeth holy.

Elizabeth's aunt, Hedwig of Silesia (d. 1243), also devoted charity to a leprosy hospital. Born into a prominent Bavarian family in the late twelfth century, Hedwig also married young, and through marriage became the duchess of Silesia. Like Radegund, Hedwig moderated her husband's rule by offering charity to prisoners, widows and orphans, and the poor. She also

assumpsit et tam in lavando quam in medicando, a quo didicerit nescio, ejus curam egit, et iste puer ea moriente stratu suo assedit'; *The Life and Afterlife of St Elizabeth of Hungary*, p. 48. On Elizabeth, see also Maurer, 'Die heilige Elisabeth und ihr Marburger Hospital'.

served as a mediator when needed. While Hedwig did not formally join an order or swear oaths of obedience as her niece Elizabeth did, she did dress as a Cistercian nun to indicate her devotion and intentions, albeit ignoring claustration (the expectation that monastic women remained enclosed within their abbey walls). Hedwig outlived all but one of her seven children, dying in 1243, and was canonized in 1267 by Clement IV.[29] Hedwig was known to care for people with leprosy, and according to her fourteenth-century anonymous *vita*, the *Legenda maior de beata Hedwigi*:

> She took special care of the leprous because of her love of He who wanted to become a leper for us. She took some leprous women living near the town of New Forum into her care, sending them money, meat, and game several times a week. She generously provided them with clothes and other necessaries, and took care of them in all things as special daughters. With a wonderful tenderness of compassion she condescended to care for those with any sort of bodily affliction, and her heart was tender toward the poor and infirm, to whom she gave both affection and a helping hand.[30]

Hedwig was also known for washing the feet of leprosy patients with her own hair, a common association of the leprous person with Christ, and the saint with the humility of Mary Magdalene.[31] Hedwig primarily offered support from afar in the manner typical for a royal woman: she sent supplies and funds to support her charity of choice. Even her more intimate service, washing the feet of leprous people, echoes the service expected of royals during Holy Week. Hedwig goes further by using her hair to solidify the reference to Christ, figuratively laying hands on him as Mary Magdalene did, as well as laying hands on the leprous, as did Christ. Unfortunately, we get no sense of the recipients' perspective on Hedwig's charity.

Hedwig, Elizabeth, and Radegund are all high-profile examples of female saints who married powerful noblemen; Hedwig and Elizabeth also bore

29 *Vita Sanctae Hedwigis*; Clement IV, bull of canonization, 1267 in *Vita Sanctae Hedwigis*; and *Das Leben der Heiligen*; Alvis, 'The Modern Lives of a Medieval Saint', pp. 3–4. On Hedwig, see also Gottschalk, *St Hedwig*; *Die Hedwigs-Predigt d. Papstes Klemens IV*, pp. 140–44.

30 *Vita Sanctae Hedwigis*, pp. 546–47: 'Leprosorum curam habuit specialem pro amore illius, qui pro nobis fieri voluit ut leprosus. Unde leprosas quasdam feminas insimul habitantes prope oppidum, quod dicitur Novum forum, sic in suam receperat curam, ut eis aliquociens in ebdomada mitteret pecunias, carnes et ferinas ac in vestibus et aliis vite necessariiis largiter providebat eisdem procurabatque ipsas in omnibus tamquam filias speciales. Mira compassionis teneritudine condescendebat afflicits qualicunque molestia corporali liquiescebatque animus eius ad pauperes et infirmos, quibus et affectum exhibebat et manum auxilii'.

31 See Luke 7.38.

children. Typical ideals of female sanctity, which stressed virginity, would not work for their *vitae*. Further, their elevated positions of wealth, power, and influence made messages of humility especially necessary in depicting them as saints. Willingness to care directly for the imprisoned, the poor, and the ill presented this image of humble sanctity, but including leprous people as a focus of these women's charity underlined their self-sacrificing humility, charity, and devotion. That this work was risky was clear from Radegund's attendant and from Conrad's reaction, but the risk of infection or social impact made the women's charity that much more powerful. The leprous body became a useful tool for these women to overcome their privileged position, and for their hagiographers to argue for their sanctity.

The Franciscan tertiary Angela of Foligno (d. 1309) took this even further when, according to her confessor Brother Arnaldo's transcription of her oral account, she fed a group of people and washed a leprous man 'whose hands were withered and decomposing'.[32] She then drank the wash-water, which she found as sweet as the communion wafer.

> And when a scab from the lepers' sores had become lodged in my throat, I tried to swallow it; and my conscience kept me from spitting it out—just as if I had received Holy Communion; and so I did dislodge it—not in order to spit it out, but so that it could go down my throat.[33]

While some may have expected Angela to spit out the scab, as the holy woman herself suggests, she refused. For Angela the leprous body became, in pieces, a manifestation of the eucharist, of Christ's physical presence. Angela's ingestion of the leprous man's flesh is an intimate gesture of accepting him as a member of her Christian community, and of understanding him metaphorically and physically as Christ. The leprous man is significant in Angela's narrative for the pieces of himself left behind for her ingestion, making him into an object of her washing, but also of her devotional practice. She seizes the power to receive communion on her own, without priestly intervention, and performs the miracle of the mass, not to consecrate the wafer, but to transform the fragmented, leprous body into Christ's flesh. By cleaning, feeding, clothing, and tending the leprous body, Elizabeth, Hedwig,

32 Angela of Foligno, *Beatae Angelae de Fulginio Visionum et instructionum liber*, p. 176: 'lavimus [...] et manus hominum, et maxime cuiusdam leprosi, qui habebat manus valde foetidas et marcidas et praepeditas et corruptas'.

33 Ibid., pp. 176–77: 'Et quia quaedam squamula illarum plagarum erat interposita in gutture meo, conata sum ad glutiendum eam, sicut si communicassem, donec deglutivi eam'. Translated in Mazzoni, *Angela of Foligno's Memorial*, p. 53.

Angela, and Radegund provided important medical treatment. They also embraced a real and lingering risk for their own bodies by ingesting scabs, kissing leprous lips, and otherwise coming into close contact with the leprous body. This vividly demonstrated their humility and lack of concern for their own safety, as they prioritized the care they provided others. Their saints' *vitae* made sure to emphasize that others found this shocking and revolting, but that these women's brave humility justified their sainthood. Such language compelled the audience to marvel at the difficulty of the saints' work, and their extraordinary piety, to understand the severity of the disease they treated and even the need for holy women's bravery in the community.

Lest we think this an entirely Western or Christian phenomenon, a legend about the eighth-century Buddhist Empress Kōmyō of Japan (d. 760) includes a similar encounter with leprosy.[34] Kōmyō was born in 701 to the influential Fujiwara family of the Nara period. She became consort of the Emperor Shōmu, and in that role was devoted to care for the sick and the poor. Her family was Buddhist and her father and grandfather were especially involved in providing state support for Buddhism. She continued their efforts by working for the creation of Hokkeji temple and of Tōdaiji temple and its Great Buddha as well as a 'national network of provincial temples', perhaps following the example of the seventh-century Empress Wu.[35] She arranged for an office that used tax money to give medicine to the poor and devoted herself to their care. The *Sequel to the Chronicles of Japan* reports that

> she cared for the people and did everything possible for their welfare. [...] The building of Tōdaiji temple and the establishment of official state temples throughout the land were initiated by the empress. She also founded both the Hiden'in to feed the starving and the Seyaku'in to care for the sick.[36]

34 I learned of this incident from Susan L. Burns's excellent plenary address, 'The Geography of Exclusion: Leprosy in Premodern Japan', presented at 'Leprosy and the "Leper" Reconsidered' at McGill University in September 2018. I am grateful to conference organizers Courtney Krolikoski and Anna Peterson, and all the presenters and attendees, for this rich and inspiring set of discussions. The address is now part of Burns, *Kingdom of the Sick*. See also Vargas-O'Bryan's chapter in the present volume, pp. 115–46, which offers a study of Gelongma Palmo, an early tenth-century Indian Buddhist nun and former leper. On Chinese Buddhism and disability, see also Jensen's chapter, pp. 87–113.

35 Daisuke, 'Empress Kōmyō's Buddhist Faith', pp. 22, 30, 33.

36 *Sequel to the Chronicles of Japan* (*Shoku Nihongi*), 760.6.7, quoted in Daisuke, 'Empress Kōmyō's Buddhist Faith', p. 22.

The *Sequel to the Chronicles of Japan* relates that Kōmyō once bathed one thousand people, described by Susan Burns as 'a merit-making activity intended to reduce the karmic burden of its sponsor'.[37] The thousandth person Kōmyō bathed suffered from leprosy, 'rai', with oozing sores.[38] She washed him carefully and then sucked out the pus from his lesions with her mouth. When she did this, the man revealed himself to be the Bodhisattva Ashuku; in Buddhism, a bodhisattva is a person with the ability to achieve nirvana who delays to help others. The story was retold by Kokan Shiren in the fourteenth century:

> The empress [...] built a warm-water bathhouse forthwith, that persons of both exalted and humble condition might be bathed. She also made a vow: 'I myself will personally cleanse the bodies of 1,000 people'. Her lord and ministers were apprehensive but the empress's powerful will was not to be checked. She had finished with 999, and there was only one last man left. The stench from the leprous eruptions that covered his entire body filled the hall. The empress was afraid to cleanse him, but thought to herself, 'I have almost completed the 1,000; how can I hold back from fulfilling my vow?' And she persevered and rubbed away at the man's back. The sick man said, 'Long ago I contracted a grievous disease, and ever since I have been afflicted with these boils. By chance, I met a healer who instructed me that by causing someone to suck the pus from them by mouth I would unfailingly be cured. But in all the world there is no one of profound compassion, and hence this stubborn illness has continued to this day. You, O empress, are revered for your unbounded mercy that you exercise. Have pity on me, I beg you!' The empress was unable to refuse, and so she sucked out the pus from his boils over his whole body, from the top of his head to his heels, and spat it out. Then she said to the sick man, 'Keep this a secret and tell no one that I have sucked your boils'. At this moment the sick man emitted a radiant light and announced, 'That your majesty has cleansed the body of the Buddha Ashuku you, too, must keep secret: tell no one'. The empress gazed at him in astonishment and saw that his marvelous form was perfect in beauty radiant, and sweetly fragrant.[39]

37 Burns, *Kingdom of the Sick*, pp. 28–29.

38 See ibid., pp. 20–22 for a discussion of 'rai' as 'leprosy'.

39 Quoted in Ury, 'Nuns and Other Female Devotees in *Genkō shakusho*', p. 194. Locating the original language for this text has proven challenging, beyond even the language barrier, and requires expertise that is also difficult to secure.

D. Max Moerman observes that in Japan 'deities who appear as lepers to test the compassion and perception of the followers' were a common literary trope in medieval narratives of curative bathing.[40] Demonstrating her commitment to her faith and her fearlessness in the face of this disease, Kōmyō proved her worthiness to be counted among the holy, just as Angela, Hedwig, Elizabeth, and Radegund had. She demonstrated humility by serving the poor and the ill as a reversal of her elevated status. And she devoted herself to her faith, which was rewarded by contact with one of the Buddhas. Kōmyō's care, devotion, humility, and willingness to sacrifice herself became a long-lasting legend about a holy woman attempting to treat leprosy. Kōmyō's holy example inspired the nuns of Hokkeji temple to see her as not just founder, but as divine, a 'manifestation of the bodhisattva Kannon'.[41] Kōmyō's story demonstrates that leprosy, a disease with global impact, similarly had resonance beyond Europe, and that care for leprous people had spiritual significance outside Christianity. It is a useful reminder that leprosy affected many cultures, and that an incurable disease provided opportunities for divine interventions. The shape of these narratives, of course, differed, with Kōmyō's example leveraging the 'Disappearing Leper' trope that kept the danger of infection from truly being present, a narrative that in Europe is much more present in the texts of male saints.[42]

For the Christian European women we have examined, however, bravery, humility, and inclusion in the face of the real presence of such danger is the recurring theme of their encounters. Many leprosy narratives depict the saint needing to overcome their revulsion at the effects of leprosy on the face and body, as Orlemanski observes:

> In Francis's and others' accounts of the leprous kiss, disgust and its concomitants provide a kind of affective heat fueling the spiritual transformations produced out of the kiss. Accounts of caring for the sick often present *two* disfigured, unruly, extraordinary bodies—one racked by the effects of disease, and one by subjective reactions to it. Face to face, infected and affected mirror one another in a moment of

40 Moerman, 'The Buddha and the Bathwater', p. 71.

41 Meeks, 'In Her Likeness', p. 360.

42 In 'Disappearing Leper' narratives the saint encounters a leprous person who requests assistance. Once the saint helps, the leprous person disappears altogether, leaving behind some sign of holiness, or transforming into Christ. Since there was no leprosy truly present, the saint was never in danger, but their humility and courage are still illustrated by the encounter. Further, the fact that the saint is worthy of attention from Christ or, in this case, a bodhisattva, further demonstrates their holiness.

> near-uncontrollable physicality, which piety takes as its opportunity for spiritual metamorphosis. Producing a certain *frisson* of disgust in the reader is also part of the rhetorical labour of such accounts. The reader's repugnance manifests the difference between his or her own reactions and the holy person's heroic feats of love.[43]

When depicting such high-status women, even the reluctance saints such as Francis were able to show and overcome could not be admitted—these holy women had no space for doubt or reluctance.

Becoming Leprous

For some Christian women, caring for leprous bodies was not enough of a sacrifice, and they looked for ways to go further, risk more, and face greater danger. Becoming leprous was a way to encounter bravely the risk of the illness, to suffer, to atone for sin, and to demonstrate Christian faith. Both male and female saints sought to experience the illness as a way of checking their pride and pursuing piety, as a way of suffering like Christ.

For the Dominican tertiary Catherine of Siena (d. 1380), contracting leprosy was a result of the same sorts of close contact with leprosy patients that Angela, Elizabeth, and Radegund had performed. After caring for a leprous woman, Raymond of Capua (d. 1399) tells us that God allowed leprosy to cover Catherine's hands,

> in order to render the triumph of his faithful spouse the more striking. [...] This misfortune did not arrest her, she preferred being covered with leprosy to renouncing her charitable functions; her body she looked upon as dust; she was not anxious concerning what might happen to it if what she did were agreeable to our Lord.[44]

After the leprous woman died and Catherine buried her, 'the disease disappeared from Catherine's body suddenly; her hands seemed to be whiter

43 Orlemanski, 'How to Kiss a Leper', p. 151.

44 AASS Apr 3:889: 'permittente Domino, pro gloriosiori sponsae suae triumph, infectionem leprae ad manus sacrae virginis deducit. [...] Sed illa in nullo propter hoc a sancto suo recedens proposito, praeligebat potius totaliter leprosa effici, quam inchoatum dimittere officium caritatis: spernebat siquidem velut lutum proprium corpus, et quidquid illi contingeret non curabat, dummodo Sponso suo aeterno grato servitio deserviret'; *Life of Saint Catharine of Sienna by the Blessed Raymond of Capua*, pp. 93–95.

than the rest of her person, as though the leprosy had imported additional delicacy to them', since the 'Lord healed instantly those hands that had been attacked with leprosy in serving [a leprous woman] during life and after death'.[45] Catherine's visible leprosy on her hands as a gift that God allowed her is an intriguing contrast to the stigmata her hands received. While leprosy marked her hands, Catherine's stigmata remained invisible. Catherine's story demonstrates that the danger of contracting leprosy for saints providing palliative care to patients was a real one, but God was willing to work a miracle for the saint's benefit.[46]

Other saints in this group followed the model of Job, whom God tested, according to the Old Testament, with many torments. Job lost his children, his home, his possessions, and his health. He developed boils 'from the sole of the foot even to the top of his head'.[47] While there is some debate about what Job's disease might have been, medieval authors depicted his boils as leprosy. Like Christ's pain, Job's sufferings in the Bible became a model for saints' lives, an example for how hagiographers might depict holy men and women who became leprous themselves.[48] His example promised medieval Christians that leprosy might be a test from God as well as an opportunity to suffer as Christ had, and that God could heal them, but that they need not—even should not—seek such healing. Instead, patience, loyalty, and endurance would demonstrate their faith and their worthiness.

This idea is most clearly represented in the life of the thirteenth-century Cistercian nun Alice of Schaerbeek.[49] Alice was 'struck' with leprosy by God, experiencing the disease 'from the sole of her foot up to the crown' of her

45 AASS Apr 3:890: 'mox de virginis manibus omnis infectio lepræ ita evanuit, ac si numquam fuissent infectæ: imo videbatur, quod manus ejus decore suo cuncta corporis ejus membra excederent, & quasi ex lepra nitorem suscepissent'; *Life of Saint Catharine of Sienna by the Blessed Raymond of Capua*, pp. 93–95.

46 It also highlights, again, the instrumentalization of the leprous in these narratives—the concern is for Catherine's experience and her reputation, leaving the leprous person as object to disappear from the story.

47 Job 2.7: 'pessimo a planta pedis usque ad verticem eius'.

48 Job 2.7: '[E]gressus igitur Satan a facie Domini percussit Job ulcere pessimo a planta pedis usque ad verticem eius'. The ulcer is cited in Leviticus as a sign of leprosy ('leprae')—see Leviticus 13. Vicchio notes that some Jewish and Muslim scholars also identified Job's illness as leprosy; *Job in the Medieval World*, p. 235. Job's illness may not have been Hansen's Disease, or Mycobacterial leprosy; Gryzbowski and Nita, 'Leprosy in the Bible', pp. 3–7. See also Rawcliffe, *Leprosy in Medieval England*, p. 57. Rawcliffe notes that Jacques de Vitry's sermons spread this message in the thirteenth century; see also Bériou and Touati, *Voluntate Dei leprosus*, pp. 24, 28–42, 101–28.

49 For more on Alice, see Spencer-Hall, 'Christ's Suppurating Wounds'. In the present volume, see the chapter by Escobedo on Alice, pp. 220–23; and on leprosy more generally, see Vargas-O'Bryan (pp. 115–46).

head, like Job.[50] Alice later died of the disease. God did not seem to be testing Alice, however. Instead, the saint's *vita* presented Alice's disease as a gift:

> What [God] did now, he did not in any vindictiveness, nor as if blaming her for some crime. He did it as might a bridegroom, minded to pay his bride a visit and bring her a token of his perfect love for her. God longed that his bride be free, be at leisure for him alone; that she linger with him in the bedroom, the bridal chamber of her mind; that there she be soothingly inebriated with a fragrance all his own. And what did he do? He struck her a heavy blow, struck her down with a disease, an incurable disease, a disease few could wish for: leprosy itself.[51]

Alice's leprous body exuded a perfume that refreshed those around her, but her body physically disintegrated in a way that horrified.[52] While many saints hold onto their wholeness even after death, Alice's *vita* emphasized her physical breakdown:

> All who caught sight of that body were shocked to a standstill, awestruck as at the sign of some horrible monster. They were convinced no creature could anywhere be found comparable with her for horror. Wholly deprived of the use of her body and of any of its members, she was committed to her bed just as a rotting corpse is committed to the earth, as if to let the rotting itself finish her off. When all such sufferings and weaknesses suddenly broke in on her, these too she welcomed with the glad delight of a bride receiving from her Groom so many long-desired gifts.[53]

50 'De B. Aleyde Scharembekana', p. 482: 'nam a planta pedis usque ad verticem, non erat in ea sanitas'.

51 'De B. Aleyde Scharembekana', p. 479: 'Post haec autem, cum ipsa virtutum augmento in annis cresceret, et tamen discretione virtutum numerum annorum superaret; volens Deus, electionis suae vas futurum, ab omni strepitu temporali, et inquinamento hujus seculi, penitus purgari; non tamen ob alicujus criminis culpam vel vindictam, sed causa visitationis et more sponsi, sponsae suae arrham tribuentis in signum perfectae dilectionis; ut soli Deo liberius posset vacare, et intra cubiculum mentis suae in thalamo secum morari, et suavitate odoris sui sponsam suam cupiens inebriari; morbo incurabili, paucis desiderabili, lepra videlicet, ipsam graviter percussit'; translation from *Life of St Alice*, p. 9.

52 'De B. Aleyde Scharembekana', p. 479, ch. 10.

53 'De B. Aleyde Scharembekana', p. 482: 'Omnes ipsum intuentes, timore quasi monstri horribilis subito steterunt perculsi et aestimabant, aliam creaturam, ei in horrore comparandam, nusquam posse reperiri. Fuit itaque ab officio, corporis scilicet et membrorum, tota destituta; et more cadaveris in terra putrescentis, in lectulo suo tradita, quasi putredine extitit consummanda. Cujusmodi passiones pariter et infirmitates, magis solito ingruentes, tanta suscepit delectatione et laetitia, ac si sponsa ab sponso acciperet munuscula diu desiderata.' *Life of St Alice*, pp. 27-28.

The *vita* lets us know Alice was grateful for her groom's gifts of torment even though—or maybe because—the disease ravaged her body. Indeed, Alice's torments were so vicious that Christ gave her comfort by allowing her to drink from his wounds: 'she would wing her way to the bosom of Christ, even as a little one to suck its mother's breasts. And how promptly she would feel her bruised members restored to soundness, thanks to the fluid from those wounds'.[54] While Angela contented herself with leprous scabs as eucharist, Alice received communion directly from Christ, her experience of leprosy granting her access without priestly intervention. This was not a healing, just a momentary comfort demonstrating God's love before she returned to her physical torments, her own passion. Alice neither sought nor desired any cure for her disease. Rather, it provided her with an opportunity to ingest Christ's body without the intervention of a priest, directly from Christ himself. She received the pain and suffering of her disease as a gift to treasure, not as a torment to erase.

Like Christ, suffering allowed Alice to be able to help others: Alice's sister, Lady Ida, was troubled by Alice's pain, which made Ida 'groan and wail and shed a whole shower of tears', but Alice told her,

> 'Do not imagine that it is for sins of my own that I am prey to these torments. Rather it is for the deceased, subject to long, excruciating detention in regions of penalty, and for the sinners of the world, already miserably trapped in the fowlers' snares and apt to be endlessly seduced. Yes, while this penalty, as you see, is rapidly consuming me, it is also having the happy effect of releasing the living, of freeing the deceased from all such snares.'[55]

For Alice, leprosy was an opportunity to redeem the souls of her community members rather than a way to atone for her own sins. Further, when she was going blind, Alice devoted one of her eyes to helping the king and the

54 'De B. Aleyde Scharembekana', p. 479: 'more parvuli causa sugendi matris ubera, ad pectus Christi convolavit et ad vulnera; quorum liquore membra sauciata sanitati concito sensit restituta'; *Life of St Alice*, p. 11. Christ also appeared in miracles, lives, and stories as a leprous man, often in the disappearing leper narrative. This image was also popular in sermons; see Jacques de Vitry and Thomas Frederick Crane, *Exempla*, cited in Spencer-Hall, 'Christ's Suppurating Wounds', p. 404 n. 60.

55 'De B. Aleyde Scharembekana', p. 481: 'non autem me putes pro peccatis meis hujusmodi exponi tormentis, sed pro defunctis in locis poenalibus diu cruciandis; et pro peccatoribus mundi, a laqueis venantium jam jam miserabiliter irretitis, et sine fine seducendis, nisi per poenam, qua me vides sic consumi, defuncti mereantur liberari; et vivi, a laqueis similiter relaxari'; *Life of St Alice*, pp. 23-24.

other to helping a count, believing that her physical disintegration directly assisted the Christian community and she could assign her body parts like boons, holy relics before she had even died. Alice's pleasure in being able to use her leprous body as gifts and her suffering to redeem sin for her community gesture at the perspective other leprous people in hagiographical texts might have held. While most texts treat the leprous as objects and instrumentalize their disease for the holy person's saintly reputation, Alice's perspective suggests that some leprous people found their position in these transactions satisfying or even fulfilling, for their own roles in redeeming sin and building saints' holy dossiers.

The opportunities presented by leprosy to suffer in imitation of Christ or to further humble oneself proved quite attractive to would-be saints. Yvette of Huy (d. 1228) and Margaret of Cortona (d. 1297) sought out the disease, wishing to be blessed by the sort of gift that God had given Alice, but neither was successful. Yvette hedged her bets, not relying only on prayer to achieve her goal; she actually joined a leprosarium, to become 'the most thoroughly miserable of all the miserable'.[56] She nursed the patients, bathed in the same water, ate and drank alongside them, courting danger as Angela of Foligno had when she drank the scabby wash-water. When she realized a blessing of leprosy was not forthcoming, she shifted tactics and became an anchoress instead, finding success in guiding others after she walled herself up in her cell. The transactional nature of Yvette's charity is revealed when she abandons the leprous people who have failed to fulfil her expectations and share leprosy with her. Finding her charity unrewarded, she switches focus, once again leaving the leprous as objects worthy only when useful to her.

According to her confessor Giunta Bevegnati, author of the *Legenda de vita et miraculis Beatae Margaritae de Cortona*, Margaret of Cortona put her faith into a dialogue with God, in which she begged him to bless her with the disease: '"Lord, infect my body with leprosy so that I will not offend again. In your compassion lead me to the cross"'.[57] God rejected her request, responding that 'her present troubles were enough. If she contracted leprosy, she might become too self-assured. But with temptations and bodily

56 AASS Jan 1:870: 'quae in meliori statu consistere secundum seculum videbatur vitae, divitiarum, et aetatis, spreta mundana gloria, tantam appetere miseriam, et miseriam omnibus miseriis graviorem, videlicet servire, et cohabitare leprosis'. See Carpenter, 'Juette of Huy'; Hugh of Floreffe, *The Life of Yvette of Huy*, trans. by McNamara; Mulder-Bakker, 'Ivetta of Huy'; Mulder-Bakker, 'Yvette of Huy'.

57 AASS Feb 3:324: 'Domine, pone in corpore meo lepram, ne de cetero te offendam, et digneris me pietate tua ad Crucem reducere'; *Life and Miracles of Margaret of Cortona*, ch. 5, p. 137.

infirmities she would continue her sense of fear and stay in the state of grace'.[58] God withheld leprosy, apparently, in order to keep Margaret from growing too confident. For Margaret the disease was a state to desire and long for, to take into her own body with simple touch supplying insufficient contact to enable her to contract the disease. Rather than bestowing charity on others, becoming leprous herself would allow Margaret to focus on her personal experience of suffering and saintliness, if only God would grant her that gift.

The disease could also guide holy men and women onto God's path. An anonymous twelfth-century Latin life of the Merovingian St Enimie (d. before 700) depicts the saint's efforts to maintain her virginity in the face of her father's determination to see her married. Enimie devoted herself to God, and 'at that moment the divine mercy that she had chosen so darkened her beauty that she was no longer to be sought in marriage, since the disease of leprosy crept through her body and her virginal flesh, infected with leprosy, was rendered disfigured.'[59] Although Enimie was cured through a ritual bath, her leprosy returned when she went back to her father, which forced her to undergo the ritual bathing repeatedly, since she became leprous each time she returned to her parents. After a series of reinfections and repeated healings, grateful for her health and finally understanding God's purpose for her, Enimie stayed away from her family, founded a double monastery, and became its abbess.[60] She decided to reject the community of her parents in favour of the monastic community and communion with God.[61] Whenever Enimie followed God's plan she was healthy, but when

58 AASS Feb 3:324: 'quod ei sufficerent poenae suae, quia cum lepra secura esset, sed cum tentationibus et infirmitate corporea ipsam conseruabat in timore et gratia'; *Life and Miracles of Margaret of Cortona*, ch. 5, p. 138.

59 'Vita, inventio et miracula sanctae Enimiae', ed. Brunel, pp. 255–56: 'Illico divina clementia que sibi eam preelegerat, ita ejus corporis fuscavit pulchritudinem ne amplius peteretur ad martiale connubium, namque elefantie morbus per eius inrepsit corpus et virginea caro infecta lepra reddita est maculosa'; translation my own.

60 Gaunt, *Gender and Genre in Medieval French Literature*, p. 192. As Gaunt has pointed out, Enimie's virginity was the focus of the life and the only justification for her holy power to work miracles, or even her sanctity. Gaunt suggested that the text reflects a woman's ability to choose a religious life over a married one, which was certainly a prominent theme in female hagiographic literature (p. 194). See also Brunel, 'Un nouveau manuscript de la vita sanctae enimiae'. For a thirteenth-century Occitan poetic version of Enemie's life by Bertran de Marseille, see Brunel and Bertran de Marseille, *La Vie de sainte Enimie*.

61 There are strong parallels between Enimie and Radegund: both were royal, both sought to avoid a marriage and devote themselves to God, both became nuns, both needed to deal with a pesky dragon troubling their abbeys, and both performed miracles through ritual bathing. In the story of Enimie's life a pilgrim also travels to Poitiers, to visit the shrine of St Hilary.

she deviated from it he struck her again. With Enimie and Alice, we finally see a saintly narrative in which the leprous person moves from object to subject, but only when the saint becomes leprous and combines both the agency of healing with the receipt of care.

For these leprosy narratives, the saints' opportunity, or desire, to contract the disease focuses not on miracle cures, but on the saints' humility, personal suffering, penitence, and imitation of Christ. We can see in the saintly desire to experience leprosy personally why the encounters with leprosy described here did not focus on miraculous cures: cure of the disease was not a universal goal for leprous people. Living with the disease held social, cultural, and spiritual meaning, for those who cared for the leprous body as well as for those who inhabited it. In Margaret's case, God warned her that she could not fulfil her desire to receive leprosy because it would compromise her humility, while Alice luxuriates in the painful breakdown of her body to linger over the living martyrdom she endured with the patience and bravery expected of a saint.

In saints' *vitae*, leprosy allowed saints to redeem sin, whether for themselves or others, to prove their devotion to God, and to follow in the path of Christ. Their examples would be instructive to medieval audiences. Alice desired no miraculous cure, as leprosy fulfilled her and was the gift she desired, on a level with receiving the stigmata.[62]

Conclusion

These holy women engaged with leprosy in ways that valued nurture and care for the leprous but did not require a healing miracle. Miraculous healing of leprosy patients was not always desirable, as the leprous served important religious, spiritual, and social purposes for the broader community. While the hagiographic record does not reveal much about the perspectives of the non-saintly leprous, the encounters discussed here suggest that leprous people accepted and even appreciated these roles as well as their opportunity to serve the Christian community.

Rather than working a miracle that quickly removed the disease and its danger, many saints (most of them women) demonstrated their charity, courage, and faith by offering palliative care to people who continued to suffer from leprosy. That female saints were the ones offering care that involved the most intimate contact and greatest personal risk is not all that

62 Spencer-Hall, 'Christ's Suppurating Wounds', p. 390.

surprising, since nursing care for the sick has long been gendered feminine and marginalized, while since the twelfth century respect for medical healing has increasingly been reserved for elite, university-educated men.[63] And yet, female saints did frequently cure other diseases, sometimes on the same pages of their saints' lives in which they did not cure leprosy.

During the current COVID-19 pandemic, we are catching a glimpse of why medieval people at the height of the leprosy crisis prioritized what we now call nursing treatment, valuing the people who sacrificed their own safety to focus attention and care on the sick. For medieval people, seeing that some high-status saints could offer cures was reassuring, but much more commonly they reminded one another that many saints put their own bodies in danger to feed, bandage, clothe, wash, and care for leprosy patients, showing us how much value caring, and especially holy women's holy labour, was accorded in medieval communities. As we applauded 'the carers' from isolation each night in New York City in Spring 2020, I was reminded that the need to feel connected is rooted deeply in our humanity as well as how much we value those who protect us. For modern communities, fearing COVID, as well as for medieval communities facing leprosy, we value the carers, especially when miracles feel short of supply. These medieval holy women received recognition for their holy labour, immortalized in text, and as saints; meanwhile, those they cared for are left in near obscurity. For our modern medical workers, especially nursing and frontline staff, the experience of stagnant pay, longer hours, terrible working conditions, infection, and death through the pandemic suggests that the emotional appreciation for caring has not translated into institutional or structural value.

Abbreviations

AASS *Acta Sanctorum*

Bibliography

Primary Sources

Angela of Foligno, *Beatae Angelae de Fulginio Visionum et instructionum liber*, ed. by J. H. Lammertz (Cologne: Heberle, 1851)

63 Green, *Making Women's Medicine Masculine*, and 'Documenting Medieval Women's Medical Practice'.

'De B. Aleyde Scharembekana, sanctimoniali Ordinis Cisterciensis, Camerae iuxta Bruxellam', *Acta Sanctorum*, ed. by Godfrey Henschen (Paris: Société des Bollandistes, 1688; repr. 1969), 2 June: 477–83

Bevegnati, Giunta, *The Life and Miracles of Saint Margaret of Cortona (1247–1297)*, trans. by Thomas Renna and Shannon Larson (St. Bonaventure: Franciscan Institute, 2012)

Bevegnati, Giunta, 'Vita, De B. Margarita Poenitente Tertii Ord. S. Francisci, Cortonae in Umbria', ed. by Godfrey Henschen, in AASS (Paris: Société des Bollandistes, 1658), 3 February: 301–57

Brunel, Clovis, and Bertran de Marseille, *La Vie de sainte Enimie* (Paris: H. Campion, 1917)

Conrad von Marburg, 'Letter to Gregory IX, 1232', in *Hessisches Urkundenbuch*, ed. by Arthur Wyss (Lezig: S. Hirzel, 1879), pp. 31–35

Die Hedwigs-Predigt d. Papstes Klemens IV. Von Jahre 1267, in *Archiv für schlesische Kirchengeschichte*, 15 (1957), 15–35

Eustratius, 'Life of Eutychios', in *Cult of Saints in Late Antiquity*, summary by Silvio Roggo, <http://csla.history.ox.ac.uk/record.php?recid=E03093> [accessed 14 February 2023]

Fortunatus, Venantius, *Vita Radegundis, Liber I*, ed. by Bruno Krusch, *Monumenta Germaniae Historica: Scriptores Rerum Merovingicarum*, 2 (Hannover: Hahn, 1888), pp. 364–77

Garton, Charles, *The Metrical Life of Saint Hugh of Lincoln: The Latin Text with Introduction, Translation, and Notes* (Lincoln: Honywood Press, 1986)

Hugh of Floreffe, 'De B. Ivetta, Sive Iutta, Vidua Relusa, Hui in Belgio', ed. by Godfrey Henschen, in AASS (Paris: Société des Bollandistes, 1902–1970), 1 January: 864–87

Hugh of Floreffe, *The Life of Yvette of Huy*, trans. by Jo Ann McNamara (Toronto: Peregrina, 1999)

Das Leben der Heiligen Hedwig, trans. by Konrad Metzger and Franz Metzger (Düsseldorf: Patmos, 1967)

Jacques de Vitry and Thomas Frederick Crane, *The Exempla or Illustrative Stories from the Sermones of Jacques de Vitry* (London: D. Nutt, 1890)

Il libro della beata Angela da Foligno: edizione critica, ed. by Ludger Thier and Abele Calufetti (Rome: Editiones Collegi S. Bonaventurae ad Claras Aquas, 1985)

The Life and Afterlife of St. Elizabeth of Hungary: Testimony from Her Canonization Hearings, trans. by Kenneth Baxter Wolf (Oxford: Oxford University Press, 2010)

Life of St Alice of Schaerbeek, trans. by Martinus Cawley (Lafayette, OR: Our Lady of Guadalupe Abbey, 2000)

'Life of Symeon Stylites the Younger', in *Cult of Saints in Late Antiquity*, summary by Lucy Parker, <http://csla.history.ox.ac.uk/record.php?recid=E04126> [accessed 13 February 2023]

Raymond of Capua, *Life of Saint Catharine of Sienna by the Blessed Raymond of Capua, Her Confessor*, ed. by E. Cartier (Philadelphia: Peter F. Cunningham, 1860)

Raymond of Capua, 'Vita de S. Catharina Senensi, Virgine de Poenitentia S. Dominici', in AASS (Antwerp: Society of Bollandists, 1675), 3 April: 853–959

'Vita, inventio et miracula sanctae Enimiae', ed. by Clovis Brunel, *Analecta Bollandiana*, 57 (1939), 237–98

Vita Sanctae Hedwigis, in *Monumenta Poloniae Historica*, vol. 4 (Krakow: Nakł. Akademii Umiejętności, 1884), pp. 501–642

Secondary Sources

Alvis, Robert E., 'The Modern Lives of a Medieval Saint: The Cult of St. Hedwig in Twentieth-Century Germany', *German Studies Review*, 36 (2013), 1–20

Bériou, Nicole, and François-Olivier Touati, *Voluntate dei leprosus: les lépreux entre conversion et exclusion aux XIIeme et XIIIeme siècles* (Spoleto: Centro Italiano di studi Sull'altro Medioevo, 1991)

Brenner, Elma, *Leprosy and Charity in Medieval Rouen* (Woodbridge, Suffolk: Boydell Press, 2015)

Brenner, Elma, 'The Leprous Body in Twelfth- and Thirteenth-Century Rouen', in *The Ends of the Body: Identity and Community in Medieval Culture*, ed. by Suzanne Conklin Akbari and Jill Ross (Toronto: University of Toronto Press, 2013), pp. 239–59

Brenner, Elma, and François-Olivier Touati, eds, *Leprosy and Identity in the Middle Ages* (Manchester: Manchester University Press, 2021)

Brunel, Clovis, 'Un nouveau manuscrit de la vita sanctae Enimiae', *Analecta Bollandiana*, 75 (1957), 366–72

Burns, Susan L., *Kingdom of the Sick: A History of Leprosy and Japan* (Honolulu: University of Hawai'i Press, 2019)

Carpenter, Jennifer, 'Juette of Huy, Recluse and Mother (1158–1228): Children and Mothering in the Saintly Life', in *Power of the Weak: Studies on Medieval Women*, ed. by Jennifer Carpenter and Sally-Beth MacLean (Urbana: University of Illinois Press, 1995), pp. 57–93

Daisuke, Mikoshiba, 'Empress Kōmyō's Buddhist Faith: Her Role in the Founding of the State Temple and Convent System', trans. by Carol Hochstedler, in *Engendering Faith: Women and Buddhism in Premodern Japan*, ed. by Barbara Ruch (Ann Arbor: University of Michigan Press, 2002), pp. 21–40

Demaitre, Luke, *Leprosy in Premodern Medicine: A Malady of the Whole Body* (Baltimore: Johns Hopkins University Press, 2007)

Edwards, A. J. M., 'An Early Twelfth Century Account of the Translation of St. Milburga of Much Wenlock', *Transactions of the Shropshire Archaeological Society*, 57 (1962–63), 134–51

Edwards, Jennifer C., *Superior Women: Medieval Female Authority in Poitiers' Abbey of Sainte-Croix* (Oxford: Oxford University Press, 2019)
Folz, R., *Les saintes reines du Moyen Age en Occident* (*Vie-XIIIe siècles*) (Brussels: Société des Bollandistes, 1992)
Gaunt, Simon, *Gender and Genre in Medieval French Literature* (Cambridge: Cambridge University Press, 1995)
Gottschalk, J., *St. Hedwig: Herzogin von Schlesien* (Cologne and Graz: Böhlau, 1964)
Green, Monica H., 'Documenting Medieval Women's Medical Practice', in *Practical Medicine from Salerno to the Black Death*, ed. by Luis García-Ballester, Roger French, Jon Arrizabalaga, and Andrew Cunningham (Cambridge: Cambridge University Press, 1994), pp. 322–52
Green, Monica H., *Making Women's Medicine Masculine: The Rise of Male Authority in Pre-Modern Gynecology* (Oxford: Oxford University Press, 2008)
Gryzbowski, Andrzej, and Malgorzata Nita, 'Leprosy in the Bible', *Clinics in Dermatology*, 34 (2016), 3–7
Kendall, Carl, et al., 'A Social Network Approach for the Study of Leprosy Transmission Beyond the Household', *Transactions of the Royal Society of Tropical Medicine and Hygiene*, 116.2 (2022), 100–07
Krolikoski, Courtney A., 'Neither Sinner nor Outcast: Leprosy in Bologna Italy, 1100–1348' (unpublished doctoral dissertation, McGill University, 2021)
Maurer, W., 'Die heilige Elisabeth und ihr Marburger Hospital', *Jahrbuch d. hessischen kirchengeschichtlichen Vereinigung*, 7 (1956), 36–69
Maurer, W., 'Zum Verständnis der heiligen Elisabeth von Thüringen', *Zeitschrift für Kirchengeschichte*, 65 (1953–54), 16–64
Mazzoni, Cristina, *Angela of Foligno's Memorial* (Woodbridge, Suffolk: Boydell & Brewer, 1999)
Meeks, Lori R., 'In Her Likeness: Female Divinity and Leadership at Medieval Chūgūji', *Japanese Journal of Religious Studies*, 34 (2007): 351–92
Mitchell, David T., and Sharon L. Snyder, *Narrative Prosthesis: Disability and the Dependencies of Discourse* (Ann Arbor: University of Michigan Press, 2000)
Moerman, D. Max, 'The Buddha and the Bathwater: Defilement and Enlightenment in the *Onsenji engi*', *Japanese Journal of Religious Studies*, 42 (2015), 71–87
Moran, Michelle T., *Colonizing Leprosy: Imperialism and the Politics of Public Health in the United States* (Chapel Hill: University of North Carolina Press, 2007)
Mulder-Bakker, Anneke B., 'Ivetta of Huy: *Mater et Magistra*', in *Sanctity and Motherhood: Essays on Holy Mothers in the Middle Ages*, ed. by Anneke B. Mulder-Bakker (New York: Garland, 1995), pp. 224–58
———, 'Yvette of Huy: The Metamorphoses of a Woman', in *Lives of the Anchoresses: The Rise of the Urban Recluse in Medieval Europe*, trans. by Myra Heerspink Scholz (Philadelphia: University of Pennsylvania Press, 2005), pp. 51–77

Orlemanski, Julie, 'How to Kiss a Leper', *postmedieval: a journal of medieval and cultural studies*, 3.2 (2012), 142–57

Peyroux, Catherine, 'The Leper's Kiss', in *Monks and Nuns, Saints and Outcasts: Religion in Medieval Society: Essays in Honor of Lester K. Little*, ed. by Sharon Farmer and Barbara H. Rosenwein (Ithaca, NY: Cornell University Press, 2000), pp. 172–88

Ploemacher, Thomas, William R. Faber, Henk Menke, Victor Rutten, and Toine Pieters, 'Reservoirs and Transmission Routes of Leprosy: A Systematic Review', *PLOS: Neglected Tropical Diseases*, 14.4 (2020), e0008276, 1–27 <https://doi.org/10.1371/journal.pntd.0008276>

Rawcliffe, Carole, *Leprosy in Medieval England* (Woodbridge, Suffolk: Boydell & Brewer, 2009)

Spencer-Hall, Alicia, 'Christ's Suppurating Wounds: Leprosy in the *Vita* of Alice of Schaerbeek (†1250)', in *Wounds and Wound Repair in Medieval Culture*, ed. by Larissa Tracy and Kelly DeVries (Leiden: Brill, 2015), pp. 389–416

Spencer-Hall, Alicia, 'Chronic Pain and Illness: Reinstating Crip-Chronic Histories to Forge Affirmative Disability Futures', in *A Cultural History of Disability in the Middle Ages*, ed. by Jonathan Hsy, Tory V. Pearman, and Joshua R. Eyler (London: Bloomsbury, 2020), pp. 51–66

Spencer-Hall, Alicia, *Medieval Saints and Modern Screens: Divine Visions as Cinematic Experience*, Knowledge Communities (Amsterdam: Amsterdam University Press, 2018)

Touati, François-Olivier, *Maladie et société au Moyen Âge: La lèpre, les lépreux et les leproseries dans la province ecclésiastique de Sens jusq'au milieu du XIVe siècle* (Brussels: De Boeck Université, 1998)

Touati, François-Olivier, 'Saint-Lazare, Fontevraud, Jérusalem', in *Robert d'Arbrissel et la vie religieuse dans l'Ouest de la France: Actes du Colloque de Fontevraud, 13–16 décembre 2001*, ed. by Jacques Dalarun (Turnhout: Brepols, 2004), pp. 199–237

Ury, Marian, 'Nuns and other Female Devotees in *Genkō shakusho*', in *Engendering Faith: Women and Buddhism in Premodern Japan*, ed. by Barbara Ruch (Ann Arbor: University of Michigan Press, 2002), pp. 189–207

Vicchio, Stephen J., *The Image of the Biblical Job: A History*, 2 vols (Eugene, OR: Wipf and Stock, 2006), II

About the Author

Jennifer C. Edwards is Professor of History at Manhattan University in Riverdale, NY, where she teaches medieval and ancient history. Her research examines medieval European women and gender, power and authority, religion, and health. She is the author of *Superior Women: Medieval Female Authority in Poitiers' Abbey of Sainte-Croix* (Oxford, 2019) and *Daily Life of Women in Chaucer's England* (ABC-CLIO, 2022). She is working currently on a book project, *Holy Healing: Medieval Saints and Leprosy*, and a Reacting to the Past game, *Christine de Pizan and the Querelle des Femmes*. She earned her PhD and MA from the University of Illinois at Urbana-Champaign and her BA from the University of Massachusetts at Amherst. She is general editor of *Medieval Feminist Forum: A Journal of Gender and Sexuality* and serves on the Advisory Board of the Society for Medieval Feminist Scholarship.

10. Healing the Unborn: Natal Disability and the Old English *Life of St Margaret* in London, British Library, Cotton MS Tiberius A.iii

Leah Pope Parker

Abstract: Medieval associations of St Margaret of Antioch with pregnancy and childbirth are well-documented, yet the hagiographical tradition associating her with preventing the birth of disabled children remains little remarked. This chapter examines London, British Library, Cotton MS Tiberius A.iii, in which an Old English *Life of St Margaret* promotes the deliverance of medieval Christians' souls through the 'healing' of disabled bodies. I argue that the manuscript and Margaret's *Life* articulate a recognizable identity category akin, though not identical, to modern notions of disability. They also witness a 'premodern eugenic logic', revealing a desire to eliminate childhood disability, and thus also excise disabled children from the family, the community, and the world.

Keywords: natal disability, childbirth, eugenics, healing, pregnancy, prognostics, St Margaret of Antioch

> Where there is the book of my martyrdom, let there not be born a child that is blind, nor halt, nor dumb, nor deaf, nor vexed by an unclean spirit, but let peace and love and truth be there.[1]

1 Parker, trans., '*Life of St. Margaret*', p. 216; 'Þær boc sy mines martyrhades, ne sy þær geboren blind cild ne healt, ne dumb, ne deaf, ne fram unclænum gaste geswenct, ac sy þær sib and lufu

Grace-Petinos, Stephanie, Leah Pope Parker, and Alicia Spencer-Hall, eds. *Disability and Sanctity in the Middle Ages.* Taylor & Francis Group, 2025
DOI 10.5117/9789463724333_CH10

According to hagiographical legend, before her execution in the early fourth century, St Margaret of Antioch prayed that a disabled child never be born wherever a copy of her martyrdom narrative is kept. During the Middle Ages, the virgin martyr came to be lauded as the patron saint of childbirth, not only because she promised to prevent the birth of disabled children, but also because she reportedly burst from the belly of a demonic dragon that consumed her in prison during her tortures.[2] Though little evidence of her historical existence can be found, St Margaret's popularity in medieval hagiography, witnessed in hundreds of medieval manuscripts, testifies to the importance of her cult.[3] Material remnants of that cult demonstrate St Margaret's pervasive presence in the lives of medieval Christians, from murals and stained glass images they would see in their churches to parchment amulets and girdles that were purported to aid women during childbirth.[4] However, little attention has thus far been paid to what appears to be a clear underlying motivator for that cult: the saint's promise to eliminate

and soþfæstnesse gast' (§ 19). All translated passages from the Tiberius *Life of St Margaret* are from Parker, trans., '*Life of St. Margaret*', and will be cited by page number; quotations from the Old English *Life of St Margaret* found in Cotton MS Tiberius A.iii are from the edition by Clayton and Magennis (*Old English Lives*); parenthetical citations refer to the paragraph numbers in this edition.

I thank Bradley Phillis, Brandy Wilcox, Cameron Hunt McNabb, and Elizabeth Bearden, as well as my co-editors Stephanie Grace-Petinos and Alicia Spencer-Hall, for support and feedback at crucial junctures in the life of this project. I am also grateful to the several graduate students at the University of Southern Mississippi—particularly Jessica Carrell, Chloé Wofford, Marisa Mills, and Morgan Brewer, as well as the participants in my Fall 2021 graduate seminar on 'Medieval Disability Studies'—whose insightful questions helped to inspire and refine parts of this essay. Any infelicities that remain are certainly my own.

2 The dragon, among other elements of the story, suggests hagiographic embellishment, which is why Margaret was withdrawn from the Roman Catholic Church's catalogue of saints in 1969; see Clayton and Magennis, *Old English Lives*, p. 3. On the hagiographic tradition of St Margaret, see ibid., pp. 3–107, as well as Di Sciacca, 'Old English Life'; Dresvina, *Maid with a Dragon*, pp. 13–52; Magennis, '"Listen Now All"'. On the association of Margaret's emergence from the dragon with childbirth, see Heyes, *Margaret's Monsters*, pp. 123–30.

3 The earliest surviving texts are ninth-century Greek *vitae*, though legends of the martyr appear to have been circulating in Rome by the fifth century. The oldest surviving vernacular *vitae* are ninth-century Old English fragments and entries in martyrologies, followed in the eleventh century by the longer prose *Life* discussed in this essay. See Dresvina, *Maid with a Dragon*, pp. 13, 15, 24–35.

4 See Bozóky, 'From Matter of Devotion', pp. 95–97; Dresvina, *Maid with a Dragon*, pp. 188–91; Egilsdóttir, 'St Margaret'; Hill, '"Leave My Virginity Alone"'; Fiddyment, et al., 'Girding the Loins?'; Jones and Olsan, 'Performative Rituals', p. 427; Larson, 'Who Is the Master?'; Morse, '"Thys Moche More"'; Skemer, 'Amulet Rolls'.

childhood disability, and thus also excise disabled children from the family, the community, and the world.[5]

Attending to the medieval pregnancy and childbirth cult of St Margaret—particularly as it is witnessed in London, British Library, Cotton MS Tiberius A.iii (hereafter T)—offers unique insight into the social role of disability in early eleventh-century England. T is a composite manuscript, likely bound together in the early modern era.[6] My interest here is in the largest unit within the compiled manuscript, folios 2–173, which Tracey-Anne Cooper suggests may have originally formed a miscellany for a churchman or archbishop.[7] This portion of T was made at Christ Church, Canterbury, likely between 1020 and 1023.[8] It contains portrait miniatures of Benedictine Reformers (added later in the eleventh century), *The Rule of St Benedict*, St Æthelwold's *Regularis concordia*, other monastic texts, prayers, homilies, prognostics, the only surviving copy of *Monasteriales indicia* (a monastic sign language manual), and one of two surviving extended forms of the *Life of St Margaret* in Old English prose.[9] Margaret's is the only saint's life in T; Cooper argues that this is because only one exemplar of Christian virtue was needed, and Margaret's story happened to fulfil both the pastoral

5 In a notable acknowledgement of disability's importance for the cult of St Margaret, Michael E. Heyes recognizes that Margaret's intervention was 'clearly tied to disability in the child rather than safety during parturiency', though he connects the prevention of disability more to preventing 'intervention by demons in the birth', than to understandings of disability beyond the text; *Margaret's Monsters*, p. 111.

6 Details regarding T's compilation are difficult to confirm due to the substantial damage to the manuscript incurred in the Cotton Library fire of 1731; on this fire and damage to the Cottonian collection now at the British Library, see Prescott, '"Their Present Miserable State"'.

7 *Monk-Bishops*, p. 263. As Neil R. Ker has noted, signs of wear and manuscript damage indicate that the original order of leaves in this unit, using present-day numbering, was 117–73, followed by 2–116, placing *The Rule of St Benedict* earliest; *Catalogue*, p. 241. The texts of interest here—namely, the *Life of St Margaret* (fols 73v–77r); 'The Development of the Foetus' (fol. 40v); a natal lunarium in Latin that is glossed in Old English (fol. 36v); another natal lunarium entirely in Old English (fols 41r–41v); and 'Omens in Pregnancy' (fols 42v–43r)—all appear in the range of leaves that originally followed, rather than preceded, *The Rule of St Benedict*.

8 Cooper argues compellingly for this unusually narrow dating based on textual and monastic contexts for the manuscript; *Monk-Bishops*, pp. 34–46. Previous palaeographic analysis typically assigned the manuscript to the broader date of the mid-eleventh century but does not rule out this slightly earlier range; see, for example, Ker, *Catalogue*, pp. 240–41. On the creation of T at Christ Church, Canterbury, see Cooper, *Monk-Bishops*, pp. 18–46.

9 The other surviving Old English prose *Life of St Margaret* witnesses a separate act of translation out of Latin in the twelfth century at Rochester; this version survives in Cambridge, Corpus Christi College, MS 303. On the Corpus *Life of St Margaret*, see Clayton and Magennis, *Old English Lives*, pp. 92–94 and 103–07 (the Old English text and translation are included at 149–80); Dresvina, *Maid with a Dragon*, pp. 28–35.

and monastic needs of the Christ Church community.[10] However, as I shall argue, patronizing the cult of St Margaret promised perks pertaining not only to pregnancy, but also to the role and existence of disability within the community. Regardless of whether T's healing miracle claims are borne out by historical reality, the very real assumptions about childbearing and disability evinced by Margaret's cult reveal a premodern eliminationist stance towards disability. I argue that this stance anticipates what disability theorist Rosemarie Garland-Thomson terms 'eugenic logic': a desire to eliminate disability from the world.[11]

The premodern eugenic logic of the cult of St Margaret applies particularly to natal disability; that is, disability appearing or originating at birth. Favouring the term 'natal disability' over 'congenital disability' helps to remove connotations of modern medicine—and particularly medical models for disability as a 'flawed' embodiment to be 'remedied'—from our consideration of medieval saints' cults. Conversations in disability studies around congenital disability often focus on heredity and outcomes for people with congenital disabilities later in life. My focus here, and the focus of the cult of St Margaret, is rather on the moments surrounding childbirth in which an unknown body (the foetus) becomes a known body (the infant), to be interpreted for its potential fit within its community. Natal disability is connected to pregnancy, childbirth, and the interpretation of foetuses or infants by adults, rather than the lived experiences of the people themselves who are born with disabilities. When the cult of St Margaret promises to eliminate natal disability, there is no potential for a disabled neonate to protest either their own elimination or a radical shift in their embodiment through 'healing', miraculous or otherwise. Thus, in the Middle Ages, as today, natal disability presented a blank screen upon which anxieties about moral and practical implications of disability could be projected, and the fantasy of a world in which disability is eliminated—a eugenic fantasy—could be entertained.

Aside from promises regarding natal disability (and Margaret's triumph over a dragon), narratives of St Margaret tend to follow a path typical of virgin martyr stories: she is abandoned by her father for being Christian; a pagan prefect desires to marry her, but when she refuses to recant her Christianity, he has her tortured and imprisoned; in prison, she faces demonic enemies; and after further ineffective torture, she is eventually executed. Studies of the Tiberius *Margaret*, with the exception of Cooper's

10 Cooper, 'Only *Life*?'.

11 Garland-Thomson, 'Case for Conserving'.

work on T, have typically focused on matters of gender, violence, or the saint's confrontations with a dragon and a devil, without attending to the text's manuscript context.[12] However, T is notable because it contains a large collection of prognostic texts—lists that purport to foretell future events based on present phenomena—in both Latin and Old English; T's quantity of prognostics is unmatched in the surviving manuscript record from early medieval England, as is its specific collection of childbirth prognostics.[13] T's prognostic contents include the only extant copies of two short Old English texts that relate childbirth to concerns of disability for the child or for the mother: 'The Development of the Foetus' and 'Omens in Pregnancy'. The correspondence between T's prognostic interests and the inclusion of a *Life of St Margaret* suggests a particular concern for the processes and outcomes of pregnancy, including the prospect of bearing children with disabilities. Much scholarship on the medieval cult of St Margaret has suggested she was not widely regarded as a patron saint of childbirth until the twelfth century, typically dating the earliest confirmation of Margaret as protector of mothers to Wace's *Vie de sainte Marguérite* (c. 1153).[14] The correspondence of the Tiberius *Margaret* and childbirth prognostics in T, however, suggests that in the early *eleventh* century, when T was made, Margaret was already closely associated with pregnancy and childbirth in England.[15]

The premodern eugenicist attitude towards disability in T was, I argue, symptomatic of larger socio-political and spiritual motivations of the late-stage Benedictine Reform, which Cooper calls 'a focused multi-generational effort to create a "Holy Society" in England'.[16] In order to earn the claim of being God's chosen people and to put an end to Danish invasions said to be earned by England's sinfulness, a 'Holy Society' in England would need to attain widespread piety and adherence to Christian moral guidelines across social classes and regional communities living in England.[17] Archbishop Wulfstan of York (d. 1023)—one of the premier political and religious

12 On gender and violence in the legend of St Margaret, see Bennett, 'Death and the Maiden'. On the saint's confrontation with the dragon and devil, see Di Sciacca, 'Old English Life', pp. 359–74; Dresvina, *Maid with a Dragon*, pp. 158–72; Heyes, *Margaret's Monsters*, pp. 15–77; Treharne, '"They Should Not Worship Devils"'.

13 See Liuzza, ed., *Anglo-Saxon Prognostics*. Claudia Di Sciacca also notes T's links to childbirth through its interest in the sacrament of baptism; 'Old English Life', pp. 383–84.

14 Cooper, 'Only *Life*?', pp. 64–68; see also Clayton and Magennis, *Old English Lives*, p. 4; Larson, 'Who Is the Master?', p. 97.

15 Heyes also notes an earlier association of Margaret with pregnancy and childbirth; *Margaret's Monsters*, p. 134 n. 19.

16 Cooper, *Monk-Bishops*, p. 48.

17 See Keynes, 'An Abbot'; Lemke, 'Fear-Mongering'.

thinkers of the early eleventh century, who served both English and Danish kings of England—laid responsibility for this task upon priests, bishops, and all clergymen in any way involved in pastoral care. **T** includes several of Wulfstan's homilies to this effect, in addition to Benedictine Reform standards such as the *Regularis concordia*.[18] **T**'s investment in childbirth not only seems to have been tied to general pastoral duties, as both Cooper and R. M. Liuzza have suggested, but also seems to reflect an overarching view of the desired 'Holy Society' as a society without disability.[19]

The remainder of this chapter explores the anxieties around disability that appear in **T**, in order to better understand early medieval considerations of disability and its role in Christian communities. Undeniably, the modern concept of disability as a collective identity group advocating for common legal protections and societal acceptance was not extant in the Middle Ages. Thus, neither did explicitly stated models exist for distinguishing impairment as a physiological reality from disability as a culturally, socially, legally, or medically constructed category.[20] Nonetheless, as Edward Wheatley has argued, religious models for disability as both an earthly physical category and a spiritual category held significance for medieval Christians.[21] Specific to early medieval England, Karen Bruce Wallace and Fay Skevington have separately identified the Old English term *unhal* ('unwhole', 'unhealthy', or 'unhale'), as a collective categorization that encompassed bodies seen as failing to meet early medieval expectations about physiological norms.[22] What remains unclear, however, is whether and to what extent individuals who experienced embodiments that we would today call disability might have considered themselves part of a community set apart from able-bodied normativity, with positive or negative consequences. We have no record of the first-hand experiences of disabled medieval neonates—imagined or real—but considering the prospects for community among adults with disabilities gives some sense of the life that would have lain before them.

By examining the healing miracle cult of St Margaret, I argue that even without a shared sense of community felt by real people with stigmatized

18 The *Regularis concordia* appears in T at fols 3r–27v. Homiletic elements attributed to Wulfstan appear between fols 88v and 93v. All of the Wulfstanian texts in T, as well as the Old English (though not the Latin) of the *Regularis concordia*, are written in the same hand as the *Life of St Margaret*; see Cooper, *Monk-Bishops*, pp. 274, 290–94.

19 Cooper, *Monk-Bishops*; Liuzza, ed., *Anglo-Saxon Prognostics*, p. 34.

20 On modern models for disability and their (in)applicability to the Middle Ages, see Eyler, 'Introduction'; Metzler, *Disability*.

21 Wheatley, *Stumbling Blocks*.

22 Bruce Wallace, '*Unhælu*'; Skevington, '*Unhal*'.

embodiments, there was indeed a medieval socio-spiritual category, comparable—albeit not identical—to modern constructs of disability. This category collected embodiments not by a hard-and-fast definition of impairment, but by assumptions of undesirability and spiritual stigma. I have argued elsewhere that in early medieval England, hagiographic narratives (as well as other genres) utilized various embodiments outside the norm in systematic assemblages of both positively and negatively coded aberrant bodies that facilitated the spiritual and narrative objectives of texts.[23] While the interconnected aberrant embodiments of saints, sinners, and ordinary Christians is certainly at play in the Tiberius *Margaret*, my primary goal here is to focus on the implications of the narrative outside the text. What did it mean for *real* people with disabilities and *real* prospective parents to hear a story such as Margaret's told in this way, or to have access to the characterization of natal disability in **T**'s prognostics? In addition to illuminating medieval perspectives on natal disability and disability generally, my second goal is to think holistically about how this particular manuscript constructs disability across its varied texts. Attending to these views of natal disability brings the prognostics and the Tiberius *Margaret* together as part of the manuscript's consistent, though nuanced, agenda to guide episcopal practice and pastoral care towards the deliverance of medieval Christians' souls—by altering the literal, physical make-up of their bodies.

A Medieval Disability Community

Disability and disabled bodies appear repeatedly throughout **T**'s *Life of St Margaret*. The text consistently associates disability with sinfulness. For example, both the narrative voice and Margaret herself refer to pagan idols and deities as 'dumb and deaf'.[24] It should be noted here, and throughout this essay, that I am using 'dumb' (*dumb*) in its medieval sense, meaning solely 'unable to speak'. Labelling pagan idols as 'dumb' or 'deaf' metaphorically associates disability with sinfulness, in much the same process that words

23 See Parker, 'Eschatology for Cannibals'; Parker, 'Embodied Lives and Afterlives'. I develop this argument further in my book, *Light of the Everlasting Life: Disability and Crip Eschatology in Old English Literature* (forthcoming 2025 from University of Michigan Press).

24 pp. 212, 213, 215. In Old English this is rendered 'dumbe and deafe' (§ 1), 'dumb and deaf' (§§ 9, 17), respectively. Lori Ann Garner observes that the phrase 'dumb and deaf' appears frequently across the Old English corpus with moral or spiritual connotations, though more nuanced approaches to deafness appear in legal and medical texts; *Hybrid Healing*, pp. 206–47, particularly at 230–31.

like 'dumb' have come to erroneously associate inability to speak with inability to learn or understand. The logic of such metaphors associates perception (often ocular, but here aural) with knowledge and faith. Speech also figures as a proxy for power in the spiritual formula wherein the word of God—i.e., Christian scripture—easily exceeds 'dumb' idols in its ability to communicate and guide human life. When Margaret is imprisoned and has just burst from the belly of the dragon, she forces a demon to confess his crimes. In response, the devil uses a similar metaphor of faith as sight and sinfulness as vision impairment when he describes luring people into sinfulness: 'I blinded them to faith'.[25] This language participates in a tradition much older than Christianity, which was nevertheless endemic to medieval Christian discourse, in which disability was metaphorically linked with sinfulness.[26] Such metaphors, though figurative, rely on literal assumptions that disability correlates to sin, whether as cause or effect of an individual's sinfulness. The stakes associated with having a child with a disability thus become eternal; if a child disabled from birth is assumed to be spiritually impaired in a way that is more significant than the original sin borne by all, then the logical goal for any Christian parent would be to not want a disabled child.

Shortly before her beheading, Margaret prays that sins be forgiven for any who contribute to her cult, specifically listing anyone who 'writes of my suffering or hears it read', 'puts a light in my church', 'might recall my name and yours [i.e., God's]', 'makes a book of my martyrdom or has one in their house', or 'builds a church in my name and there writes my martyrdom or purchases it through their labour'.[27] As a whole, this prayer promotes the textual transmission of the *passio*. While building a church dedicated to St Margaret, putting a light in her church, and simply evoking the saint's name are mentioned, all of the remaining actions by which one might earn the saint's intercession are related to her textual, hagiographic cult, most notably simply having the book present at the scene of childbirth. The emphasis on the narrative and the physical object of a hagiographical book transforms manuscripts like **T** itself into objects of curative power.[28]

25 p. 214. 'Ic hig ableonde fram geleafan' (§ 15).

26 Parker, 'Embodied Lives and Afterlives', *passim*, but see especially pp. 30–96 and 162–201.

27 pp. 215–16. Margaret describes her supplicants as anyone who 'writeþ mine þrowunga oþþe hi geheraþ rædan', 'leoht deþ on minum cirican', 'si gemindig minum naman and þines', 'macað boc mines martirhades oþþe on his huse hæbbe', or 'cyrcan timbrige on minum naman and þær awrite mine þrowunge oþþe of his gewinne gebicge' (§ 19).

28 A fifteenth-century golden bead in the shape of an open book—likely representing a Book of Hours or a hagiographic collection, not a Bible as has been reported—was discovered in York

Margaret's request for her devotees to receive special protections relating to pregnancy and childbirth specifically names several disabilities, quoted more fully in the epigraph to this chapter: 'let there not be born a child that is blind, nor halt, nor dumb, nor deaf, nor vexed by an unclean spirit'.[29] Margaret uses the phrasing, 'let there not *be born* a child' (emphasis added), rather than asking for such a child never to be conceived, quickened (which refers to the first detectable movement of the foetus *in utero*), or go through any other part of the procreative process. She likewise makes no mention of children not acquiring disability during or after birth. As a result, there are only two processes by which this prayer might be fulfilled: either through prenatal healing or the selective spontaneous abortion of foetuses developing with disabilities. Miscarriage and even intentional abortion were certainly realities in early medieval England, but the importance of healing in the remainder of the saint's life suggests that prenatal healing was the primary implication of the prayer, even if the offer of selective abortion remains a possibility. The notion of healing disabled neonates coexists with the prospective extermination of disabled neonates; the eugenic logic of eliminating disability from the world permits both possibilities.[30]

Margaret's prayer correlates the forgiveness of sins and the healing of the body, as if to suggest that forgiving the parents' sins in turn also prevents the disability of their child(ren). Granted, the forgiveness of sins is a ubiquitous intercessory perk of venerating any Christian saint, and healing is certainly not uncommon, as the essays in this volume demonstrate. The prevention of natal disability, however, is quite unique. In Margaret's prayer and in a Christian moral framework, the forgiveness of sins and healing of the body are distinguished from one another, though very much related as parallel desirable outcomes. Just as Christians are expected to repent and desire forgiveness for their sins, they are also expected to want to be healed and for their children to be preventatively healed.

in 2021. The bead depicts St Margaret emerging from a dragon, as well as St Leonard (another patron of childbirth). The form of this object suggests that Margaret's call for the creation of books of her martyrdom was well-received by her cult, such that even a bead, perhaps meant to be worn during pregnancy and childbirth, would be shaped like a book containing an image of the saint. See Donohoe, 'Locating Childbirth Devotion', pp. 736–37.

29 p. 216. 'Ne sy þær geboren blind cild ne healt, ne dumb, ne deaf, ne fram unclænum gaste geswenct' (§ 19).

30 As Maeve Callan has shown, other medieval saints venerated in the British Isles also reportedly provided miraculous abortions, albeit not so closely tied to disability as the cult of St Margaret promises. See Callan, *Sacred Sisters*, p. 28.

After Margaret's prayer, a voice from heaven, accompanied by thunder and a dove bearing a cross, says,

> Your body will be venerated among mankind, that whosoever touches your relics, at that time will be healed from any impairment [*untrumnesse*] that he has. And where your relics are or the book of your martyrdom, neither evil nor unclean spirit will draw near there.[31]

The heavenly voice seems to disregard Margaret's request for the healing or prevention of natal disabilities that are physical. Instead, the voice affirms that where Margaret's relics or book are present, 'neither evil nor unclean spirit will draw near there', picking up on the language Margaret had used of no newly born child being 'vexed by an unclean spirit', potentially as a way of describing mental illness, cognitive impairment, or other forms of neurodivergence.[32] The omission of other potential natal disabilities (i.e., blindness, deafness, speech and mobility impairments) suggests that 'evil or unclean spirit[s]' might have been understood as the cause of physical and sensory impairments as well as neural differences, underscoring a spiritual aetiology of disability as being reflective of or caused by sinfulness and proximity to evil.

Margaret only asks to heal the unborn, but the larger scene in the *vita* also depicts the healing of born humans who appeal to her cult. After Margaret is beheaded and her head carried up into heaven by angels, 'All those who were in poor health [*wannhale*], halt and blind, dumb and deaf, if they would touch the holy woman's body, they were entirely healed'.[33] The heavenly voice had promised that any who touch Margaret's relics will be healed from 'any impairment [*untrumnesse*]'.[34] Old English *untrumnesse* (a state of being *untrum*: literally 'un-trim' or 'misarranged') and *wannhale* (from *wanhal*: literally 'lacking with respect to health') are catch-all terms that appear widely in Old English medical and spiritual texts, particularly in healing miracle narratives, as ways of grouping those who request or receive healing

31 p. 216. 'Þin lichama biþ wurþful mid mannum, þæt swa hwa swa ahrineþ þine reliquias, of þære tide fram swa hwylcre untrumnesse swa he hæfþ he biþ gehæld. And þær þine reliquias beoþ oþþe boc þines martirhades, ne genealæcþ þær naþor ne yfel ne se unclæne gast' (§ 20).

32 p. 216. The voice promises that 'naþor ne yfel ne se unclæne gast' (§ 20) will be permitted near Margaret's relics or book of her martyrdom, while Margaret had prayed that a child at whose birth she is invoked not be afflicted by an 'unclænum gaste' (§ 19).

33 p. 216. 'Ealle þa þe wannhale wæron, healtte and blinde, dumbe and deafe, and hi onhrinon þære halgan fæmnan lichaman, ealle hi wurdon gehælde' (§ 23).

34 p. 216. 'Swa hwylcre untrumnesse' (§ 20).

and describing only vaguely the actual living human experience of having such an impairment.[35] The attention to various impairments as a collective of embodied experiences, albeit at the expense of nuance and specificity in such generalizing terms, suggests the possibility of framing disability as a collective experience—a *shared* experience—in early medieval England, and perhaps in Western Christendom more broadly. Moments like these in healing narratives suggest a particularly medieval Christian definition of 'disability'—even without a single, unifying label or term—as embodiments that a saint might heal or be asked to heal, including embodiments that saints themselves might experience.[36] This collectivism is a far cry from the unifying disability identity of twentieth- and twenty-first-century disability activism—and it is not clear from this text whether it could have been an affirming, productive, or positively experienced community—but it is nonetheless a much more recognizable solidarity rooted in embodied difference than has previously been identified in premodern Christendom.

Prognosticating Pregnancy in Cotton MS Tiberius A.iii

Healing miracles promised inclusion in the Christian salvation community for medieval people with disabilities. The manuscript context of the Tiberius *Margaret* gives unique insight, however, into the relationship between disability and salvation in the context of pregnancy and childbirth. **T** contains the largest number, as well as the 'richest and most complex' collection, of prognostics of any manuscript surviving from early medieval England.[37] The prognostics in **T** make predictions of future events predominantly based on lunar cycles, visions in dreams, days of the week, and the timing of thunder. **T** also witnesses two texts that are otherwise unattested in Old

35 For example, in Ælfric of Eynsham's late-tenth-century *Lives of Saints*, variations of *untrum* and *wanhal* are used to describe those about to be miraculously healed in the *vitae* of SS Sebastian, Agnes, Mark, and Swithun, to name a few. See Ælfric of Eynsham, *Old English Lives of Saints*, I, pp. 164–67; I, 238–39; II, pp. 70–71; and II, pp. 214–17, respectively.

36 See, for example, Easterling (pp. 63–86); Gillibrand (pp. 165–85); Holtan (pp. 147–63); Trembinski (pp. 39–62); and Vargas-O'Bryan (pp. 115–46) in the present volume.

37 Liuzza, ed., *Anglo-Saxon Prognostics*, p. 3. T contains twenty-two distinct prognostic texts, while the next largest set—the personal prayer book of Abbot Ælfwine of New Minster, Winchester (d. 1057), now London, British Library, Cotton MS Titus D.xxvi/xxvii—contains seventeen. These include some parallel childbirth prognostics, though Liuzza points out that there is no evidence T was directly or indirectly copied from Titus D.xxvi/xxvii. On the prognostic contents of early English manuscripts, see Liuzza, 'Prognostics in Context', pp. 213–30; see also Chardonnens, *Anglo-Saxon Prognostics*.

English, which articulate the course of pregnancy and outcomes associated with various characteristics of the gestational parent; the manuscript thus uniquely combines pregnancy and childbirth prognostics with a *Life of St Margaret*, burgeoning patroness of childbirth. Liuzza writes that T's prognostics

> chart the health of the physical body seen as a theatre of cosmic influence, a fluid system whose ebbs and flows—whether in the blood, in the course of good and bad fortune, or in the shifting images found in dreams—must be recognized in order to be managed.[38]

Moreover, Liuzza notes that in manuscripts from early medieval England, 'the most common prognostic texts, whether lunar or calendrical, are those devoted to medical matters'.[39] Prognostics for the outcome of sickness based on the day a person falls ill would have been quite valuable for managing the flow of pilgrims seeking healing from saints venerated at Christ Church, Canterbury, where T was made. For example, if a person falls ill on the fifteenth day of the month and the patient or their caregiver are informed that this indicates the patient 'will be in danger', it would be perfectly reasonable to pursue various courses for healing, such as an appeal for intervention at the shrine of a nearby saint.[40] In this way, T's concerns with health, impairment, and disability are not unusual among the nineteen manuscripts from early medieval England that contain prognostic texts; rather, they are unique in their particular commitment to childbirth and natal disability.

Just as a prognostic indicating levels of risk for an ill adult could prompt a pilgrimage for healing, childbirth lunaria (predictions based on the night of the lunar month within which a child is born) could help inspire devotion to the childbirth cult of St Margaret. The birth lunarium in T that appears on fols 41r–41v includes several nights of the lunar month that would be risky for the health of a child born on that night. Birth on the eighth, fifteenth, seventeenth, or twentieth nights all suggest an early death, but more intriguingly, 'if he is born on the second night [of the lunar month], he will always be sick [*seoc*] and unhealthy [*unhal*]'.[41] The Old English word *unhal*, which,

38 Liuzza, 'Prognostics in Context', p. 209.

39 Ibid., p. 202.

40 'He dyrfð'; this is the Old English gloss on a Latin medical lunarium on fol. 37r, glossing 'periclitat' in the Latin. Liuzza, ed. and trans., *Anglo-Saxon Prognostics*, pp. 166/167.

41 'Gif he bið on tweigra nihta acenned. se bið a seoc ⁊ unhal'; Liuzza, ed. and trans., *Anglo-Saxon Prognostics*, pp. 202/203, 204/205. Notably, births on the ninth and twenty-seventh nights of the lunar month associate peril with the birth itself, though not necessarily for the neonate.

as noted above, literally means 'unwhole', 'unhale', or 'unhealthy', is the nearest semantic equivalent in Old English to modern 'disability'.[42] In this context, the presence of *unhælu* (in the adjectival form *unhal*), suggests chronic illness and a reasonably long life with a physical impairment. To be *unhal* is distinguished from being *seoc*; the precise distinction is unclear, but might refer to different effects of impairment or perhaps the distinction between repeated acute illnesses (*seocness*) and a singular chronic illness (*unhælu*). Unlike other nights of the lunar month, birth on the second night does not forebode an early death, but rather a life lived with a disabling sickness, impairment, or other health concern.

These prognostics suggest that live births of children with disabilities generated significantly different concerns than foetal or infant mortality. Crucially, this signals that the births of disabled infants were not held as equivalent to an outcome with no living infant at all. This perhaps seems obvious—the difference is literally life and death—but the distinction also had spiritual implications for the infant's afterlife. Neonates with disabilities were considered living members of the community, whose spiritual prospects (i.e., their possibility of salvation) were of very real concern. That disabled infants were conceptualized differently from stillborn foetuses or victims of infant mortality affirms that the lives and afterlives of infants with disabilities were meaningful in early medieval Christian conceptions of salvation. Disabled neonates invited questions of whether and how someone born disabled might attain salvation, because their prospects for salvation signalled the holiness of the community.

T's childbirth lunarium states that a child born on the second night of the lunar month 'will always [*a*] be sick and unhealthy'.[43] The use of Old English *a*—meaning 'always' or 'forever'—invests this prognostic with both earthly and eternal weight. A child's earthly life lived with chronic illness or disability would have familial, social, and economic consequences.[44] The word *a* in Old English, though, commonly appears as part of a characterization of the afterlife, as in the conclusion to T's *Life of St Margaret*, in which the author prays, 'To him [Christ] may there be glory and love and honor and majesty and power and greatness in the world of all worlds, truly eternal [*a*] without any end. Amen'.[45] The semantic range of Old English *a* contains

42 Bruce Wallace, '*Unhælu*'; Skevington, '*Unhal*'.

43 'Se bið a seoc ⁊ unhal'; Liuzza, ed. and trans., *Anglo-Saxon Prognostics*, pp. 202/203.

44 See, for example, Easterling (pp. 63–86, esp. 64–66, 70–71) in the present volume.

45 p. 217. 'Þam sy wuldor and lof and wurðmynt and þrym and anweald and micelnys on ealra worulda woruld, soþlice a butan ænigum ende. Amen' (§ 24).

both the prospect of an earthly life with prolonged disability and also the possibility of continued disabling effects from a given embodiment even after death in the Christian afterlife, by implying a predestination towards sin and damnation from the moment a child is born with a disability—that is, unless there is some intervention to prevent that disability from coming into the child's life in the first place.

A variation on the prognostics' terminology describing health and disability—*wannhale*, meaning 'incompletely healthy' or 'in poor health'—appears in the Tiberius *Margaret* describing those who are healed by touching the saint's recently deceased body: 'And all those who were in poor health [*wannhale*], halt and blind, dumb and deaf, if they would touch the holy woman's body, they were entirely healed'.[46] This line appears across folios 77r–77v of **T**, dozens of manuscript leaves away from the childbirth lunarium that warns of *unhælu* in the future of a child born the second night of a lunar month. Nonetheless, their coexistence in this manuscript testifies to the shared ideological community present in and around Christ Church in the eleventh century. A concerned parent going into labour just after a new moon might be particularly motivated to venerate St Margaret through any number of means, in order to secure the birth of a child on the second night of the lunar month without any form of *unhælu*—that is, a child without disability.

According to **T**, the need for saintly intervention into a child's prospects for (dis)ability might also be anticipated before the date of the child's birth could even be known. Immediately prior to the childbirth lunarium just discussed, **T** contains the unique Old English witness to a text known as 'The Development of the Foetus', which lists the corporeal and spiritual components of the foetus that develop, month by month.[47] The foetus develops its 'brain' (*brægen*), 'veins' (*ædran*), 'limbs' (*limum*), 'ribs' (*ribb*), 'skin' (*he byþ gehyd*), 'bones' (*ban*), 'toes and fingers' (*tan* and *fingras*), and 'organs' (*breostþing*).[48] The only mention in this text of any potential irregularity in the development of the foetus comes in the tenth month, in which 'the woman will not escape with her life if the child is not born, because it turns into a deadly disease [*feorhadle*] in her belly, most often on

46 p. 216. 'And ealle þa þe wannhale wæron, healtte and blinde, dumbe and deafe, and hi onhrinon þære halgan fæmnan lichaman, ealle hi wurdon gehælde' (§ 23).

47 In T, the text spans fols 40v–41r. 'The Development of the Foetus', the subsequent natal lunarium, and most of 'Omens in Pregnancy' are written in T in the hand Cooper identifies as the same scribe that copied the *Life of St Margaret* into the manuscript; *Monk-Bishops*, p. 278.

48 Liuzza, ed. and trans., *Anglo-Saxon Prognostics*, pp. 200/201. Liuzza titles this text 'Note on the Growth of the Fetus, English'.

a Tuesday night'.[49] The transformation of a foetus into *feorhadle*—literally a 'life-sickness'—focuses anxieties over a healthy birth not on the neonate, but on the life-or-death stakes for the person who is giving birth.[50] Sequencing of foetal development, meanwhile, asserts the legibility of the prenatal, foetal body and claims both a normative process by which foetal bodies develop and also a knowable expectation that foetal bodies are necessarily not yet the complete, 'able' bodies of postnatal infants. Even a foetus that is developing 'normally' is not yet 'complete'.

While 'The Development of the Foetus' tracks only the progression of foetal development, a slightly later prognostic in **T**, 'Omens in Pregnancy', gives additional predictions about the fate of a foetus.[51] The majority of the text interprets observable signs for whether a child will be male or female (e.g., a high or a low expanded midriff or the gait of the gestational parent). Its final two signs, however, warn of disability outcomes based on eating habits during pregnancy:

> If the woman is four or five months pregnant and frequently eats nuts or acorns or fresh fruits, then it sometimes turns out that because of that the child will be foolish. [...] If she eats the flesh of bulls or rams, or bucks or boars, or cocks or ganders, or of any animal that can engender, then it sometimes happens that because of that the child will be hunchbacked and deformed.[52]

These lines suggest a maternal cause for disability, both cognitive (a child being 'foolish [*disig*]') and physical (a child being 'hunchbacked [*hoforode*] and deformed [*healede*]').[53] If a pregnant person were known to have done

49 'Þæt wif hit ne gedigð hyre feore. gif þæt bearn accenned ne biþ. forþam þe hit in þam magan wyrð hire to feorhadle oftost on tiwesniht'; Liuzza, ed. and trans., *Anglo-Saxon Prognostics*, pp. 200/201.

50 As Caroline (Caz) R. Batten has shown, Old English medical texts indicate a broad recognition of pregnancy as a period of 'vulnerability and marginality', as well as an 'increased proximity to death'; '"Lazarus, Come Forth"', p. 142, but see passim. On parturient mortality in early medieval England, see also Sayer and Dickinson, 'Reconsidering'.

51 In T, 'Omens in Pregnancy' appears at fols 42v–43r.

52 'Gif wif biþ bearneacen feower monoð oþþe fife ⁊ heo þonne gelome eteð hnyte oþþe æceren oþþe ænige niwe bleda þonne gelimpeð hit hwilum þurh þæt þæt þæt cild biþ disig. [...] Gef heo eteð fearres flæsc oððe rammes oþþe buccan oþþe bæres oþþe hanan oþþe ganran oþþe æniges þara neata. þe strynan mæg þonne gelimpeð hit hwilum þurh þæt þæt þæt cild bið hoforode ⁊ healede'; Liuzza, ed. and trans., *Anglo-Saxon Prognostics*, pp. 212/213.

53 This suggestion that one's behaviour during pregnancy might influence the formation of the foetus anticipates the placement of responsibility for 'monstrous' births on the behaviour

such things, perhaps without realizing the 'risks', it would be logical to seek to remedy the situation with the procedures located later in the manuscript: the veneration of the cult of St Margaret at the scene of the child's birth. As the Tiberius *Margaret* suggests, having a book of Margaret's *Life* present when a child is born should prevent even a child whose gestational parent ate fresh fruit in the second trimester of pregnancy from becoming 'foolish [*disig*]' as the prognostic says, or 'vexed by an unclean spirit' as the Tiberius *Margaret* says.[54] With Margaret's aid, even a child whose gestational parent ate the meat of a rooster or bull while pregnant should not be born 'deformed [*healede*]', as the prognostic warns, nor, in the words of Margaret's prayer, 'halt [*healt*]'. Thus, even accounting for the apparently misguided eating habits of pregnant individuals, the cult of St Margaret could promise to bring only able-bodied infants into the world.

Texts such as 'The Development of the Foetus' and 'Omens in Pregnancy' purport to discern and diagnose the corporeal status of a foetus. These texts claim to read the pregnant body and know what occurs within, and to know how and when a foetus becomes a human, answering questions similar to those that motivate prenatal ultrasounds today: 'What does my foetus's face look like? What kind of genitalia are they developing? Are they what I define as "healthy"? Is there more than one? When does a foetus stop being "it" and start being "he", "she", or "they"?' Soon-to-be parents in the Middle Ages asked these same questions. For medieval audiences, the piecemeal development of the foetal body is crucial to the articulation of how a foetus becomes a human. The imagined foetal body was little like the familiar images of modern sonograms; rather, they were gradual accumulations of parts, without soul, without ribs, without skin until the appropriate month for those parts to develop. Where 'The Development of the Foetus' claims knowledge of the expected progression of prenatal development, 'Omens in Pregnancy' also claims to know bio-social markers that will impact the postnatal embodied existence of the child. Anticipating the sex of the foetus, as well as its prospect of disability, gives expectant parents opportunities to prepare for a given outcome: a male child versus a female child; an able-bodied child versus one who is disabled. Such knowledge certainly serves the purpose of benevolent anticipation of one's child's arrival. However, when combined in T with a text such as the Tiberius *Margaret*, which promises to prevent the existence of a disabled child,

of the mother that has been observed in later periods. See Geil, 'Monstrous Womb'; Park and Daston, 'Unnatural Conceptions', p. 53; Rajendran, 'E(race)ing the Future'.

54 p. 216. 'Fram unclænum gaste geswenct' (§ 19).

prognostic information about the development of the foetal body takes a tone verging on eugenic. The pregnancy prognostics necessarily offer not just diagnosis, but also prognosis, which as Garland-Thomson argues, 'extends future knowing into future making', and in turn makes possible the very idea of a eugenic societal programme.[55]

The Eleventh-Century Pregnancy Cult of St Margaret

Several other prognostic texts in **T** have obstetric concerns. Clearly, as Liuzza suggests, '[t]he compilers of the collection had a special interest in addressing the anxieties surrounding childbirth; one assumes this was for pastoral reasons'.[56] Even if monastics were generally not themselves carrying pregnancies or giving birth, childbirth prognostics and the childbirth cult of St Margaret were integral parts of monastic life at Christ Church. By the third generation of the Benedictine Reform in England, a major item on the ecclesiastical agenda was the education of priests, who could then pass knowledge on to the laity. Thus, the inclusion of pregnancy prognostics and the Tiberius *Margaret* in **T** plausibly reflects an effort to model for priests (and through them, the laity) proper approaches to pregnancy, childbirth, and natal disability, as they pertained to individual salvation: another central interest of the Benedictine Reformers. If disability signified sin, then the creation of a 'Holy Society' in England called for the elimination of disability; one use of **T**, it seems, was to aid that purpose.

The promotion of St Margaret and stigmatizing of natal disability potentially also promised economic benefits for the monks of Christ Church, Canterbury, because those same monks may well have possessed relics thought to be St Margaret's when **T** was compiled.[57] The litany in **T** capitalizes her name, along with the names of SS Dunstan and Augustine of Canterbury, saints whose remains certainly were buried at Christ Church.[58] Cooper hypothesizes that a purported girdle of St Margaret that was recorded in the fourteenth century at Waltham Abbey may have accompanied relics of SS Dunstan and Ælfheah as gifts from another priory at Canterbury, St Gregory's.[59] A girdle would have been a particularly potent contact relic

55 Garland-Thomson, 'Human Biodiversity Conservation', p. 14.

56 Liuzza, ed., *Anglo-Saxon Prognostics*, p. 34.

57 Cooper, 'Only *Life*?', pp. 77–80. On the importance of Margaret's relics at Christ Church, see also Cooper, *Monk-Bishops*, p. 40.

58 Cooper, 'Only *Life*?', p. 78.

59 Ibid.

from the patroness of childbirth, as it could in dire cases be used to adorn the body of a person undergoing a difficult labour, surrounding the pregnant person with the protection of the saint, both literally and figuratively.[60] If any relics of St Margaret were possessed at Christ Church in the eleventh century, their veneration might easily have provided sufficient motivation for the adaptation of the Tiberius *Life of St Margaret* and its inclusion in **T**.[61]

Moreover, an eleventh-century cult of St Margaret at Canterbury—and specifically a pregnancy and childbirth cult—helps to explain why an episcopal manual such as **T** would contain so many texts about pregnancy, foetal development, and childbirth. Canterbury's bishops needed to know how to talk to, or at least about, the pregnant people coming to seek the aid of St Margaret. Many of the texts in **T** suggest that the manuscript was made, as Cooper argues, as a collection of 'sound, practical advice that might be welcomed by a new monk-bishop who was about to combine his monastic vocation with new duties in the secular church'.[62] Such a monk, being elevated to a bishopric, would newly have cause to interact with questions of pregnancy and childbirth. Transitioning to a more pastoral role would involve the new bishop in 'churching': the ceremonial cleansing of postpartum parishioners and welcoming them back into both the physical space of the church and the Christian spiritual community. In general, the bishop would interact much more closely with life outside the monastery than he had previously done as a monk.[63] *Monasteriales indicia*, the monastic sign language manual contained in **T**, supports this notion. As Cooper notes, it contains two separate lists of signs for varieties of people: the first list groups together typical figures of the monastery: 'abbot, dean, provost, cellarer, master, and sacrist'; the other, however, adds non-monastic personages with whom monk-bishops would be likely to interact: 'king, queen, priests who are not monks, deacons, celibate priests and lay men and women who are not in orders'.[64] This extended set of social roles relevant to monk-bishops (rather than just monks) notably includes

60 Recent non-invasive sampling of residues on a fifteenth-century birthing girdle has demonstrated that such items were indeed used in childbirth; see Fiddyment, et al., 'Girding the Loins?'. On birthing girdles, see also Donohoe, 'Birth Amulets'; Sexon, 'Gender-Querying Christ's Wounds'. Christine Voth and Dana M. Oswald are presently engaged in exciting new work on birthing girdles in medieval England, which I benefitted from learning about at the 2022 Southeastern Medieval Association Conference.

61 The presence of Margaret's relics in the region might also have motivated the creation of the Corpus *Life of St Margaret* in the twelfth century at nearby Rochester.

62 Cooper, *Monk-Bishops*, p. 161.

63 Cooper, 'Only *Life*?', pp. 65–66.

64 Cooper, *Monk-Bishops*, p. 150.

women not among the professional religious; that is, the largest category of people likely to become pregnant and give birth.

Cooper argues that England's monk-bishops at the time of T's production had goals that 'focused on the spiritual health of the nation, addressing practical and obtainable objectives from their key leadership positions, rather than enforcing sweeping changes to the organizational structure of the English Church'.[65] Based on this assumption, the process of preventing natal disability, as it is inscribed in the Tiberius *Margaret*, provides a clear strategy for readers such as monk-bishops to give pastoral advice and work to eliminate natal disability one childbirth prayer at a time. The copying of the Tiberius *Margaret* into T at Christ Church, Canterbury suggests there may have been a concerted effort to spread this strategy for disability prevention—even elimination—as part of the project to build a 'Holy Society' in England.

Conclusion: Premodern Eugenic Logic

The anxieties evident in T about disability and sin resonate with Rosemarie Garland-Thomson's concept of 'eugenic logic', which 'tells us that our world would be a better place if disability could be eliminated. [...] Why—eugenic logic asks—should the world we make and occupy together include disability at all?'[66] I agree with Garland-Thomson's assertion that eugenic logic, as she describes it, is 'distinctly modern'—at least in part.[67] She writes:

> Disability is one of the adversaries over which modernity strives to triumph. The notion of progress, in its requirement for the constant change that propels it forward, gets its teeth in part from this fantasy of wiping out disability. Purging disability has become one emblem of the achievement of progress and its twin, improvement. [...] Those who are supposedly incurable frustrate modernity's will to change the world.[68]

Certainly, eugenic logic plays into particular notions of 'progress and its twin, improvement', that are distinctly modern. However, it is one of the myths of modernity that such drives were newly conceived in the modern

65 Ibid., p. 161.
66 Garland-Thomson, 'Case for Conserving', pp. 339–40.
67 Ibid., p. 351.
68 Garland-Thomson, 'Cultural Logic', p. 781.

world. The desire for societal 'improvement' existed—albeit in different forms—in the *pre*modern world, long before the modern term 'eugenics' came into existence, as the desire to eliminate disability in Margaret's prayer and in **T** demonstrates. Margaret's prayer and Old English pregnancy prognostics prefigure the eugenic logic of modernity, evidencing anxieties about disability as a collective category in the Middle Ages, and a desire to prevent disability from entering the world, heading it off before a child is even born. The shift between medieval Christian and modern Western attitudes towards disability is not so much a shift from non-eugenic to eugenic logics, but rather a shift with respect to means. At least some medieval Christians looked to saints and God for the elimination of disability; some modern Christians and adherents of other religions still do. However, to a much greater extent, modern eugenic logics look also to science, pseudo-science, and medicine.

There is no reason to believe that any eleventh-century monk-bishops actually expected to completely eliminate disability from their world or even just from England. However, the collection of texts assembled in **T**, which form the underpinnings for a pregnancy cult of St Margaret, reveal a premodern eugenic logic that if such elimination were possible, it would be desirable. In envisioning a world without disability, medieval theologians could take advantage of a timeline that generally exceeds that of modern medicine: the eternal timeline of Christian salvation history. Where modern eugenic logics fixate on healing in life or elimination of disability *through* death (that is, murder and so-called 'euthanasia'), medieval eschatologies of disability could fixate on healing in life or elimination of disability *after* death.[69] Indeed, this was the promise of the Christian Resurrection, as Augustine of Hippo affirmed in the fifth century:

> There will be no deformity produced by unharmonious parts, in that place where both anyone that is distorted shall be straightened, and those with little of what is seemly will be made whole from a source that the Creator knows, and moreover those with more beyond what is seemly will have that excess removed, while protecting the completeness of bodily matter.[70]

69 On medieval Christian Resurrection theology and the anticipated form of the Resurrection body, essential reading is Bynum, *Resurrection of the Body*.

70 Augustine of Hippo, trans. by Parker, '*City of God*', p. 159. 'Nulla erit deformitas quam facit incongruentia partium ubi et quae prava sunt corrigentur, et quod minus est quam decet unde Creator novit inde supplebitur, et quod plus est quam decet materiae servata integritate detrahetur'; Augustine of Hippo, *City of God*, XXII.19.

In the pregnancy cult of St Margaret, we can recognize the desire for that 'harmonious', 'straightened', and 'complete' body of the afterlife spilling over into a desire to eliminate non-normative embodiments in the earthly life of eleventh-century England.

Abbreviations

T London, British Library, Cotton MS Tiberius A.iii

Bibliography

Manuscripts

Cambridge, Corpus Christi College, MS 303
London, British Library, Cotton MS Tiberius A.iii
London, British Library, Cotton MS Titus D.xxvi/xxvii

Primary Sources

Ælfric of Eynsham, *Old English Lives of Saints*, ed. by Mary Clayton and Juliet Mullins, Dumbarton Oaks Medieval Library, 58–60, 3 vols (Cambridge, MA: Harvard University Press, 2019)

Augustine of Hippo, '*The City of God Against the Pagans* (413–26)', trans. by Leah Pope Parker, in *The Medieval Disability Sourcebook*, ed. by Cameron Hunt McNabb (Earth, Milky Way: punctum books, 2020), pp. 157–61

Augustine of Hippo, *The City of God Against the Pagans: Books 21–22*, trans. by William M. Green, Loeb Classical Library, 417, 7 vols (Cambridge, MA: Harvard University Press, 1972), VII

Clayton, Mary, and Hugh Magennis, eds, *The Old English Lives of St Margaret* (Cambridge: Cambridge University Press, 1994)

Liuzza, R. M., ed., *Anglo-Saxon Prognostics: An Edition and Translation of Texts from London, British Library MS Cotton Tiberius A.iii* (Woodbridge, Suffolk: Boydell Press, 2011)

Parker, Leah Pope, trans., 'The *Life of St. Margaret of Antioch* (11th c.)', in *The Medieval Disability Sourcebook: Western Europe*, ed. by Cameron Hunt McNabb (Earth, Milky Way: punctum books, 2020), pp. 210–19

Secondary Sources

Batten, Caroline (Caz) R., '"Lazarus, Come Forth": Pregnancy and Childbirth in the Life Course of Early Medieval English Women', in *Early Medieval English*

Life Courses, ed. by Thijs Porck and Harriet Soper (Leiden and Boston: Brill, 2021), pp. 140–58

Bennett, Judith M., 'Death and the Maiden', *Journal of Medieval and Early Modern Studies*, 42.2 (2012), 269–305

Bozóky, Edina, 'From Matter of Devotion to Amulets', *Medieval Folklore*, 3 (1994), 91–107

Bruce Wallace, Karen, '*Unhælu*: Anglo-Saxon Conceptions of Impairment and Disability' (unpublished doctoral dissertation, Ohio State University, 2014)

Bynum, Caroline Walker, *The Resurrection of the Body in Western Christianity, 200–1336* (New York: Columbia University Press, 1995)

Callan, Maeve, *Sacred Sisters: Gender, Sanctity, and Power in Medieval Ireland*, (Amsterdam: Amsterdam University Press, 2019)

Chardonnens, László Sándor, *Anglo-Saxon Prognostics, 900–1100: Study and Texts* (Leiden: Brill, 2007)

Cooper, Tracey-Anne, *Monk-Bishops and the English Benedictine Reform Movement: Reading London, BL, Cotton Tiberius A.iii in Its Manuscript Context* (Toronto: Pontifical Institute of Mediaeval Studies, 2015)

Cooper, Tracey-Anne, 'Why Is Margaret's the Only *Life* in London, BL, Cotton MS Tiberius A.iii?', in *Writing Women Saints in Anglo-Saxon England*, ed. by Paul Szarmach (Toronto: University of Toronto Press, 2013), pp. 55–81

Di Sciacca, Claudia, 'The Old English Life of Saint Margaret in London, British Library, Cotton Tiberius A. III: Sources and Relationships', *Journal of English and Germanic Philology*, 118.3 (2019), 354–89

Donohoe, Róisín, 'Birth Amulets', in *The Palgrave Encyclopedia of Medieval Women's Writing in the Global Middle Ages*, ed. by Michelle M. Sauer, Diane Watt, and Liz Herbert McAvoy (Cham: Springer International, 2022), <https://doi-org.lynx.lib.usm.edu/10.1007/978-3-030-76219-3_11-1>

Donohoe, Róisín, 'Locating Childbirth Devotion in the English Parish Church, 1450–1580', *The Historical Journal*, 66.4 (2023), 725–45

Dresvina, Juliana, *A Maid with a Dragon: The Cult of St Margaret of Antioch in Medieval England* (Oxford: Oxford University Press, 2016)

Egilsdóttir, Ásdís, 'St Margaret, Patroness of Childbirth', in *Mythological Women: Studies in Memory of Lotte Motz, 1922–1997*, ed. by Rudolf Simek and Wilhelm Heizmann (Vienna: Fassbaender, 2002), pp. 319–30

Eyler, Joshua R., 'Introduction: Breaking Boundaries, Building Bridges', in *Disability in the Middle Ages: Reconsiderations and Reverberations*, ed. by Joshua R. Eyler (Farnham, Surrey: Ashgate, 2010), pp. 1–8

Fiddyment, Sarah, Natalie J. Goodison, Elma Brenner, Stefania Signorello, Kierri Price, and Matthew J. Collins, 'Girding the Loins? Direct Evidence of the Use of a Medieval English Parchment Birthing Girdle from Biomolecular Analysis', *Royal Society Open Science*, 8.3 (2021), <https://doi.org/10.1098/rsos.202055>

Garland-Thomson, Rosemarie, 'The Case for Conserving Disability', *Journal of Bioethical Inquiry*, 9.3 (2012), 339–55

Garland-Thomson, Rosemarie, 'The Cultural Logic of Euthanasia: "Sad Fancyings" in Herman Melville's "Bartleby"', *American Literature*, 76.4 (2004), 777–804

Garland-Thomson, Rosemarie, 'Human Biodiversity Conservation: A Consensual Ethical Principle', *The American Journal of Bioethics*, 15.6 (2015), 13–15

Garner, Lori Ann, *Hybrid Healing: Old English Remedies and Medical Texts* (Manchester: Manchester University Press, 2022)

Geil, Melissa Hull, 'The Monstrous Womb of Early Modern Midwifery Manuals', in *Monstrosity, Disability, and the Posthuman in the Medieval and Early Modern World*, ed. by Richard H. Godden and Asa Simon Mittman (New York: Palgrave Macmillan, 2019), pp. 249–66

Heyes, Michael E., *Margaret's Monsters: Women, Identity, and the Life of St Margaret in Medieval England* (London and New York: Routledge, 2019)

Hill, Carole, '"Leave My Virginity Alone": The Cult of St Margaret of Antioch in Norwich: In Pursuit of a Pragmatic Piety', in *Medieval East Anglia*, ed. by Christopher Harper-Bill (Woodbridge, Suffolk: Boydell Press, 2005), pp. 225–45

Jones, Peter Murray, and Lea T. Olsan, 'Performative Rituals for Conception and Childbirth in England, 900–1500', *Bulletin of the History of Medicine*, 89.3 (2015), 406–33

Ker, N. R., *Catalogue of Manuscripts Containing Anglo-Saxon* (Oxford: Clarendon Press, 1957)

Keynes, Simon, 'An Abbot, an Archbishop, and the Viking Raids of 1006–7 and 1009–12', *Anglo-Saxon England*, 36 (2007), 151–220

Larson, Wendy R., 'Who Is the Master of This Narrative?: Maternal Patronage and the Cult of St Margaret', in *Gendering the Master Narrative: Women and Power in the Middle Ages*, ed. by Mary C. Erler and Maryanne Kowaleski (Ithaca, NY: Cornell University Press, 2003), pp. 94–104

Lemke, Andreas, 'Fear-Mongering, Political Shrewdness or Setting the Stage for a "Holy Society"?—Wulfstan's *Sermo Lupi ad Anglos*', *English Studies*, 95.7 (2014), 758–76

Liuzza, R. M., 'Anglo-Saxon Prognostics in Context: A Survey and Handlist of Manuscripts', *Anglo-Saxon England*, 30 (2001), 181–230

Magennis, Hugh, '"Listen Now All and Understand": Adaptation of Hagiographical Material for Vernacular Audiences in the Old English *Lives of St Margaret*', *Speculum*, 71.1 (1996), 27–42

Metzler, Irina, *Disability in Medieval Europe: Thinking about Physical Impairment during the High Middle Ages, c. 1100–1400* (New York: Routledge, 2006)

Morse, Mary, '"Thys Moche More Ys Oure Lady Mary Longe": Takamiya MS 56 and the English Birth Girdle Tradition', in *Middle English Texts in Transition: A*

Festschrift Dedicated to Toshiyuki Takamiya on His 70th Birthday, ed. by Simon Horobin and Linne Mooney (York: York Medieval Press, 2014), pp. 199–219

Park, Katharine, and Lorraine Daston, 'Unnatural Conceptions: The Study of Monsters in Sixteenth- and Seventeenth-Century France and England', *Past and Present*, 92 (1981), 20–54

Parker, Leah Pope, 'Embodied Lives and Afterlives: Disability and the Eschatological Imaginary in Early Medieval England' (unpublished doctoral dissertation, University of Wisconsin–Madison, 2019)

Parker, Leah Pope, 'Eschatology for Cannibals: A System of Aberrance in the Old English *Andreas*', in *Monstrosity, Disability, and the Posthuman in the Medieval and Early Modern World*, ed. by Richard H. Godden and Asa Simon Mittman (New York: Palgrave Macmillan, 2019), pp. 227–48

Parker, Leah Pope, *Light of the Everlasting Life: Disability and Crip Eschatology in Old English Literature* (Ann Arbor: University of Michigan Press, forthcoming 2025)

Prescott, Andrew, '"Their Present Miserable State of Cremation": The Restoration of the Cotton Library', in *Sir Robert Cotton as Collector: Essays on an Early Stuart Courtier and His Legacy*, ed. by C. J. Wright (London: British Library Publications, 1997), pp. 391–454

Rajendran, Shyama, 'E(race)ing the Future: Imagined Medieval Reproductive Possibilities and the Monstrosity of Power', in *Monstrosity, Disability, and the Posthuman in the Medieval and Early Modern World*, ed. by Richard H. Godden and Asa Simon Mittman (New York: Palgrave Macmillan, 2019), pp. 127–43

Sayer, Duncan, and Sam D. Dickinson, 'Reconsidering Obstetric Death and Female Fertility in Anglo-Saxon England', *World Archaeology*, 45.2 (2013), 285–97

Sexon, Sophie, 'Gender-Querying Christ's Wounds: A Non-Binary Interpretation of Christ's Body in Late Medieval Imagery', in *Trans and Genderqueer Subjects in Medieval Hagiography*, ed. by Alicia Spencer-Hall and Blake Gutt (Amsterdam: Amsterdam University Press, 2021), pp. 133–53

Skemer, Don C., 'Amulet Rolls and Female Devotion in the Late Middle Ages', *Scriptorium*, 55 (2001), 197–227

Skevington, Fay, 'The *Unhal* and the Semantics of Anglo-Saxon Disability', in *Social Dimensions of Medieval Disease and Disability*, ed. by Sally Crawford and Christina Lee (Oxford: Archaeopress, 2014), pp. 7–13

Treharne, Elaine M., '"They Should Not Worship Devils … Which Neither Can See, nor Hear, nor Walk": The Sensibility of the Virtuous and *The Life of St Margaret*', in *Proceedings of the PMR Conference, 15*, ed. by Phillip Pulsiano (Villanova, PA: Villanova University, 1991), pp. 221–36

Wheatley, Edward, *Stumbling Blocks before the Blind: Medieval Constructions of a Disability* (Ann Arbor: University of Michigan Press, 2010)

About the Author

Leah Pope Parker is Assistant Professor of English and English Undergraduate Coordinator at the University of Southern Mississippi. Parker's research explores disability and religion in medieval English literature and has been published in the *Journal of English and Germanic Philology* and *Early Middle English*. Her monograph, *Light of the Everlasting Life: Disability and Crip Eschatology in Old English Literature*, is forthcoming in 2025 from University of Michigan Press.

Epilogue: Curative Time and Crip Ancestorship

Richard H. Godden

Abstract: This epilogue reflects on the explicit and implicit engagements with crip time throughout the present volume. In particular, I locate, in the complex relationship between disability and sanctity, a vital opportunity to explore crip time in the Middle Ages. I focus on two episodes of miraculous healing—an encounter between King Edward the Confessor and an Irish cripple named Ghillie Michael, and the story of a paralytic named Humbert who is cured at the shrine of St Foy—in order to recognize crip ancestorship and the opportunity for cross-temporal identification. Although these episodes function according to a teleological temporality that prioritizes cure and restoration, we can identify in them moments of resistance to normativity, and we can glimpse the lived experience of disabled people in the Middle Ages.

Keywords: crip time, crip ancestorship, episodes of miraculous healing, King Edward the Confessor, St Foy

In the Acknowledgments to the present volume, the editors describe an alternative history where there would have been two volumes, and not just one. 'We are haunted by our second "ghost" volume', they state. Moved by this frank declaration, I want to open my own contribution with the recognition that I have an essay in that graveyard. Originally intent on being a contributor, I withdrew for a myriad of reasons, including the time pressures of beginning a new job, worry that I might need the chapter for my monograph, and other concerns that I did not state at the time. Looking back, even though this was pre-pandemic, I am cognizant now that what I was feeling was crip time, a disturbance, a disruption, or rejection of linear, teleological time. To put it another way, I was tired, and feeling in my body

Grace-Petinos, Stephanie, Leah Pope Parker, and Alicia Spencer-Hall, eds. *Disability and Sanctity in the Middle Ages.* Taylor & Francis Group, 2025
DOI 10.5117/9789463724333_EPI

that I needed to slow down, something not often allowed for within the forward momentum of academic time. As a wheelchair user, medievalist, and a scholar working in Critical Disability Studies, I have slowly, if painfully, begun to make my peace with the vagaries of crip time.

As many have noted, crip time is more than a simple rejection of normative time—it is highly individualized, an embodied experience of time that starts and stops, recurs and disrupts.[1] More than anything, it is an opportunity for disabled people to write and rewrite their own narratives, and for those working in medieval disability studies (and other fields), it is an opportunity to locate and embrace crip ancestorship. In this short epilogue, I argue that interrogating the relationship between disability and sanctity provides a vital opportunity to explore crip time in the Middle Ages. Not only do the many episodes of miraculous healing provide documentary material of lived experience, they also allow for the possibility of cross temporal identifications that resist otherwise normative temporalities.

As a category and an identity position, disability almost always finds itself set in opposition: the opposite of health, of normal, of powerful, and of so many other terms that attach a name to those states of being to which societies grant value. In their Introduction, Stephanie Grace-Petinos, Leah Pope Parker, and Alicia Spencer-Hall describe how *disability* and *sanctity* appear to be set in such an opposition. Given the widespread assumption that disability and deformity was tied to sin within medieval cultural frameworks, we can easily see how these terms might be opposed.[2] If disability comes from sinfulness, then possessing such embodied difference would stand in stark contrast to the perfection of sanctity. However, as the essays in this volume attest—and especially the chapters by Rachael Gillibrand, Donna Trembinski, and Aidan Holtan—while disability *could* be a signifier of sin, it could also gesture towards sanctity, or could just be a testimony to lived experience with illness and impairment. For instance, as Trembinski examines, figures like St Francis of Assisi were, themselves, disabled.[3] And yet, disability and sanctity are often distinguished by the bodily imperfection of one group, and the perfection of the other. The impaired or debilitated body bears the marks of mortality and earthly corruption, whereas the body of the saint most often does not bear those marks, instead being perfect,

1 See Samuels, 'Six Ways'; Kafer, *Feminist, Queer, Crip*; Spencer-Hall, 'Chronic Pain'; Godden, 'Neighboring Disability'.

2 For important discussions on the relationship between sin and disability, see Metzler, *Disability in Medieval Europe*; Wheatley, *Stumbling Blocks*.

3 See Trembinski, pp. 39–62.

incorruptible. Of course, several essays in this volume trouble such a neat dichotomy. In fact, despite the diversity of primary sources, geographical contexts, and disciplinary approaches in this volume, one stable thread of analysis throughout these chapters—especially those by Christopher Jensen, Jennifer C. Edwards, Leah Pope Parker, Ivette Vargas-O'Bryan, and Joshua S. Easterling—is the relative instability of any easily legible opposition between disability and sanctity. Further, while these two categories are mutually constitutive, an ever-collapsing binary, they also represent two different embodied orientations towards temporality. On the one hand, there is the imperfect, non-normative body that ineluctably reminds one of finitude, of mortality, and postlapsarian time. On the other, there is the perfect, inviolate body, one that gestures towards the eternal. Notably, the word 'perfect' occurs several times in this volume, both in the language of the contributors, but also appearing in the various primary sources under analysis. It would be worthwhile to remember that not only does perfect mean flawless, whole and pristine, it also refers to an orientation towards time: for instance, the perfect tense. It means that which is completed, as opposed to the imperfect, which is still in motion.

The essays here take a varied approach to questions of disability and sanctity, but my particular focus is on the episodes of miraculous healing that can be found in histories, medieval romance, drama, and the documents supporting the canonization of saints. Despite a great variety in impairments, healing outcomes, and manners of supplication, such episodes follow a basic grammar: someone impaired in their body or mind encounters or seeks out a sanctified figure, and after some act of supplication, the disabled figure may be healed. The relationship between supplicant and saint resembles that of the patient and physician, suggesting a power dynamic where one figure has the power to act, and the other is acted upon. As an example, we might look briefly to the encounter between King Edward the Confessor (r. 1042–1066) and an Irish cripple named Ghillie Michael in *The History of Saint Edward the King* by Matthew Paris, written around the 1230s.[4] I have returned often to this episode in my own work because, as Jonathan Hsy and I observe, this scene exhibits a 'thick temporality' to be unpacked:

4 Although outside of my specific focus here, it is worthwhile noting that the disabled figure King Edward encounters is Irish. As several scholars have demonstrated, there are links between racialization and disability in the Middle Ages, both generally and to Irishness specifically. For example, see Heng, *The Invention of Race*, pp. 33–42. For an important discussion of race, monstrosity and disability in Gerald of Wales's writings on Ireland, see Newman-Stille, 'Morality and Monstrous Disability'.

It happened that King Edward was in his palace in London. He went to the nearby chapel of Saint Peter to hear mass, accompanied by knights of high rank, among them Hugh, his chamberlain. Sitting in the road was a poor, crippled man, ever so needy and wretched. His name was Ghillie Michael, and he was Irish by race. He was thin, deformed, feeble, and weak. He cried out:

'Alas! Alas! Here I am, a poor unfortunate, twisted and disfigured, for whom no one has pity. Alas! Why was I ever born?'

His face was wrinkled and dark, and everyone took pity on his lament. His feet were twisted, his muscles were numb, and his legs were thin and nearly without flesh. From the knees down his legs turned unnaturally toward his back, and his withered feet, which also turned backwards, stuck to his buttocks. The poor wretch pulled himself along the muddy road with the help of ingeniously made hand trestles that he held against his chest.

[...]

[Edward] sent for the poor man and bundled him onto his back, making him his load, and thus he carried the weary invalid. Those who did not know why he was doing this taunted him, saying:

'Stop that: Why are you carrying that stinking wretch? The pus from his wounds is running down your clothing and soiling you and your robe, wetting you to your garters!'

But Edward would not put the man down. And at that the man's dead flesh began to stretch and his joints relaxed, correcting his deformities. The sinews that had been turned front to back were restored to their proper position.[5]

5 Godden and Hsy, 'Analytical Survey', p. 333. Citation from Paris, *The History of Saint Edward the King*, pp. 78–79. 'Il avint ke Aedward li reis / A Lundres fu en sun paleis. / A la chapele ala seint Pere / Oir messe, ke pres ere, / E des chivalers grant rencs / U fu Huges li chamberlencs. / Un povre sëet eu chemin, / Cuntrait, mendifs e orfanin. / Guil Michel avoit cist nun, E fu Irais de nacïun, / Megres, cuntraiz, febles e las, / Ki s'escrieit: "Allas, allas! / Jo sui ci un povre dolent / De ki nus hum pité ne prent, / Ki tort sui e desfigurez. / Las, purquei fu jo unc nez?" / La face avoit fruncie e teinte. / Tut unt pité de sa pleinte. / Les pez out tortz, nerfs engurdiz, / Gambes sanz brahun, engresliz, / Si ke dé genoilz la junture / Au dos se tuert cuntre nature. / Li pé besturné, flestriz, / As nages s'aerdent revertiz. / A uns eschameus feitiz / K'il teneit cuntre sun piz / Se trait li povre frarin / Par cel enboué chemin. [...] Atant ad mandé le povre humme, / Au dos le trusse, si en fait summe, / S'enporte le malade las. / Li nunsavant s'en funt lur gas. / Dient li: "Lessez atant! / Ke portez tu le las puant? / De ses boces la quiture / Desent par vostre vesture, / Vostre cors e robe soille / E gesk'as garetz vus moille." / Mais ne laist k'il ne l'enporte. / Atant es vus ke la char morte / S'estent, e laschent les junctures, / S'adrescent les cuntrefaitures. / Li nerfs ki furent besturnee / En lur droit liu sunt redrescee'; Paris, *La Estoire de Seint Aedward Le*

During this encounter, we can see the familiar contours of the episode of miraculous healing, where an impaired individual is healed through contact with the divine, in this case, physical touch between the cripple and the King who will one day be sanctified. Further, this short narrative neatly demonstrates why David T. Mitchell and Sharon L. Snyder's concept of narrative prosthesis has been so generative within the field of medieval studies.[6] Mitchell and Snyder present a schematic wherein disabled figures are introduced, brought from the periphery to the centre, and then 'the remainder of the story rehabilitates or fixes the deviance in some manner.'[7] The temporality introduced here is a decidedly normative one, where impairment gives way to health, the corruptible to the eternal. In most instances when a disabled character shows up in medieval literature and culture, they almost always seem to exist in order to be healed. Healing episodes, therefore, are teleological, reinforcing ideas of perfection and normative embodiment.

However, as many of the essays collected here do, we can follow the call of Julie Orlemanski and practice 'reading tendentiously', that is, 'reading genres that seem to resist the project of disability studies but doing so equipped with a partisan solidarity extended to disabled figures.'[8] In other words, despite the drive towards normalcy that narrative prosthesis always seems to herald, we can instead claim solidarity not with the physician or miraculous healer, but with the impaired. As I have written elsewhere, 'by centering disabled bodies, dwelling in those moments before prostheticization, other possibilities for community and selfhood become legible.'[9] To read tendentiously, to resist the narrative drive towards wholeness or normalcy, we can perceive how disability and sanctity are not precisely set in opposition here, but are instead intermingled, co-constitutive. As Christopher Baswell observes, this moment 'enact[s] Edward's definitive move from corruptible mortality to sanctity, yet they embody the insufficiencies, the permanent breakages, and the uncanny, queer affiliations such a move involves.'[10] And, as Hsy and I argue, 'What begins as asynchrony, a clash of embodied difference, becomes a new kind of synchrony where the two bodies, in an

Rei, pp. 55–57, ll. 1919–46, 1975–1990. With thanks to Amanda J. Langley for her invaluable help in sourcing the Anglo-Norman text.

6 Mitchell and Snyder, *Narrative Prosthesis*. For an excellent example of such work, see Pearman, *Women and Disability*.

7 Mitchell and Snyder, *Narrative Prosthesis*, p. 53.

8 Julie Orlemanski, 'Literary Genre', p. 1254.

9 Godden, 'Neighboring Disability', p. 244.

10 Baswell, 'King Edward and the Cripple', p. 28.

interdependent embrace, affect each other.'[11] At first glance, then, the figure of Ghillie Michael appears to be the one who benefits the most from this encounter, but Edward himself moves from 'corruptible mortality to sanctity', demonstrating how the sanctified depend upon the impaired.[12] In a similar vein, Elizabeth A. Wiedenheft's contribution to this volume demonstrates the socioeconomic networks in which shrines and saints operate within medieval communities.[13] And, as Ghillie Michael's pus stains and mingles with both the royal vestments and the sanctified body of King Edward, we can further see the porosity of the threshold between disability and sanctity, much like in the cases that Aidan Holtan describes, where marks of bodily vulnerability and injury are still present on the incorrupt corpse of the saint.[14]

Medieval literature is full of such stories. As one further example, I turn to the story of a man named Humbert, whose health is accounted as one of the miracles attributed to St Foy:

> With his parents' help, a person named Humbert was brought from the Agenais so that he might gain the holy virgin's favors. His mother's livid [*livida*] nature had sent him forth from her womb in a condition in which his lower body, from the kidneys down, lay lifeless [*premortuum*]. He lived there for a great many years, supported through the compassion of pious people, when finally, after the solemn feast day of the Holy Mother of God's Assumption, he was visited by divine pity. On the night after the Feast he was keeping vigil before the glorious martyr's shrine along with many others, when intense pains shot through his useless limbs and he began to wail and cry out. But even in the midst of these pains he did not stop bellowing out his prayer to Sainte Foy; he sobbed as he begged her to cast her merciful gaze upon him. Suddenly there was a cracking sound and his twisted limbs were stretched out straight. Through his invocation of the holy virgin the disabled body [*debilia*] he had dragged around since he left his mother's womb was now healed. And so he cast aside the crutches [*scabellis*] of a paralytic, which he had formerly used when he needed to go somewhere, and moved across the ground leaping like a grasshopper [*locusteos*]. Now he took pleasure in running through the crowds, scampering nimbly to and fro.[15]

11 Godden and Hsy, 'Analytical Survey', p. 333.

12 Baswell, 'King Edward and the Cripple', p. 28.

13 See Wiedenheft, pp. 189–206.

14 See Holtan, pp. 147–63.

15 *The Book of Sainte Foy*, p. 201. 'Non multum huic dissimile aliud restat miraculum, quod expectanti pagine nobis videtur inserendum. Ad sancte virginis promerenda beneficia quidam

This episode fits the familiar pattern of acts of miraculous healing attributed to a saint. As such, it does end with the supplicant being healed. It also notably mentions an aetiology for Humbert's condition, which was his mother's 'livid' nature. *Livida* here could refer to a spiteful or malicious nature. Rather than being infirm because of his own sinful nature, his paralytic condition is, instead, attributed to the humoral and physiological status of his parents at the moment of his conception. And yet, we can also glimpse instances of crip time, especially with his regular and persistent vigil-keeping before the shrine of St Foy. Prior to the eventfulness of his receipt of 'divine pity', this episode details the years and years he spent in the community, receiving aid and care from others.[16] We can only assume that his holding vigil at the shrine was a recurring factor in his life. It is also worth noting that, after Humbert is healed, he leaves behind his *scabellis*, or crutches, another common occurrence in these episodes. Reinforcing Wiedenheft's analysis of the economic dimensions of healing shrines, abandoned crutches serve as proof and advertisement of the efficacy of a particular shrine. Although the crutch serves as a sign of the triumph of normative temporalities in these episodes, it is also a reminder that there will be more discarded objects because there will be more impaired supplicants, more disabled people living in the community.

In *Feminist, Queer, Crip*, Alison Kafer describes 'prognosis time', which is 'a liminal temporality, a casting out of time; rather than a stable, steady progression through the stages of life, time is arrested, stopped.'[17] Similarly, Ghillie Michael and Humbert, and so many other figures like them, appear to be living in such a time prior to miraculous healing. But most importantly, we can see here the workings of 'curative time', a restless temporality of

ex territorio Agennensium, nomine Humbertus, ope parentum advehitur, quem a renibus usque deorsum livida natura matris ab alvo exposuerat premortuum. Qui cum devotorum misericordia plurimis annis ibi sustentaretur, tandem divina pietate visitatus est post celeberrimum sancte Dei genitricis Assumptionis diem. Subsequuta nocte, dum ante gloriose martyris propiciatorium in vigiliis cum multis aliis pernoctaret, dolore nimio per languida membra corripitur, atque cum ingentibus cepit clamoribus emittere planctus. Quos inter dolores, sancte Fidis non desinit cum clamore suffragia, et ut ei propicietur cum lacrimis exorat. Inde subito fragore contracta in directum extenduntur membra, et que maternis a visceribus traxerat debilia, per sancte virginis invocationem suscipit valida. Sicque spretis scabellis, quibus locusteos saltus, si quando alias tenderet, per terram emittere solebat, solidis gressibus inter ceteras turbas discurrere congaudet'; *Liber miraculorum sancte Fidis*, p. 198. On St Foy, see also, in this volume, Wiedenheft, pp. 189–206.

16 For further discussion of the communal aspects of care, see Rawcliffe, *Urban Bodies*. Rawcliffe describes how 'informal and generally elusive networks based on kinship, gender, neighbourhood and parish helped the sick and disabled with *ad hoc* support, which, by its very nature, remains unquantifiable' (p. 314).

17 Kafer, *Feminist, Queer, Crip*, p. 36.

travel, of vigil, seeking not just cure, but also care.[18] Kafer also uses the term 'curative time', which she describes as a form of 'compulsory able-bodiedness/able-mindedness', and 'an understanding of disability that not only *expects* and *assumes* intervention but also cannot imagine or comprehend anything other than intervention.'[19] I purposefully use the same term here, but with a difference: Kafer's analysis perfectly captures the normative temporalities of episodes of miraculous healing, but I would suggest that we can also locate a counternarrative amidst the orientation towards cure, by the disabled figure, that makes legible the lived experience of disability. The medical model of disability might prioritize intervention, and in episodes of miraculous healing intervention always seems possible, but whether or not these figures were truly healed by the intervention of saintly intercessors, these records and histories demonstrate the experience of crip time by individuals as well as the existence of interdependent communities of care. In other words, we can read these instances of curative time tendentiously.

Dwelling with these figures in curative time, that is to say, the time prior to the moment of miraculous healing, we can see many ways to claim crip ancestorship. In addition to the inescapable moments of pain and the labour involved in simply being disabled, we can also observe instances of care, community, and interdependent webs of relationship. By reading tendentiously, we are complicating the assumed structures and relationship between categories like disability and sanctity, and to a degree, we are doing so by reading anachronistically, reading the medieval concepts of infirmity and debility through the modern construction of disability. Foundational to the work of medieval disability studies is Irina Metzler's observation that there was no word for *disability* in the Middle Ages.[20] As such, we are always working through anachronism. As a potent example of this, Rachael Gillibrand's essay in this volume explores visual impairment as disability.[21] In a modern context, wearing eyeglasses is not necessarily a sign of disability, yet the need to wear spectacles in the Middle Ages most certainly would have been. This reminds us of the constructedness and elasticity of categories we often take for granted.

In order to further locate crip ancestorship and solidarity with Humbert, I would like to close by looking once more at the very end of his story. After

18 For a discussion of the surprising mobility and travel of disabled individuals in the Middle Ages, see Irina Metzler, 'Have Crutch, Will Travel'.

19 Kafer, *Feminist, Queer, Crip*, p. 27 (emphasis in original).

20 Metzler, *Disability in Medieval Europe*, p. 5.

21 See Gillibrand, pp. 165–85.

abandoning his crutches, he 'moved across the ground leaping like a grasshopper [*locusteos*]. Now he took pleasure in running through the crowds, scampering nimbly to and fro.' Firstly, I must admit that the description of him leaping like a grasshopper is thoroughly charming, and gives a feeling of joy that we may not always glimpse in some of these episodes. Further, although this joy comes after being cured, I recognize in this something different. Where before he moved slowly and ploddingly, he now takes pleasure in his ability to move with alacrity and dexterity. This reminds me powerfully of my own experience first using a power wheelchair, after only using a manual. Until coming across this episode, I never fully saw a description that so mirrored my own elation at sudden movement. Of course, this recognition on my part is anachronistic, and perhaps extends past the usual remit of the scholar. And yet, though my reading is highly individualized at this moment, it continues the work of resisting normative and teleological understandings of impairment. I would also note that the comparison of Humbert to a grasshopper scampering gives a powerful sense of non-normativity. Although no further details are given, I can only imagine that his movements, in those first moments of being healed, are atypical. Perhaps he is going on all fours, or just violating some sense of able-bodied decorum. Regardless, even in the triumph of normativity we can perceive the presence of nonnormative embodiment. Resistance reverberates in his crip joy.[22] By reading disability and sanctity alongside each other, as this volume so nimbly does, we can make legible the lives and experiences of those crip ancestors.

Bibliography

Primary Sources

Paris, Matthew, *La Estoire de Seint Aedward Le Rei*, ed. by Kathryn Young Wallace (London: Anglo-Norman Text Society, 1983)

Paris, Matthew, *The History of Saint Edward the King*, trans. by Thelma S. Fenster and Jocelyn Wogan-Browne (Tempe: Arizona State University, 2008)

The Book of Sainte Foy, trans. by Pamela Sheingorn (Philadelphia: University of Pennsylvania Press, 1995)

Liber miraculorum sancte Fidis, publié d'après le manuscrit de la Bibliothèque de Schlestadt avec une introduction et des notes par M. l'abbé A. Bouillet, ed. by Auguste Bouillet (Paris: Alphonse Picard et Fils, 1897)

22 Barbarin, 'Joy is advocacy too'.

Secondary Sources

Barbarin, Imani, 'Joy is advocacy too' [Twitter] (@Imani_Barbarin, 16 June 2023)

Baswell, Christopher, 'King Edward and the Cripple', in *Chaucer and the Challenges of Medievalism*, ed. by Donka Minkova and Theresa Tinkle (Frankfurt: Peter Lang, 2003), pp. 15–29

Godden, Richard H., 'Neighboring Disability in Medieval Literature', *Exemplaria: A Journal of Theory in Medieval and Renaissance Studies*, 32.3 (2020), 229–47

Godden, Richard H., and Jonathan Hsy, 'Analytical Survey: Encountering Disability in the Middle Ages', *New Medieval Literatures*, 15 (2013), 313–39

Heng, Geraldine, *The Invention of Race in the European Middle Ages* (Cambridge: Cambridge University Press, 2018)

Kafer, Alison, *Feminist Queer Crip* (Bloomington: Indiana University Press, 2013)

Metzler, Irina, *Disability in Medieval Europe: Thinking about Physical Impairment during the High Middle Ages, c. 1100–1400* (New York: Routledge, 2006)

Metzler, Irina, 'Have Crutch, Will Travel: Disabled People on the Move in Medieval Europe', in *Travels and Mobilities in the Middle Ages: From the Atlantic to the Black Sea*, ed. by Felicitas Schmieder and Marianne O'Doherty (Turnhout: Brepols, 2015), pp. 91–117

Mitchell, David T., and Sharon L. Snyder, *Narrative Prosthesis: Disability and the Dependencies of Discourse* (Ann Arbor: University of Michigan Press, 2000)

Newman-Stille, Derek, 'Morality and Monstrous Disability in *Topographia Hibernica*', in *The Treatment of Disabled Persons in Medieval Europe: Examining Disability in the Historical, Legal, Literary, Medical, and Religious Discourses of the Middle Ages*, ed. by Wendy Turner and Tory Vandeventer Pearman (Lewiston, NY: Edwin Mellen Press, 2010), pp. 231–57

Orlemanski, Julie, 'Literary Genre, Medieval Studies, and the Prosthesis of Disability', *Textual Practice*, 30.7 (2016), 1253–72

Pearman, Tory Vandeventer, *Women and Disability in Medieval Literature* (New York: Palgrave, 2010)

Rawcliffe, Carole, *Urban Bodies: Communal Health in Late Medieval English Towns and Cities* (Woodbridge, Suffolk: Boydell Press, 2013)

Samuels, Ellen, 'Six Ways of Looking at Crip Time', *Disability Studies Quarterly*, 37.3 (2017), <https://dsq-sds.org/article/view/5824/4684>

Spencer-Hall, Alicia, 'Chronic Pain and Illness: Reinstating Chronic-Crip Histories to Forge Affirmative Disability Futures', in *A Cultural History of Disability in the Middle Ages*, ed. by Jonathan Hsy, Tory V. Pearman, and Joshua R. Eyler (London: Bloomsbury, 2020), pp. 51–66

Wheatley, Edward, *Stumbling Blocks Before the Blind: Medieval Constructions of a Disability* (Ann Arbor: University of Michigan Press, 2010)

About the Author

Richard H. Godden is Assistant Professor of English at Louisiana State University. He works primarily on medieval romance, Chaucer, and representations of disability and monstrosity in the Middle Ages. His monograph-in-progress, *Material Subjects: An Ecology of Prosthesis in Medieval Literature and Culture*, focuses on the material objects with which medieval bodies were so intimate, including not only recognizable prosthetics that serve as assistive devices such as spectacles and crutches, but also more common literary and cultural objects such as armour, clothing, and religious relics. He is co-editor of the collections *Monstrosity, Disability, and the Posthuman in the Medieval and Early Modern World* and *The Open Access Companion to The Canterbury Tales.*

Index